Diagnostic Atlas
of Renal Pathology

Commissioning Editor: Michael Houston
Project Development Manager: Sheila Black
Project Manager: Kathryn Mason
Editorial Assistant: Gemma Lawson
Senior Designer: Sarah Russell
Illustration Manager: Mick Ruddy
Illustrator: Dominic Doyle
Medical Photographer: Brent Weedman
Marketing Managers (UK/USA): Lucy Everest/Ethel Cathers

Diagnostic Atlas of Renal Pathology

A Companion to Brenner & Rector's
The Kidney, 7th edition

Agnes B Fogo MD
Professor of Pathology, Medicine and Pediatrics
Director, Renal/Electron Microscopy Laboratory
Department of Pathology
Vanderbilt University Medical Center
Nashville, TN
USA

Michael Kashgarian MD
Professor of Pathology and Molecular, Cellular, and Developmental Biology
Director, Diagnostic Electron Microscopy and Renal Pathology
Department of Pathology
Yale University School of Medicine
New Haven, CT
USA

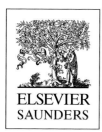

ELSEVIER
SAUNDERS

ELSEVIER
SAUNDERS

An imprint of Elsevier Limited

First published 2005
 Reprinted 2005

ISBN 1 4160 2871 4

British Library Cataloguing in Publication Data
A catalogue record for this book is available from the British Library

Library of Congress Cataloging in Publication Data
A catalog record for this book is available from the Library of Congress

Notice
Medical knowledge is constantly changing. Standard safety precautions must be followed, but as new research and clinical experience broaden our knowledge, changes in treatment and drug therapy may become necessary or appropriate. Readers are advised to check the most current product information provided by the manufacturer of each drug to be administered to verify the recommended dose, the method and duration of administration, and contraindications. It is the responsibility of the practitioner, relying on experience and knowledge of the patient, to determine dosages and the best treatment for each individual patient. Neither the Publisher nor the editors/contributor assumes any liability for any injury and/or damage to persons or property arising from this publication.

The Publisher

ELSEVIER   your source for books,
           journals and multimedia
           in the health sciences

www.elsevierhealth.com

Working together to grow
libraries in developing countries

www.elsevier.com | www.bookaid.org | www.sabre.org

ELSEVIER   BOOK AID   Sabre Foundation
           International

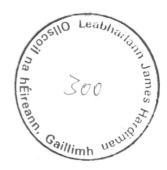

The
Publisher's
policy is to use
**paper manufactured
from sustainable forests**

Printed in Spain

Last digit is print number: 9 8 7 6 5 4 3 2

Contents

CHAPTER 1
GLOMERULAR DISEASES

CHAPTER 2
VASCULAR DISEASES

CHAPTER 3
TUBULOINTERSTITIAL DISEASES

CHAPTER 4
RENAL TRANSPLANTATION

CHAPTER 5
CYSTIC DISEASES OF THE KIDNEY

CHAPTER 6
RENAL NEOPLASIA

Preface

The approach used in organizing material for this book is unique in that it is specifically designed to be a companion book to *The Kidney* by Brenner and Rector, one of the towering classics in the field of nephrology. We have followed the organization of topics to expand and illustrate in greater detail renal biopsy findings in those diseases discussed in Brenner and Rector. Thus, the book is organized into primary glomerular diseases, secondary glomerular diseases, vascular diseases, tubulointerstitial diseases, renal transplantation, cystic diseases of the kidney and renal neoplasia. Within the glomerular diseases section, the organization again follows that of *The Kidney*, grouping diseases that cause nephrotic syndrome, those that cause nephritic syndrome, and further subdividing according to pathogenetic mechanisms. This is primarily an Atlas, where emphasis is placed on illustration of pathologic lesions. The format of the Atlas allows in-depth and detailed illustration of a spectrum of morphologic lesions characteristic for each of the entities discussed. However, we have also added focused discussion, outlining key characteristic pathologic findings, and prognostic, pathogenetic and etiologic information. We have brought in the newest information regarding categorization and classification of diseases, and emphasized how this relates to the various morphological lesions illustrated and their clinical significance. The references are representative and focused rather than inclusive. For in-depth discussion of clinical presentations, pathophysiology of those manifestations and treatment, comprehensive references are detailed in *The Kidney*, and the reader is referred to this nephrology text for in-depth discussion of these aspects of renal diseases.

Agnes Fogo
Michael Kashgarian
2005

Acknowledgements

Renal pathology is the ultimate teamwork exercise, with communications with nephrologists, pathologists, and highly skilled laboratory technicians to allow optimal communications, clinicopathological correlations, and diagnoses which give specific categorization of disease, and prognostic and etiologic information. This book also represents such teamwork. It has been a pleasure and an honor to work with Dr Michael Kashgarian, whose vision initially inspired this Atlas, with illustration of characteristic lesions, and emphasis on new classifications and insights into pathogenesis. I would also like to thank my renal pathology laboratory team, my fellows and colleagues, without whom it would not have been possible to produce this work. In particular I would like to acknowledge the efforts of Dr Paisit Paveksakon, Dr Xochi Geiger, Dr Patricia Revelo, and Dr Michele Rossini, for help in identifying beautiful, photogenic lesions. Lastly, but not leastly, I would like to thank my husband, Byron, and my children, Katherine, Michelle, and Kristin for their patient support and encouragement.

Agnes Fogo

The production of this Atlas is the result of our love of the craft of renal pathology. It required commitment to the making of a product that we hope will be a positive addition to the field of nephrology. It would not have been possible without the diligence, patience and organizational abilities of my co-author Agnes Fogo who kept me focused on our goal. The material presented is really the contribution of the many clinical nephrologists with whom I have had the pleasure to work and to whom I am deeply indebted for their collaboration over the years. The presentation of the images would not have been possible without the expert help of the staff of the Yale Department of Pathology Graphics and Imaging section whose advice and assistance was essential to the fruition of this work.

Michael Kashgarian

Glomerular Diseases

Chapter

1

References to **Brenner & Rector's** *The Kidney* **7th edition** are given in parentheses below.

Normal growth and maturation

The normal glomerulus consists of a complex branching network of capillaries originating at the afferent arteriole and draining into the efferent arteriole (Figs 1.1–1.3). The glomerulus contains three resident cell types: mesangial, endothelial, and epithelial cells. The visceral epithelial cells (also called podocytes) cover the urinary surface of the glomerular basement membrane (GBM) with its foot processes, with intervening slit diaphragms. Endothelial cells are opposed to the inner surface of the GBM and are fenestrated (Figs 1.4, 1.5). At the stalk of the capillary, the endothelial cell is

Fig. 1.1 In the normal glomerulus, the capillary loops are open, the mesangial areas have no more than three nuclei each, and foot processes are intact, without any deposits or proliferation.

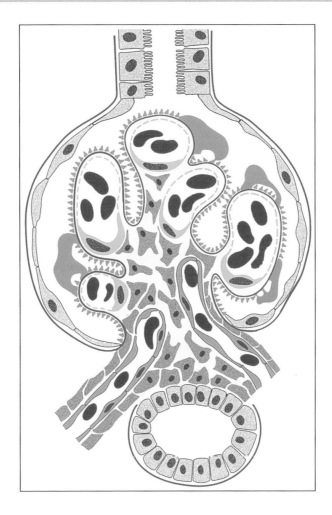

separated from the mesangial cells by the intervening mesangial matrix. The term *endocapillary* is used to describe proliferation filling up the capillary lumen, contributed to by proliferation of mesangial, endothelial and infiltrating inflammatory cells. In contrast, *extracapillary* proliferation refers to proliferation of the parietal epithelial cells that line Bowman's capsule. Specific lesions are described according to their distribution as being segmental vs. global, or diffuse vs. focal. Specialized terminology is also used to describe the specific lesions. A list of commonly used terms and their definitions are provided in Table 1.1.

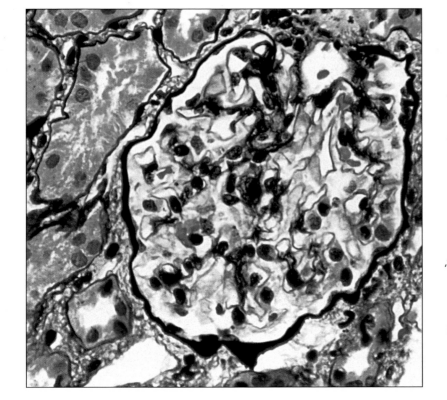

Fig. 1.2 The normal glomerulus has thin, delicate glomerular basement membranes, three or fewer mesangial cell nuclei per mesangial area, and is surrounded by Bowman's capsule. The adjacent tubules show a thin delicate tubular basement membrane without lamellation or surrounding interstitial fibrosis. The vascular pole shows surrounding extraglomerular mesangial cells. The apparent mesangial cellularity of the glomerulus is highly dependent on the thickness of the section, and it is recommended that renal biopsies be cut at 2 μm thickness. This plastic embedded section is cut at 1 μm (Jones' silver stain, ×400).

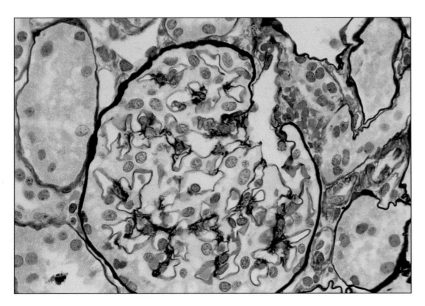

Fig. 1.3 This paraffin-embedded 2 μm section illustrates a normal glomerulus with normal vascular pole with minimal periglomerular interstitial fibrosis and surrounding intact tubules. Mesangial cellularity and matrix are within normal limits (Jones' silver stain, ×400).

Fig. 1.4 The normal glomerular basement membrane in the adult is approximately 325-375 nm in thickness. Overlying podocytes show intact foot processes with minimal effacement in this case. The mesangial matrix surrounds mesangial cells without expansion or hypercellularity. Endothelial cells show normal fenestration. The parietal cells lining Bowman's capsule are flat and squamous in appearance (transmission EM, TEM, ×1500).

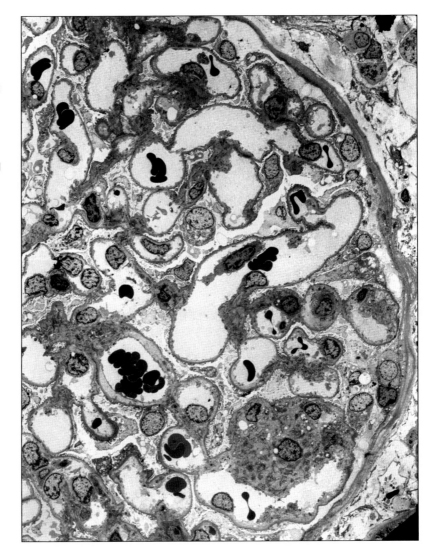

The mesangial cell is a contractile cell that lies embedded in the mesangial matrix in the stalk region of the capillary loops, attached to anchor sites at the ends of the loop by thin extensions of its cytoplasm. Normally up to three mesangial cell nuclei per lobule are present. The glomerular basement membrane consists of three layers distinguished by electron microscopy (EM), the central broadest lamina densa and the less electron-dense zones of lamina rara externa and interna (Figs. 1.4, 1.5).

Fig. 1.5 This glomerulus shows only minimal abnormalities by electron microscopy, with rare vacuoles and blebs in the podocytes. The foot processes are largely intact. The glomerular basement membrane is of normal thickness. Red blood cells and rare platelet fragments are found within capillary lumina. The mesangial areas show mesangial cells surrounded by matrix (TEM, ×3000).

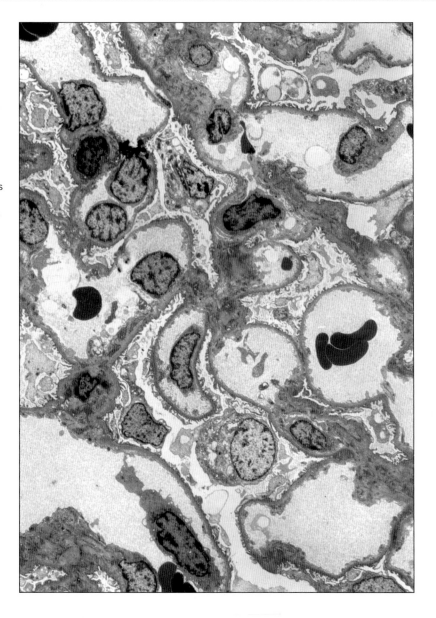

The glomerulus is surrounded by Bowman's capsule, which is lined by parietal epithelial cells. These are continuous with the proximal tubule, identifiable by its PAS-positive brush border. The efferent and afferent arterioles can be distinguished morphologically in favorably oriented sections or by tracing their origins on serial sections. Segmental, interlobular and arcuate arteries may also be present in

TABLE 1.1   Definitions of Common Terms To Describe Morphological Lesions

Light microscopic

Focal	Involving some glomeruli
Diffuse	Involving all glomeruli
Segmental	Involving part of glomerular tuft
Global	Involving total glomerular tuft
Lobular	Simplified, lobular appearance of capillary loop architecture due to endocapillary proliferation (defined below) (seen in e.g. MPGN)
Nodular	Relatively acellular areas of mesangial matrix (seen in e.g. diabetic nephropathy)
Glomerular sclerosis	Obliteration of capillary loop and increased matrix
Crescent	Proliferation of parietal epithelial cells
Spikes	Projections of glomerular basement membrane intervening between subepithelial immune deposits (seen in e.g. membranous glomerulopathy)
Endocapillary proliferation	Proliferation of mesangial and/or endothelial cells and infiltrating inflammatory cells, filling up and distending capillary lumens (seen in e.g. proliferative lupus nephritis)
Hyaline	Descriptive of glassy, smooth appearing material
Hyalinosis	Hyaline-appearing insudation of plasma proteins (seen in e.g. focal segmental glomerulosclerosis)
Mesangial area	Stalk region of capillary loop with mesangial cells surrounded by matrix
Subepithelial	Between visceral epithelial cell and glomerular basement membrane
Subendothelial	Between endothelial cell and glomerular basement membrane
Tram-track	Double contour of glomerular basement due to deposits and/or CMIP (see EM definitions below)
Wire loop	Thick, rigid appearance of capillary loop due to subendothelial deposits
Activity	Description encompassing possible treatment-sensitive lesions, e.g. extent of cellular crescents, cellular infiltrate, necrosis, proliferation
Chronicity	Description of probable irreversible lesions, e.g. extent of tubular atrophy, interstitial fibrosis, fibrous cresents, sclerosis

Immunofluorescence

Granular	Discontinuous flecks of staining producing granular pattern; seen along capillary loop in membranous glomerulopathy
Linear	Smooth continuous staining, seen along capillary loop in e.g. anti-GBM antibody-mediated GN, or along TBM in anti-TBM nephritis

TABLE 1.1—cont'd	
Electron Microscopy	
Foot process effacement	Flattening of foot processes so that they cover the basement membrane, with loss of slit diaphragms
Microvillous transformation	Small extensions of visceral epithelial cells with villus-like appearance
Circumferential mesangial interposition (CMIP)	Extension of mesangial cell or infiltrating monocyte cytoplasm with interposition between endothelial cell cytoplasm and basement membrane, often with underlying new basement membrane formation
Reticular aggregates	Organized arrays of membrane particles within endothelial cells
Immunotactoid GP	Large, organized microtubular deposits, >30 nm diameter
Fibrillary GN	Fibrils 14–20 nm diameter without organization

Abbreviations: GP, glomerulopathy; GN, glomerulonephritis; GBM, glomerular basement membrane; TBM, tubular basement membrane; MPGN, membranoproliferative GN.

the renal biopsy specimen. The cortical biopsy also allows assessment of the tubulointerstitium. Proximal tubules are readily identified by their PAS-positive brush border, lacking in the distal tubules. Collecting ducts show cuboidal, cobblestone-like epithelium. The medulla may also be included in the biopsy.

During fetal maturation, the glomerular capillary tufts are initially covered by large, cuboidal, darkly staining epithelial cells with only small lumina visible (Figs 1.6–1.8). The cells lining Bowman's space undergo similar change from initial tall columnar to cuboidal to flattened epithelial cells, except for those located at the opening of the proximal tubule, where cells remain taller. Immature nephrons may occasionally be seen in the superficial cortex of children up to 1 year of age (Figs 1.6–1.9). Glomerular growth continues until adulthood, with average normal glomerular diameter approximately 95 μm in a group of patients less than 5 years old (average age 2.2 years) and 140 to 160 μm in adulthood. Thickening of the GBM also occurs normally with maturational growth. Normal ranges are from 220 to 260 nm at 1 year of age, 280 to 327 nm at age 5 years, 329 to 370 nm at age 10 years and 358 to 399 nm at age 15 years, the latter similar to adult normal thickness (Figs 1.4, 1.5). Global glomerulosclerosis may occur without renal disease as a part of normal maturation aging and repair. Less than 5% global glomerulo-sclerosis is expected in children and young adults, and less than (age divided by 2, minus 10) per cent in aged normal individuals.

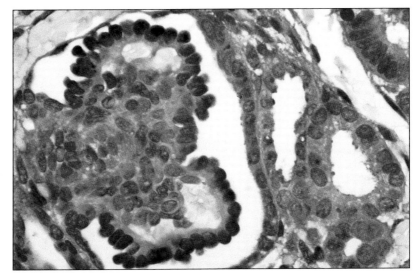

Fig. 1.6 During development, various stages of immature glomeruli may be found at different cortical levels within the kidney. The deep juxtamedullary glomeruli mature first. This immature glomerulus is from the mid-cortical level of a 28-week gestation premature baby. There is prominent mesangium and very simple capillary branching with overlying plump, cuboidal glomerular visceral epithelial cells. The parietal epithelial cells lining Bowman's capsule are also more cuboidal than in the mature state (periodic acid Schiff (PAS), ×400).

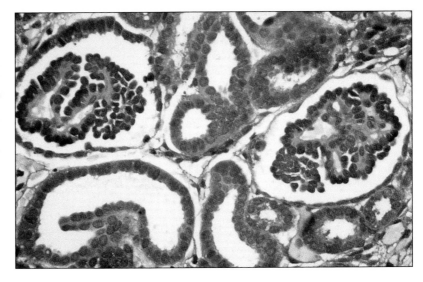

Fig. 1.7 These glomeruli are from the same 28-week gestation baby as shown in Figure 1.3. They have more complex capillary branching pattern, but maintain immature, plump glomerular visceral epithelial cells. In one glomerulus, the parietal epithelial cells are flattened and more mature in appearance (PAS, ×200).

Fig. 1.8 This deep juxtamedullary glomerulus is from the same 28-week gestational baby as shown in the previous figures. There is a complex capillary branching pattern with overlying plump, still immature glomerular visceral epithelial cells. Bowman's space is pouching out to form a junction with the proximal tubular epithe-lium on the right (PAS, ×400).

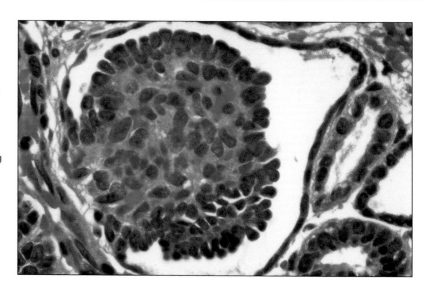

Fig. 1.9 The small, but completely mature glomerulus of a normal term baby is illustrated, with complex capillary branching pattern and mature, pale-gray flattened podocytes overlying the capillary loops. The normal vascular pole is seen at the upper left. Normal proximal tubules with PAS positive brush border with interven-ing peritubular capillaries are also illustrated. Although glomeruli do not increase in number with maturational growth, they increase in size. Normal glomerular diameter in children less than five years old in our biopsy practice is <95 μm. Individual laboratories must establish their own normal parameters since fixation and processing conditions may influence this parameter (PAS, ×100).

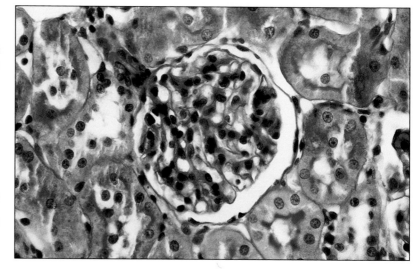

Fig. 1.10 The more super-ficial glomeruli are less mature than the deeper juxtamedullary glomeruli in this term infant. There is persistence of immature podocytes of the more superficial glomeruli, although capillary branching pattern already is complex (PAS, ×100).

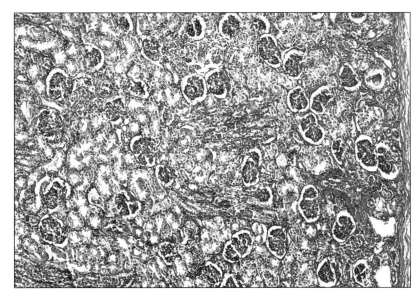

Fig. 1.11 Immature glomeruli from a three-day old infant show immature, plump cuboidal podocytes, with moderately complex capillary branching pattern of the glomerulus on the right, and more simple branching pattern of the glomeruli on the left (PAS, ×100).

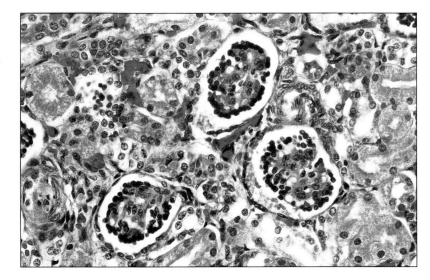

Selected reading

Fogo A, Hawkins E P, Berry P L et al 1990 Glomerular hypertrophy in minimal change disease predicts subsequent progression to focal glomerular sclerosis. Kidney International 38:115–123.

Kaplan C, Pasternack B, Shah H et al 1975 Age-related incidence of sclerotic glomeruli in human kidneys. American Journal of Pathology 80:227–234.

Kappel B, Olsen S 1980 Cortical interstitial tissue and sclerosed glomeruli in the normal human kidney, related to age and sex. A quantitative study. Virchows Archiv (Pathological Anatomy) 387:271–277.

Morita M, White R H R, Raafat F et al 1988 Glomerular basement membrane thickness in children. A morphometric study. Pediatric Nephrology 2:190–195.

Shindo S, Yoshimoto M, Kuriya N et al 1988. Glomerular basement membrane thickness in recurrent and persistent hematuria and nephrotic syndrome: correlation with sex and age. Pediatric Nephrology 2:196–199.

Smith S M, Hoy W E, Cobb L 1989 Low incidence of glomerulosclerosis in normal kidneys. Archives of Pathology and Laboratory Medicine 113:1253–1256.

Primary glomerular diseases

Glomerular diseases that cause nephrotic syndrome: non-immune complex

Minimal change disease and focal segmental glomerulosclerosis

Minimal change disease (MCD) and focal segmental glomerulosclerosis (FSGS) both typically present as the nephrotic syndrome, and cannot be readily distinguished based solely on clinical presentation. In children, nephrotic syndrome is presumed to be due to MCD and biopsy is only done if the child is steroid unresponsive or has clinical features suggesting another etiology of the nephrotic syndrome. In adults, MCD accounts for 10–15% of nephrotic syndrome. FSGS is increasing in incidence, and in the USA in adults has surpassed membranous glomerulonephritis as a cause of nephrotic syndrome (18.7% incidence), especially in African Americans and in Hispanics. Similar increases have also been reported in children with nephrotic syndrome. Serologic studies, including complement levels, are typically within normal limits in both MCD and FSGS. Renal biopsy is essential to determine the etiology of nephrotic syndrome in adults, and also in children who are not steroid responders. The ultimate prognosis differs dramatically, with complete recovery the rule in MCD, contrasting progressive renal insufficiency in FSGS. Several variants of FSGS have also been investigated for their prognostic significance. A working classification proposal is given in Table 1.2. Each of the subtypes will be discussed below.

Minimal change disease

Minimal change disease (MCD) is named for the apparent structurally normal glomeruli by light microscopy (Figs 1.12, 1.13). There are no specific vascular or tubulointerstitial lesions in idiopathic MCD. However, MCD may also occur in the middle-aged or older adult who has nonspecific focal areas of tubulointerstitial scarring and mild vascular lesions (arteriosclerosis, arteriolar hyaline related to hypertension, or other unrelated disease. Global glomerulosclerosis, in contrast to the segmental lesion, is not of

TABLE 1.2   **FSGS Variants**

Type	Defining feature
FSGS, not otherwise specified	Discrete segmental sclerosis
FSGS, perihilar variant	Perihilar sclerosis *and* hyalinosis
FSGS, cellular variant	Endocapillary hypercellularity
FSGS, tip variant	Sclerosis at tubular pole with adhesion at tubular lumen/neck
FSGS, collapsing variant (Collapsing glomerulopathy)	Segmental or global collapse *and* podocyte hyperplasia/hypertrophy

Fig. 1.12   The glomeruli are normal by LM, but with diffuse effacement of foot processes by EM.

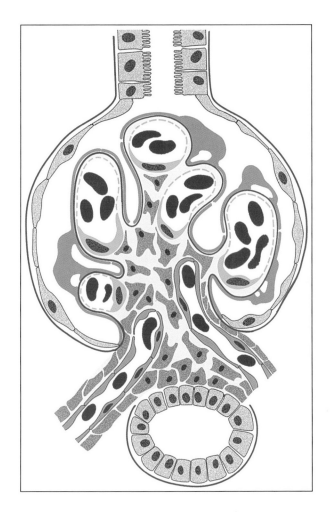

Fig. 1.13   Minimal change disease. Glomeruli appear unremarkable by light microscopy, and in young patients there is no tubulointerstitial fibrosis, as in this patient. In older patients, MCD may occur on a background of nonspecific scarring of the tubulointerstitium (Jones' silver stain, ×200).

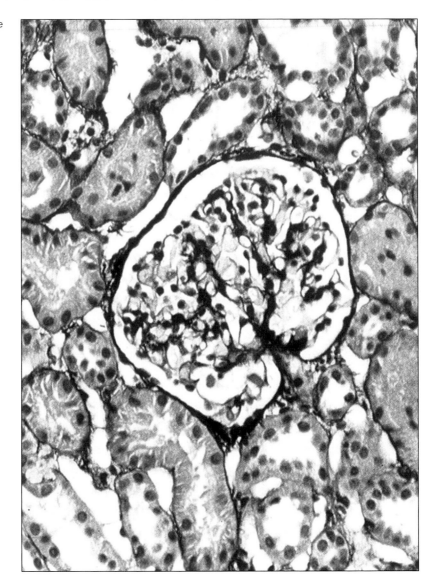

Fig. 1.14 Minimal change disease. Foot process effacement is extensive, often complete, in minimal change disease, although extent of foot process effacement cannot be used as a definitive criterion to differentiate this entity from FSGS. The glomerular basement membrane is unremarkable, and there are no deposits (TEM, ×3000).

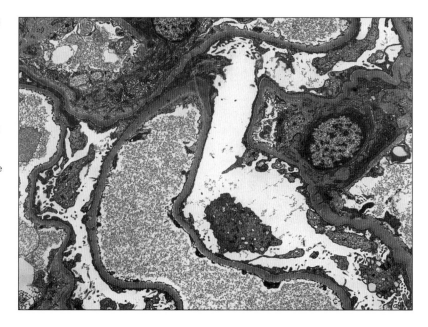

special diagnostic significance in considering the differential of MCD vs. FSGS. Globally sclerotic glomeruli may be normally seen at any age, and are thought to result from normal 'wear and tear,' and not specific disease mechanisms in most cases. Up to 10% of glomeruli may be normally totally sclerosed in people younger than 40 years. The extent of global sclerosis increases with aging, up to 30% by age 80 (estimate by calculating half the patient's age, minus 10).

Associated acute interstitial nephritis (AIN), which is characterized by edema and interstitial lymphoplasmacytic infiltrate, often with eosinophils, suggests a drug-induced hypersensitivity reaction. This combined syndrome of MCD and AIN is classically due to nonsteroidal anti-inflammatory drugs (NSAIDs). This condition is usually reversible with discontinuation of the drug.

Immunofluorescence studies are typically negative in MCD. The presence of IgM staining in otherwise apparent MCD biopsies has been a source of previous controversy, with some authors considering this a specific entity, so-called 'IgM nephropathy' (see below).

Electron microscopy shows extensive foot process effacement, vacuolization and microvillous transformation of epithelial cells in MCD (Figs 1.14, 1.15).

Fig. 1.15 Minimal change disease. Extensive foot process effacement and microvillous transformation of visceral epithelial cells in MCD. Although the endothelial cells are mildly swollen, the glomerular basement membrane is unremarkable, and there are no deposits (TEM, ×8000).

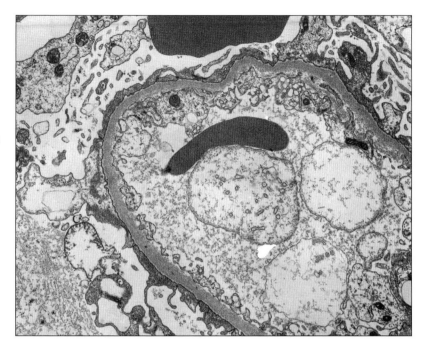

Selected reading

Fogo A, Ichikawa I 1996 Focal segmental glomerulosclerosis – a view and review. Pediatric Nephrology 10:374–391.

Gulati S, Sharma AP, Sharma RK et al 1999 Changing trends of histopathology in childhood nephrotic syndrome. American Journal of Kidney Disease 3:646–650.

Focal segmental glomerulosclerosis

In FSGS of usual type (not otherwise specified, NOS, Table 1.2), sclerosis involves some, but not all glomeruli (focal), and the sclerosis affects a portion of, but not the entire, glomerular tuft (segmental) (Figs 1.16, 1.17). The morphologic diagnosis of focal segmental glomerulosclerosis is a light microscopic description of this pattern of scarring, which may occur in many settings. Differentiation of MCD (see above) from FSGS relies upon a large enough sample to detect the sclerotic glomeruli, since the detection of even a single glomerulus involved with segmental sclerosis is sufficient to invoke a diagnosis of FSGS rather than MCD. Thus, it is apparent that the distinction of MCD and FSGS may be difficult, especially with the smaller and smaller samples obtained with current biopsy guns and smaller needles. A sample of only 10 glomeruli has a 35%

Fig. 1.16 FSGS. There is sharply defined segmental sclerosis, defined as obliteration of capillary loops and increased matrix, without deposits and with diffuse foot process effacement by EM. Adhesions can also be present.

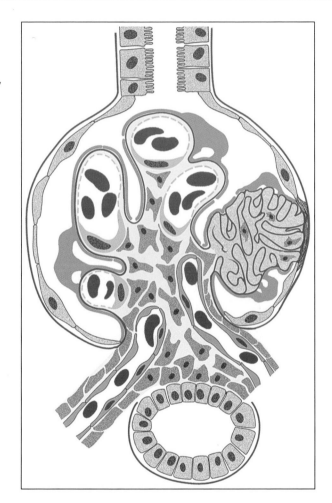

Fig. 1.17 FSGS. Early in FSGS, lesions are very focal, involving initially the juxtamedullary glomeruli. Tubulointerstitial fibrosis in a given section may be a clue to adjacent early segmental sclerotic lesions, which can be detected by careful serial section examination. In this field, one of four glomeruli shows early segmental sclerosis of usual type, with an adjacent area of tubulointerstitial fibrosis (Jones' silver stain, ×100).

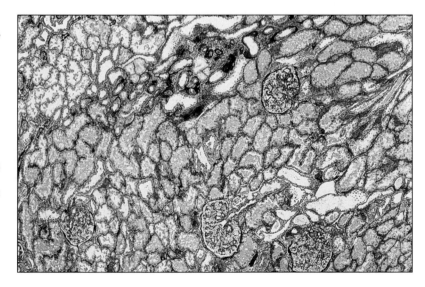

probability of missing a focal lesion that affects 10% of the nephrons, decreasing to 12% if 20 glomeruli are sampled. The initial sclerosis is in the juxtamedullary glomeruli, and this region should be included in the sample (Fig. 1.17). Conversely, sampling on one section by definition cannot identify all of the focally and segmentally distributed scars. Three-dimensional studies examining serial sections of glomeruli in cases of idiopathic FSGS have demonstrated that the process indeed is focal, i.e. glomeruli without any sclerosis exist even when disease is well established (Figs 1.18, 1.19).

Because of these limitations in detection of sclerotic lesions, other diagnostic features in glomeruli uninvolved by the sclerotic process have been sought to suspect FSGS even without sclerosed glomeruli. Abnormal glomerular enlargement (see below) appears to be an early indicator of the sclerotic process even before overt sclerosis can be detected. The presence of marked glomerular enlargement in a biopsy of otherwise apparent MCD would therefore rather suggest an early, incipient stage of FSGS. Diffuse mesangial hypercellularity may be a morphological feature superimposed on changes of either MCD or FSGS, with or without IgM deposits, without defined prognostic significance (see below).

The PAS-positive acellular material in the segmental sclerotic lesions of the glomerulus may have different composition depending upon the diverse pathophysiologic mechanisms discussed below. The sclerotic process is defined by glomerular capillary collapse

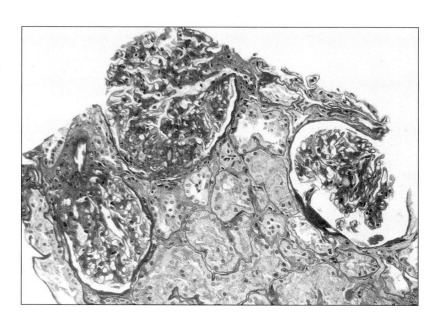

Fig. 1.18 FSGS. There is early segmental sclerosis that involves the periphery in one glomerulus, and the hilar area in another glomerulus, but without significant hyalinosis. This is characteristic of FSGS (PAS, ×200).

Fig. 1.19   FSGS. There are more advanced segmental sclerotic lesions affecting two of the three glomeruli in this field, with surrounding proportionate tubulointerstitial fibrosis. The sclerosis is characterized by increased matrix and obliteration of capillary lumens, and is of the usual type of FSGS (Jones' silver stain, ×200).

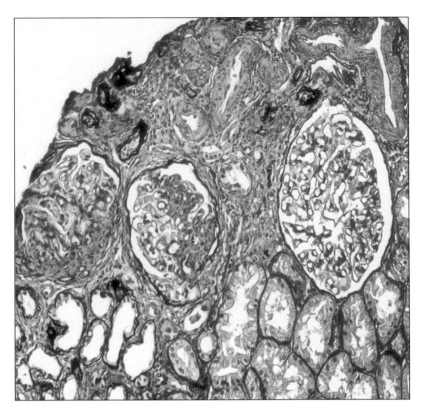

Fig. 1.20   FSGS. Near end-stage FSGS is present, with global or near global sclerosis of all glomeruli and extensive tubulointerstitial fibrosis and vascular thickening (Jones' silver stain, ×200).

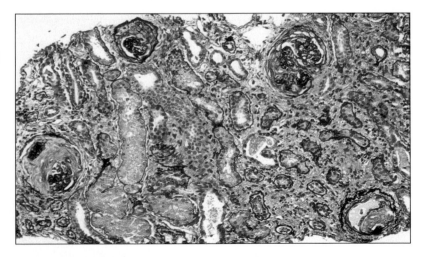

with increase in matrix, and varies from small, early lesions to near global sclerosis (Fig. 1.20–1.23). The segmental sclerosis lesions are discrete, and may be located in perihilar and/or peripheral portions of the glomerulus. There may be associated global glomerulosclerosis, which has no specific diagnostic significance. Uninvolved

Fig. 1.21 FSGS. The typical segmental sclerotic lesion in FSGS is characterized by increased matrix and obliteration of capillary lumina, frequently with hyalinosis and adhesions, as illustrated here. There is surrounding tubulointerstitial fibrosis. The uninvolved segment of the glomerulus appears unremarkable (Jones' silver stain, ×200).

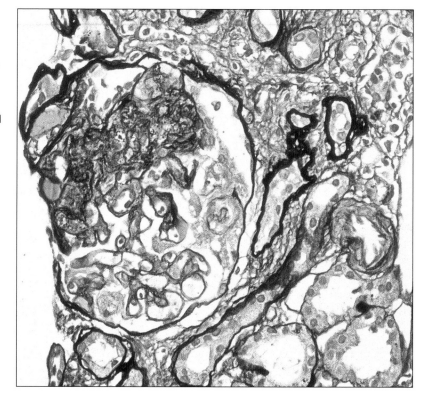

Fig. 1.22 FSGS. An advanced segmental sclerotic lesion of FSGS is shown, with only minimal hyaline droplets. There is increased mesangial matrix and obliteration of capillary lumina involving the majority of the glomerulus. The uninvolved portion of the glomerulus has mild increase in mesangial matrix. The adjacent tubule shows atrophy and a proteinaceous cast (PAS, ×400).

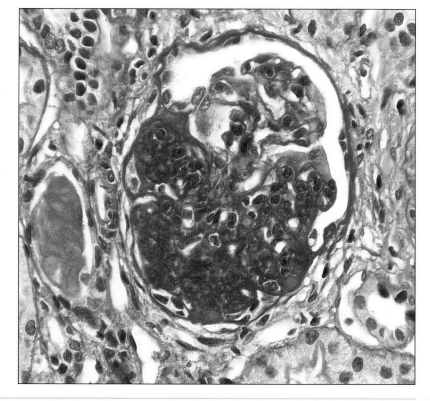

Fig. 1.23   FSGS. The segmental sclerotic lesion of FSGS is illustrated, with increased mesangial matrix and obliteration of capillary lumina. The remnants of the glomerular basement membrane in the sclerosed segment can be seen as wrinkled lines on this silver stain. The uninvolved portion of the glomerulus shows minimal mesangial matrix increase. Although this sclerotic lesion involves the vascular pole, there is not associated hyalinosis, and the lesion is therefore best classified as FSGS, NOS (Jones' silver stain, ×400).

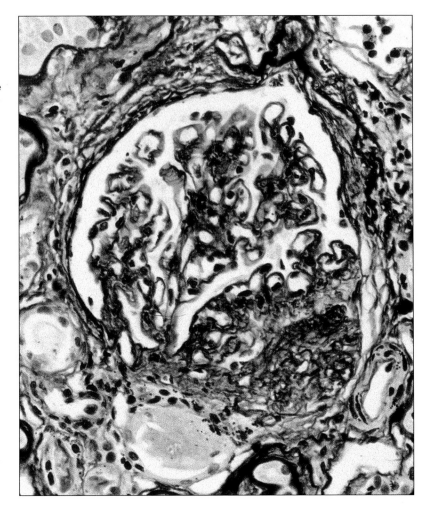

glomeruli show no apparent lesions by light microscopy, but may appear enlarged, as do glomeruli with early stage segmental sclerosis. The glomerulosclerosis may be associated with hyalinosis, resulting from insudation of plasma proteins, producing a smooth, glassy (hyaline) appearance (Fig. 1.24). This occurs particularly in the axial, vascular pole region. Of note, arteriolar hyalinosis may occur with hypertensive injury and should not be taken *per se* as evidence of a sclerotic lesion (see hilar type FSGS below). Vascular thickening may be prominent late in the course of FSGS. Adhesion of the podocyte to Bowman's capsule (synechiae) can be an early manifestation of sclerosis (Fig. 1.25). The glomerulosclerosis is accompanied by tubular atrophy, interstitial fibrosis with interstitial lymphocytes, proportional to the degree of scarring in the glomerulus (Fig. 1.22).

Fig. 1.24 FSGS. In this case of FSGS, there was extensive hyalinosis in the sclerotic areas, which are characterized by increased mesangial matrix and obliteration of capillary lumina. There are also adhesions of the sclerotic segments to Bowman's capsule, with thickened and disrupted Bowman's capsule. The hyalinosis represents an insudation of plasma proteins, reflecting endothelial injury (Jones' silver stain, ×400).

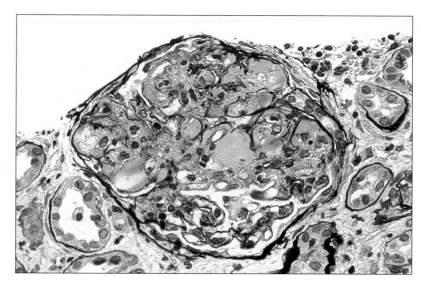

Fig. 1.25 FSGS. Early lesion of FSGS with adhesion of glomerular tuft to Bowman's capsule and small segmental area of hyalinosis and intracapillary foam cells (Jones' silver stain, ×400).

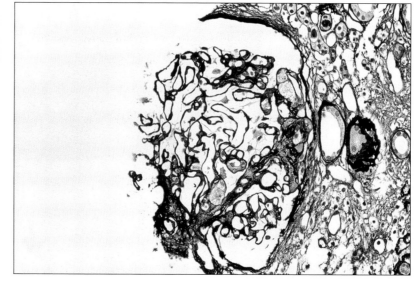

Of note, in HIV-associated nephropathy (HIVAN) and collapsing nephropathy, tubular lesions are disproportionally severe (see below).

Immunofluorescence may show non-specific entrapment of IgM and C3 in sclerotic areas or areas where mesangial matrix is increased (Fig. 1.26).

Electron microscopy shows foot process effacement that often is not complete in FSGS (Fig. 1.27). However, extent of foot process

Fig. 1.26 FSGS. Immuno-fluorescence studies in FSGS do not show immune complexes, but may show IgM in sclerotic areas or in areas of mesangial expansion (anti-IgM antibody immunofluorescence, ×400).

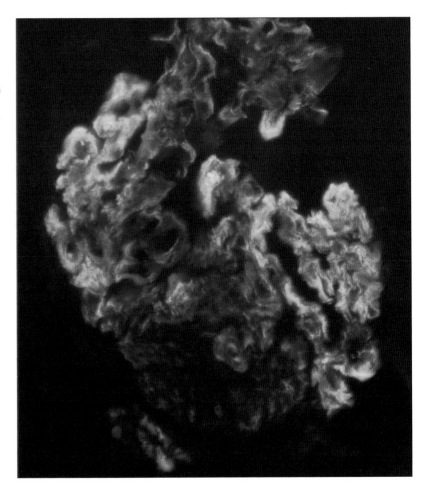

effacement does not allow precise distinction between MCD and FSGS in individual cases. Foot process effacement tends to be more extensive in primary FSGS compared with secondary FSGS, however, the overlap between these two categories does not allow one to use this as a diagnostic feature in individual cases. The absence of any foot process effacement should cast doubt on the diagnosis of FSGS. There are no immune deposits in idiopathic FSGS, but mesangial matrix is increased in sclerotic areas (Fig. 1.28). Areas of hyalin may be present in the sclerotic segments and appear dense by EM, but should be readily recognized as hyalin by correlating with scout section light microscopic appearance (Fig. 1.29). The presence of numerous reticular aggregates in endothelial cells in the setting of segmental glomerulosclerosis with collapsing features suggests possible HIV-associated nephropathy (see below).

Fig. 1.27 FSGS. By electron microscopy, there is extensive foot process effacement in FSGS. However, it may not be complete, as illustrated here. If there is less than approximately 50% foot process effacement, the diagnosis of primary FSGS is in doubt. There is also mesangial matrix expansion, without immune deposits (TEM, ×3000).

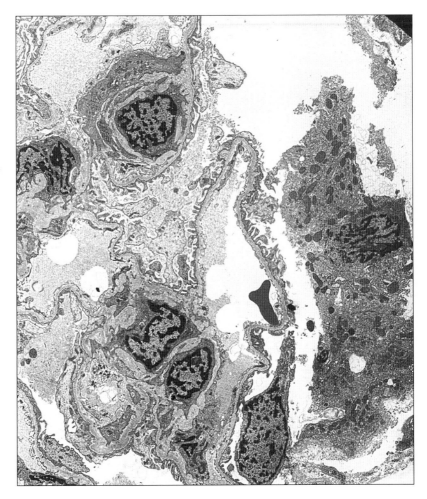

Diagnosis of recurrence of FSGS in the transplant

Most recurrences occur within the first months after transplantation, although proteinuria may recur immediately after the graft is implanted. Foot process effacement is present at time of recurrence of proteinuria and precedes the development of sclerosis, typically by weeks to months. Glomerular enlargement at this stage of recurrent FSGS is prominent in children, who otherwise do not undergo glomerular enlargement when receiving an adult kidney. (In contrast, an adult recipient of a single kidney will normally have marked renal and glomerular growth to provide adequate glomerular filtration rate (GFR)). Overt sclerosis is not noted until weeks to

Fig. 1.28 FSGS. Segmental increase in matrix with obliterated capillary lumens is apparent in this case of FSGS. The overlying visceral epithelial cells show vacuolization, microvillous transformation and extensive foot process effacement. The corrugated, collapsed glomerular basement membrane is evident. There are no immune deposits (TEM, ×5000).

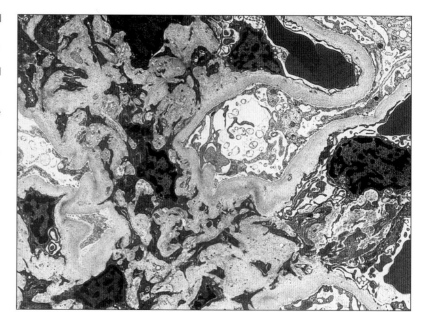

Fig. 1.29 FSGS. Hyaline deposit within a segmentally sclerotic area in FSGS. Hyaline is smooth, homogeneous, usually located in areas of sclerosis, and frequently contains lipid (clear, round areas). The sclerotic segment is characterized by increased matrix and obliteration of the capillary lumen, with dense adhesion to the overlying fibrotic Bowman's capsule (TEM, ×3000).

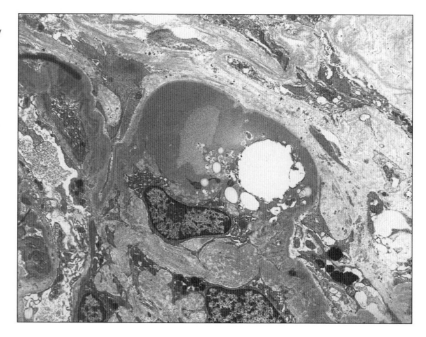

even months after recurrence of nephrotic syndrome. Thus, during this time interval in the setting of the FSGS patient with nephrotic syndrome in the transplant, foot process effacement alone without detectable segmental sclerosis, is evidence of recurrent FSGS.

Differential diagnosis of MCD vs. FSGS

Some investigators have felt that the common clinical presentation and similar findings in intact glomeruli indicate that MCD and FSGS are two manifestations of the same disease. Our data and those from others rather support differences even at the earliest time points. Much evidence has pointed to the participation of abnormal glomerular adaptation and growth factors in the pathogenesis of glomerulosclerosis. Several studies have shown that glomerular enlargement precedes overt glomerulosclerosis, both in pediatric and adult patients who otherwise had apparent MCD initially. Patients with abnormal glomerular growth even on initial biopsies that did not show overt sclerotic lesions, subsequently developed overt glomerulosclerosis, documented in later biopsies. A cut-off of >50% larger glomerular area than normal for age was a sensitive indicator of increased risk for progression in one series of children with nephrotic syndrome. Of note, glomeruli grow in size until approximately age 18 years, although no new glomeruli are formed after birth, so age-matched controls must be used in the pediatric population to assess normal glomerular size.

The finding of mesangial hypercellularity (more than 80% of glomeruli with >3 cells per mesangial region) has been proposed to indicate a subtype of primary MCD with poorer prognosis and increased risk for development of FSGS. However, several series have failed to confirm a definite clinical correlation of this morphologic variant. Thus, in several series, patients with this manifestation on renal biopsies that otherwise show apparent MCD despite decreased initial response to steroids, had ultimate good prognosis. Lack of uniform application of criteria for morphologic definition of mesangial hypercellularity makes it difficult to assess impact of this feature on prognosis. Children with FSGS and mesangial hypercellularity did not show worse prognosis than those with typical FSGS. Thus, diffuse mesangial hypercellularity does not appear to impart a specific prognostic significance in either MCD or FSGS, or to differentiate between apparent MCD and unsampled FSGS.

IgM deposits by IF in association with mesangial hypercellularity may indicate a poorer response to steroids, and some patients have shown histological FSGS on second biopsy after an initial biopsy showed 'IgM nephropathy'. However, the significance of IgM deposits by IF in the setting of normal glomeruli by light microscopy has been difficult to assess. Again, series of biopsies from children with FSGS and nephrotic syndrome have failed to show a specific predictive value of the IgM staining with or without diffuse mesangial hypercellularity. If deposits are present by EM as well as by IF, a mesangiopathic immune complex glomerulonephritis should be diagnosed.

In summary, the diagnosis of FSGS cannot be completely excluded when segmental sclerotic lesions are not detected, even with an adequate size biopsy. It is therefore best to include the possibility of undersampled FSGS in biopsies from patients with nephrotic syndrome, no immune complexes and foot process effacement, especially when glomerular number is less than 25, or other morphologic findings indicative of probability of undersampled FSGS are present. These include glomerular enlargement and interstitial fibrosis (in young patients).

Etiology/pathogenesis

The pathogenesis of MCD appears related to abnormal cytokines which only affect glomerular permeability, and do not promote sclerogenic mechanisms. MCD has been associated with drug-induced hypersensitivity reactions. MCD also has been associated with Hodgkin's disease, bee stings, and other venom exposure, implicating immune dysfunction as an initiating factor.

Primary FSGS is thought to result from an undefined circulating factor or factors, which mediate abnormal glomerular permeability and ultimately sclerosis. Recent studies have pointed to epithelial cell injury and dedifferentiation of its phenotype in the pathogenesis of nephrotic syndrome.

New studies of the molecular biology of the podocyte and identification of genes mutated in rare familial forms of FSGS (α-actinin-4 and podocin) or in congenital nephrotic syndrome of Finnish type (nephrin, NPHS1), have given important new insights into mechanisms of progressive glomerulosclerosis and nephrotic syndrome. Nephrin localizes to the slit diaphragm of the podocyte and is tightly associated with CD2-associated protein (CD2AP). Nephrin functions as a zona occludens-type junction protein, and along with CD2AP provides a crucial role in receptor patterning and cytoskeletal polarity, and perhaps signaling. Mice engineered to be deficient in CD2AP develop congenital nephrotic syndrome, similar to congenital nephrotic syndrome of Finnish type. Autosomal dominant FSGS is caused by mutation in α-actinin 4 (ACTN4). This is hypothesized to cause altered actin cytoskeleton interaction, causing FSGS through a gain-of-function mechanism, contrasting the loss-of-function mechanism implicated for disease caused by the nephrin mutation. Patients with α-actinin 4 mutation progress to end-stage by age 30, with rare recurrence in the transplant. Podocin, another podocyte specific gene (NPHS2) is mutated in autosomal recessive FSGS that has an early onset in childhood with rapid progression to end-stage. Podocin is an integral stomatin protein family member and interacts with the CD2AP-nephrin complex, indicating that podocin could serve in the structural organization of the slit diaphragm. Acquired disruption of some of these complexly interacting podocyte molecules has been demonstrated in experimental models and in human proteinuric diseases. Thus, it is possible that novel molecular and immunostaining techniques to detect abnormalities in these genes will become of diagnostic and prognostic utility, although there currently are no specific morphologic findings recognized to distinguish the FSGS cases due to mutations in these genes from other types of FSGS.

Selected reading

General

Braden G L, Mulhern J G, O'Shea M H et al 2000 Changing incidence of glomerular diseases in adults. American Journal of Kidney Disease 35:878–883.

Corwin H L, Schwartz M M, Lewis E J 1988 The importance of sample size in the interpretation of the renal biopsy. American Journal of Nephrology 8:85–89.

D'Agati V 1994 The many masks of focal segmental glomerulosclerosis. Kidney International 46:1223–1241.

D'Agati V D, Fogo A B, Bruijn J A, Jennette J C 2004 Pathologic classification of focal segmental glomerulosclerosis: a working proposal. American Journal of Kidney Disease 43:368–382.

Fogo A, Hawkins E P, Berry P L et al 1990 Glomerular hypertrophy in minimal change disease predicts subsequent progression to focal glomerular sclerosis. Kidney International 38:115–123.

Fogo A, Ichikawa I 1996 Focal segmental glomerulosclerosis – a view and review. Pediatric Nephrology 10:374–391.

Gulati S, Sharma A P, Sharma R K et al 1999 Changing trends of histopathology in childhood nephrotic syndrome. American Journal of Kidney Disease 3:646–650.

Haas M, Spargo B, Coventry S 1995 Increasing incidence of focal-segmental glomerulosclerosis among adult nephropathies: A 20-year renal biopsy study. American Journal of Kidney Disease 26:740–750.

Smith S M, Hoy W E, Cobb L 1989 Low incidence of glomerulosclerosis in normal kidneys. Archives of Pathology and Laboratory Medicine 113:1253–1256.

Genetics

Boute N, Gribouval O, Roselli S et al 2000 NPHS2, encoding the glomerular protein podocin, is mutated in autosomal recessive steroid-resistant nephrotic syndrome. Nature Genetics 24:349–354.

Kaplan J M, Kim S H, North K N et al 2000 Mutations in ACTN4, encoding alpha-actinin-4, cause familial focal segmental glomerulosclerosis. Nature Genetics 24:251–256.

Karle S M, Uetz B, Ronner V et al 2002 Novel mutations in NPHS2 detected in both familial and sporadic steroid-resistant nephrotic syndrome. Journal of the American Society of Nephrology 13:388–393.

Collapsing glomerulopathy

Collapsing glomerulopathy has a poor prognosis with marked proteinuria, rapid loss of renal function and virtually no responsiveness to corticosteroids alone. This lesion occurs in both Caucasians and in African Americans, although some series show strong African American preponderance. The incidence of this lesion varies in different geographic regions. In New York, the incidence has increased from 11% of all cases of idiopathic FSGS from 1979 to 1985, to 20% of this group from 1986 to 1989, to 24% of idiopathic FSGS from 1990 to 1993. In a large renal biopsy practice centered in Chicago, the collapsing variant accounted for only 4.7% of FSGS biopsies.

By light microscopy there is glomerular tuft collapse (segmental or global) *and* overlying visceral epithelial cell hyperplasia and hypertrophy (Fig. 1.30). Collapsing lesions are more often global than segmental (Table 1.2, Figs 1.31, 1.32). Segmental lesions may involve perihilar and/or peripheral portions of the glomerulus (Fig. 1.33). There are frequent marked protein droplets in the hypertrophied visceral epithelial cells (Fig. 1.34). Adhesions and hyalinosis are uncommon in the early stage of the lesion, as are mesangial hypercellularity and glomerulomegaly. Involvement of even a single glomerulus with this collapsing lesion is proposed to warrant classification as collapsing glomerulopathy, with its attendant poor prognosis (Fig. 1.35). Other types of segmental sclerosis (Table 1.2) may coexist. Differentiation of cellular or collapsing type FSGS from usual, nos FSGS, may be difficult in some cases (Fig. 1.36). Vessels do not show specific lesions. Tubules show injury disproportionate to the sclerosis, with microcystic change (Fig. 1.37), and there is interstitial inflammation.

Immunofluorescence may show IgM and C3 in sclerotic segments. Electron microscopy shows the wrinkled, collapsed TBM and overlying visceral epithelial cell hypertrophy/hyperplasia with frequent

Fig. 1.30 Collapsing GP. There is segmental or global collapse of the capillary tuft with overlying visceral epithelial cell hyperplasia, without deposits.

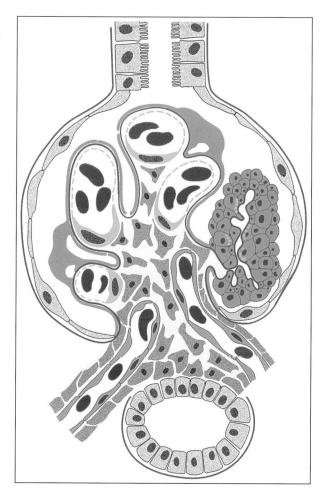

Fig. 1.31 Collapsing GP. Collapsing glomerulopathy is charac-terized by collapse of the glomerular tuft with marked proliferation of overlying glomerular visceral epithelial cells, often with prominent protein droplets. The collapse may be global, or more segmental (Jones' silver stain, ×400).

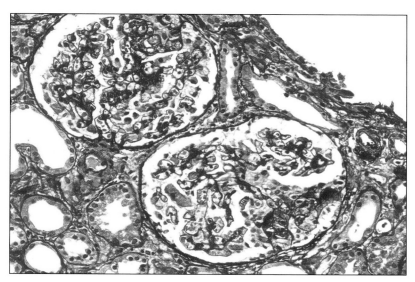

Fig. 1.32   Collapsing GP. Extensive collapse with marked visceral epithelial cell hyperplasia in collapsing glomerulopathy (Jones' silver stain, ×400).

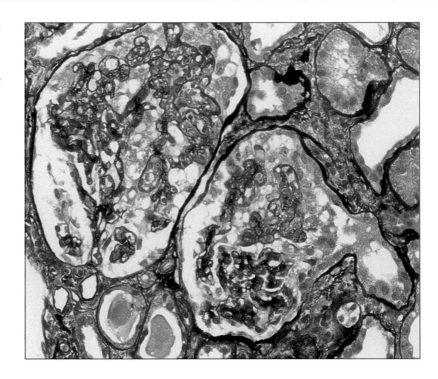

Fig. 1.33   Collapsing GP. Occasionally the collapse in collapsing glomerulopathy may be quite segmental, with the remainder of the glomerular capillary tuft showing no alterations. There is marked segmental collapse with overlying visceral epithelial cell hyperplasia in this case of collapsing glomerulopathy (Jones' silver stain, ×200).

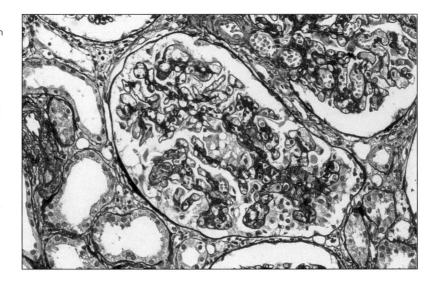

Fig. 1.34 Collapsing GP. There is collapse of the glomerular tuft and overlying hyperplasia of the visceral epithelial cells, with prominent protein reabsorption droplets (Jones' silver stain, ×400).

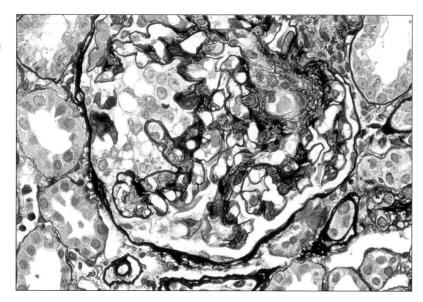

Fig. 1.35 Collapsing GP. There are some overlap features between the cellular type of FSGS and collapsing glomerulopathy, as illustrated here. There is collapse in areas, and segmental endocapillary hypercellularity, with occasional neutrophils and foam cells, with overlying visceral epithelial cell hyperplasia. However, the endocapillary hypercellularity is not quite prominent enough to classify as a cellular lesion, and this lesion would best be classified as collapsing glomerulopathy (Jones' silver stain, ×400).

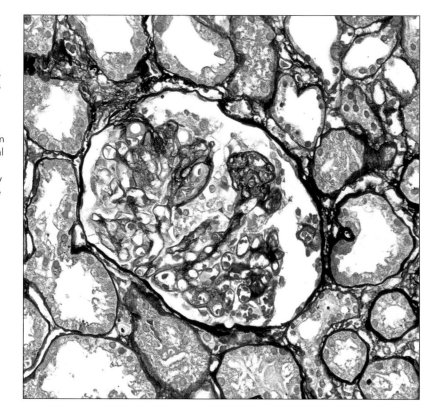

Fig. 1.36 Complex FSGS. This glomerulus shows an early, complex sclerosing lesion with varying features. There is a segmental area of adhesion with hyalinosis (left), with mild overlying visceral epithelial cell hypertrophy/hyperplasia. In the adjacent lobule, there is an early cellular lesion with mild endocapillary hypercellularity, but without the typical foam cells of FSGS, cellular variant. There is not well-established collapse, and the cellular lesion occupies only a very small portion of the tuft. This is therefore best classified as FSGS, NOS, although it shows some overlapping features with both the cellular and collapsing variants of FSGS (endocapillary hypercellularity and visceral epithelial cell hypertrophy/hyperplasia). This most likely represents an early sclerosing lesion (Jones' silver stain, ×400).

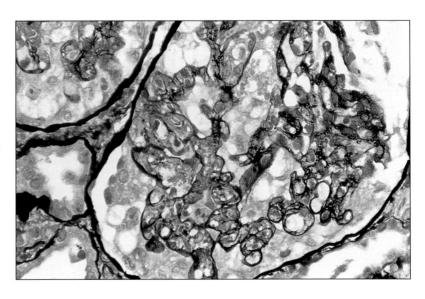

vacuoles and protein droplets. No immune complexes are present (Fig. 1.38). Reticular aggregates are not present in idiopathic collapsing glomerulopathy.

Etiology/pathogenesis

Mature podocytes do not usually proliferate due to high expression of cyclin-dependent kinase inhibitor p27kip1. In collapsing glomerulopathy and HIVAN, p27kip1 expression is lost in areas of collapse, with proliferation and dedifferentiation. These observations point to a dysregulated phenotype of the podocyte in the pathogenesis of

Fig. 1.37 Collapsing GP. Collapsing glomerulopathy is often associated with disproportionate tubulointerstitial injury with microcystic change with proteinaceous casts, as shown here (Jones' silver stain, ×200).

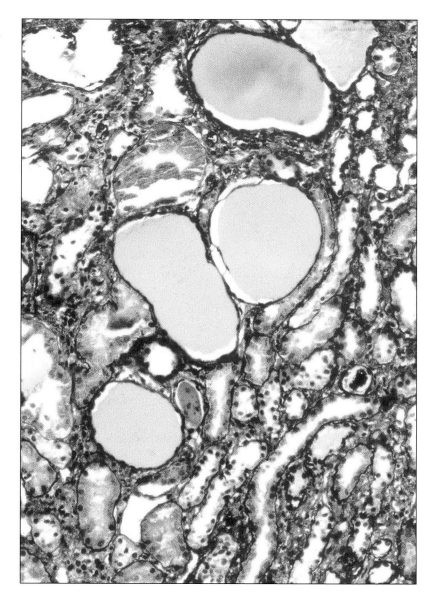

these disorders. The etiology has not yet been defined, however, a possible viral agent has been proposed. Evidence of parvovirus infection was more frequent in patients with collapsing glomerulopathy compared with controls, usual type FSGS or HIVAN, suggesting an association. Treatment with pamidronate also has been linked to

Fig. 1.38 Collapsing glomerulopathy. There is corrugation of the GBM with segmental areas of collapse by electron microscopy, without any deposits. Glomerular visceral epithelial cells show extensive foot process effacement, vacuolization, and microvillous transformation as illustrated here. In idiopathic collapsing glomerulopathy, there are no reticular aggregates, in contrast to HIVAN, where they are frequent (TEM, ×7000).

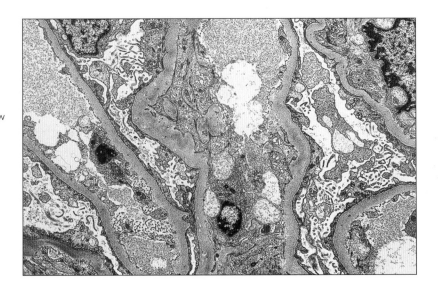

development of collapsing glomerulopathy. Recurrence in the transplant has been reported. De novo collapsing glomerulopathy has also been noted in the transplant, linked to cyclosporine toxicity. Collapsing glomerular lesions also occur in native kidneys in a zonal distribution associated with severe vascular injury.

Selected reading

Barisoni L, Kriz W, Mundel P et al 1999 The dysregulated podocyte phenotype: a novel concept in the pathogenesis of collapsing idiopathic focal segmental glomerulosclerosis and HIV-associated nephropathy. Journal of the American Society of Nephrology 10:51–56.

Detwiler R K, Falk R F, Hogan S L et al 1994 Collapsing glomerulopathy: A clinically and pathologically distinct variant of focal segmental glomerulosclerosis. Kidney International 45:1416–1424.

Laurinavicius A, Hurwitz S, Rennke H G 1999 Collapsing glomerulopathy in HIV and non-HIV patients: a clinicopathological and follow-up study. Kidney International 56:2203–2213.

Markowitz G S, Appel G B, Fine P L et al 2001 Collapsing focal segmental glomerulosclerosis following treatment with high-dose pamidronate. Journal of the American Society of Nephrology 12:1164–1172.

Moudgil A, Nast C C, Bagga A et al 2001 Association of parvovirus B19 infection with idiopathic collapsing glomerulopathy. Kidney International 59:2126–2133.

Valeri A, Barisoni L, Appel G B et al 1996 Idiopathic collapsing focal segmental glomerulosclerosis: a clinicopathologic study. Kidney International 50:1734–1746.

Tip lesion variant of FSGS

Patients with tip lesion present with nephrotic syndrome. This lesion was proposed to represent an early lesion with good prognosis similar to MCD. However, later follow-up has revealed a less than benign prognosis in some patients.

The tip lesion is defined as glomerulosclerosis involving only the tubular pole of the glomerulus (Fig. 1.39). The collapsing glomerulopathy variant must be excluded to diagnose tip variant FSGS (Table 1.2). It is defined as the presence of at least one segmental lesion involving the outer 25% of the glomerulus next to the proximal tubule pole with adhesion between the tuft and Bowman's capsule at the tubule lumen or neck (Figs 1.40, 1.41). Thus, the proximal tubule pole must be identified in order to recognize and

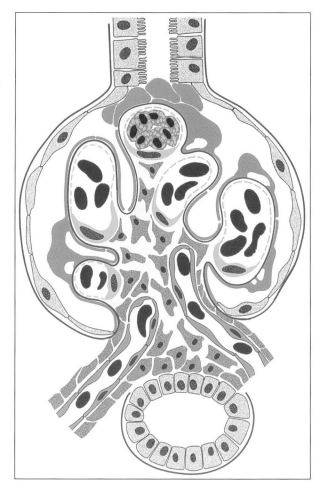

Fig. 1.39 FSGS, tip lesion. Segmental sclerosis is confined to the proximal tubular pole, and often has endocapillary proliferation with foam cells and overlying visceral epithelial cell hyperplasia. Foot processes are diffusely effaced, without deposits.

Fig. 1.40 FSGS, tip lesion. The localized sclerotic lesion that only involves the proximal tubular pole of the glomerulus is classified as the tip variant of FSGS (PAS, ×100).

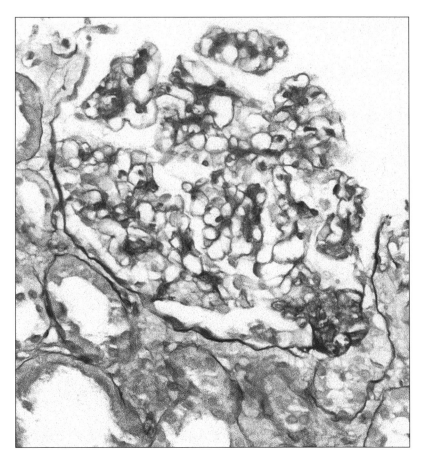

Fig. 1.41 FSGS, tip lesion. The adhesion between the glomerular tuft and the neck of the proximal tubule with intracapillary foam cells is evident in this tip lesion variant of FSGS (Jones' silver stain, ×400).

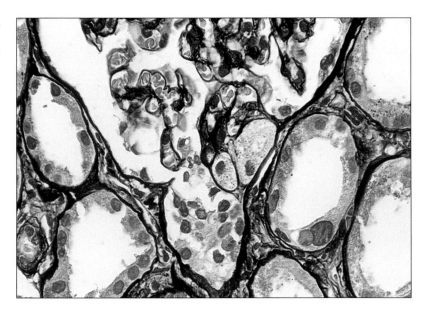

diagnose the lesion. The segmental lesion may be characterized by either endocapillary hypercellularity (involving <50% of the tuft) or sclerosis (involving <25% of the tuft). Foam cells are common, but hyalinosis is variable. The involved area often shows podocyte hypertrophy/hyperplasia. Mesangial hypercellularity, glomerulomegaly and arteriolar hyalinosis are variable. Other glomeruli may show usual segmental lesions or cellular lesions. IF and EM findings are as in usual type FSGS.

Etiology/pathogenesis

The etiology and pathogenesis are unknown.

Selected reading

Howie A J, Brewer D B 1985 Further studies on the glomerular tip lesion: Early and late stages and life table analysis. Journal of Pathology 147:245–255.
Stokes M B, Markowitz G S, Lin J et al 2004 Glomerular tip lesion: a distinct entity within the minimal change disease/focal segmental glomerulosclerosis spectrum. Kidney International 65:1690–1702.

Cellular variant of FSGS

Patients with the cellular variant of FSGS present with abrupt onset of nephrotic syndrome. To diagnose the cellular variant of FSGS, we

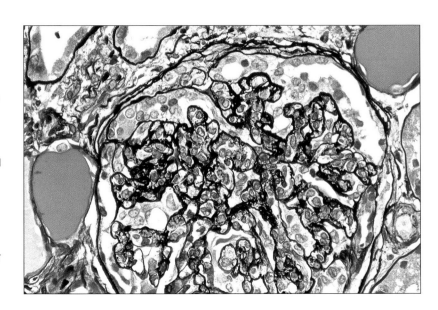

Fig. 1.42   FSGS, cellular. There is extensive endocapillary hyper-cellularity with frequent mononuclear cells and multifocal, early adhesions of the tuft to Bowman's capsule in this cellular variant of FSGS. There is mild prominence of the overlying visceral epithelial cells, but not frank hyperplasia, and no collapse of the glomerular tuft to indicate collapsing glomerulopathy. Immune complexes were excluded by IF and EM (Jones' silver stain, ×400).

Fig. 1.43   FSGS, cellular. There is only a segmental area of endocapillary hypercellularity with hypertrophy of overlying visceral epithelial cells in this cellular variant of FSGS. Immune complexes were excluded by IF and EM (Jones' silver stain, ×400).

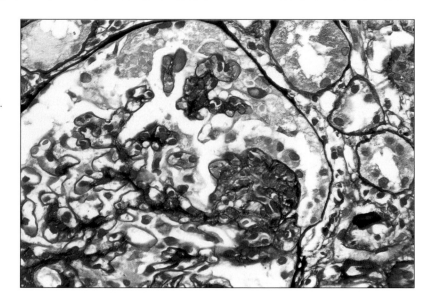

propose that tip lesion and collapsing glomerulopathy must be excluded (Table 1.2). The cellular variant of FSGS is then defined as at least one glomerulus with endocapillary proliferation involving at least 25% of the tuft and occluding the lumen (Figs 1.42, 1.43). The endocapillary cells typically include foam cells, macrophages and endothelial cells. Neutrophils and lymphocytes may also be present. There may be podocyte hyperplasia/hypertrophy overlying this lesion, but unlike in collapsing glomerulopathy, this is not a required feature. These lesions may develop into progressively less cellular, more sclerotic lesions, becoming indistinguishable clinically and morphologically from classical FSGS (Fig. 1.36). Thus, other glomeruli in the biopsy may contain usual type of segmental or global glomerulosclerosis. IF and EM findings are as in usual type FSGS.

Etiology/pathogenesis

This cellular lesion may be an early abnormality seen by LM when FSGS recurs in the transplant. Thus, this morphologic variant is postulated to represent an early, active FSGS lesion.

Selected reading

Schwartz M M, Evans J, Bain R et al 1999 Focal segmental glomerulosclerosis: prognostic implications of the cellular lesion. Journal of American Society of Nephrology 10:1900–1907.

Fig. 1.44 Secondary FSGS. Segmental sclerosis may also be seen secondary to other conditions, or be associated with hypertensive arterionephrosclerosis, as in this case. The diagnosis of primary FSGS was excluded by very limited foot process effacement, disproportionate vascular sclerosis, extensive global sclerosis, and most importantly, the clinical course with long-standing hypertension preceding any evidence of renal dysfunction (Jones' silver stain, ×100).

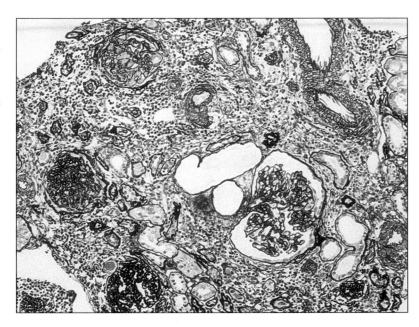

Perihilar variant of FSGS

Patients present with proteinuria. Patients may have hypertension or other underlying conditions linked to renal scarring (Fig. 1.44). To diagnose this type, cellular, tip variants of FSGS and collapsing glomerulopathy must first be excluded (Table 1.2). Perihilar type FSGS is defined by perihilar sclerosis and hyalinosis involving >50% of involved glomeruli. Glomerulomegaly and adhesions are common. There is often arteriolar hyalinosis, but arteriolar hyalin alone is insufficient for diagnosis (Figs 1.45, 1.46). Mesangial hypercellularity is usually absent, and podocytes do not typically show hyperplasia/hypertrophy. IF and EM findings are as in usual type FSGS.

Etiology/pathogenesis – secondary forms of FSGS

Predominantly perihilar lesions of sclerosis have been proposed to represent a response to reduced renal mass. This variant may occur in idiopathic FSGS and is also common in patients with secondary forms of FSGS related to adaptive responses to reduced nephron mass and/or glomerular hypertension. Many insults to the kidney may result in secondary FSGS, either as the sole manifestation of injury, or superimposed on other renal disease manifestations.

Fig. 1.45 FSGS, perihilar. The perihilar type of FSGS shows vascular pole sclerosis with hyalinosis, often with hyalin extending into the arteriolar pole, as seen on these adjacent sections of a glomerulus with perihilar variant of FSGS. This may often be secondary to other conditions or associated with arterionephrosclerosis, or be idiopathic (a, PAS; b, Jones' silver stain, ×200).

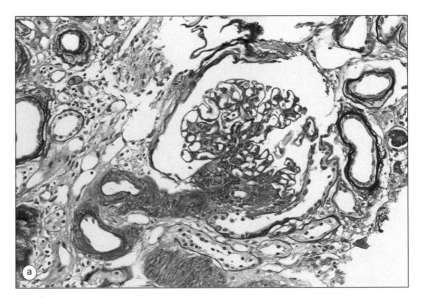

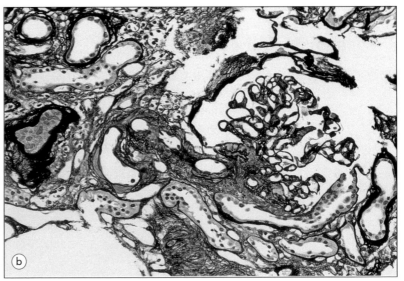

Lesions of FSGS may be seen in association with diseases with abnormal, maladaptive responses of glomerular growth and pressures, e.g. in diabetes, obesity, HIV infection, heroin abuse, cyanotic heart disease, or sickle cell disease. Thus, secondary sclerosis occurs in the chronic stage of many immune complex or proliferative diseases. In some of these settings, the morphologic appearance of sclerosis can indicate the nature of the initial insult: Obesity-associated FSGS shows mild changes related to glucose intolerance (mesangial expansion, GBM thickening), subtotal foot process

Fig. 1.46 FSGS, perihilar. This glomerulus shows a more extensive perihilar lesion of FSGS, associated with hyalinosis and periglomerular fibrosis.
In this case, the lesion was likely due to arterionephrosclerosis associated with hypertension (Jones' silver stain, ×400).

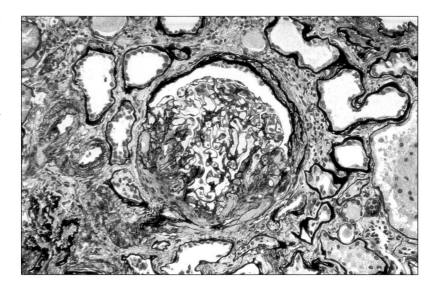

effacement and marked glomerulomegaly. The course is more indolent than for idiopathic FSGS with less frequent nephrotic syndrome. In FSGS secondary to reflux nephropathy, there is frequently prominent periglomerular fibrosis and thickening of Bowman's capsule and patchy, 'geographic' pattern interstitial scarring, in addition to the heterogeneous glomerulosclerosis. FSGS associated with heroin use does not show pathognomonic features, although global glomerulosclerosis, epithelial cell changes, interstitial fibrosis and tubular injury tend to be more prominent than in idiopathic cases of FSGS. FSGS also can develop in association with decreased renal mass. The best example is oligomeganephronia, where nephron number is greatly reduced, with resulting markedly enlarged remaining glomeruli, and occurrence of FSGS. Patients with unilateral renal agenesis show apparent higher risk of FSGS than the general population. Loss of one kidney later in life does not elicit the same degree of growth response in the remaining kidney as in the young and has a lesser association with scarring in the remaining kidney. However, when one kidney and a portion of the other are lost in the adult, patients appear to have increased risk of developing FSGS.

Selected reading

Kambham N, Markowitz G S, Valeri A M et al 2001 Obesity-related glomerulopathy: an emerging epidemic. Kidney International 59:1498–1509.

Rennke H G, Klein P S 1989 Pathogenesis and significance of nonprimary focal and segmental glomerulosclerosis. American Journal of Kidney Disease 13:443–456.

C1q nephropathy

C1q nephropathy is an immune complex-mediated glomerulopathy, defined by the presence of mesangial immunoglobulin and complement deposits, with C1q immunofluorescence staining intensity being greater than or equal to that of other components. C1q nephropathy is a disorder primarily of children and young adults. Patients typically present with nephrotic syndrome, and may have an active urinary sediment, but do not have SLE clinically. Some of those with sclerosis at time of biopsy have developed end stage renal disease. The prognosis of those without sclerosis at time of biopsies awaits further follow-up studies. In our opinion, C1q nephropathy may be viewed as an unusual lesion related to MCD-FSGS.

By light microscopy, there is a spectrum of possible glomerular alterations, including no histologic abnormalities, mesangial proliferation, focal or diffuse proliferative glomerulonephritis, or focal segmental glomerulosclerosis with or without associated mesangial proliferation (Figs 1.47, 1.48).

Immunofluorescence microscopy typically shows predominant C1q, along with C3 and immunoglobulins (Fig. 1.49).

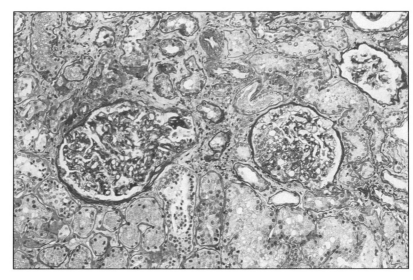

Fig. 1.47 C1q nephropathy. C1q nephropathy may show a variety of lesions by light microscopy, from nearly normal, to mesangial or focal proliferative or segmental sclerosis. The glomerulus on the left shows a small area of segmental sclerosis with adhesion at proximal tubular pole, whereas the glomerulus on the right shows segmental proliferation. There is associated mild tubulointerstitial fibrosis (PAS, ×200).

Fig. 1.48 C1q nephropathy. There is mild mesangial proliferation and early sclerosis of portions of the tuft, with mild periglomerular fibrosis (Jones' silver stain, ×400).

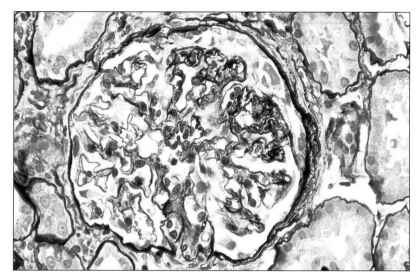

Fig. 1.49 C1q nephropathy. The defining feature of C1q nephropathy is dominant C1q staining by immuno-fluorescence, typically in a mesangial pattern. Focal peripheral capillary loop extension may also be present (anti-C1q antibody immunofluorescence, ×400).

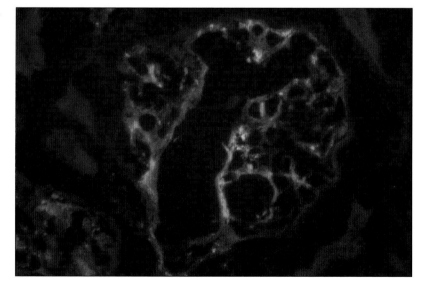

Electron microscopy typically shows deposits confined to the mesangium. Notably, reticular aggregates, a common feature in patients with lupus nephritis, are absent (Fig. 1.50).

Fig. 1.50 C1q nephropathy. There is predominant mesangial dense deposits by electron microscopy. There may be variable foot process effacement, as in this case. Importantly, reticular aggregates, a characteristic feature of lupus nephritis, are not present in C1q nephropathy (TEM, ×5000).

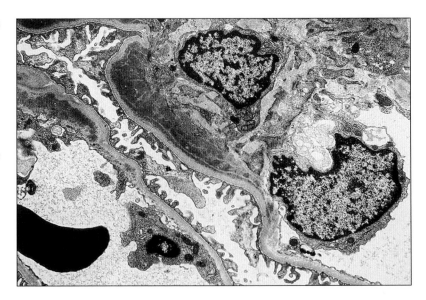

Selected reading

Jennette J C, Hipp C G 1985 C1q nephropathy: A distinct pathologic entity usually causing nephrotic syndrome. American Journal of Kidney Disease 6:103–110.

Markowitz G S, Schwimmer J A, Stokes M B et al 2003 C1q nephropathy: a variant of focal segmental glomerulosclerosis. Kidney International 64:1232–1240.

Congenital nephrotic syndrome of Finnish type

Congenital nephrotic syndrome of Finnish type (CNF) is an inherited autosomal recessive disease due to mutation of nephrin gene (NPHS1), located on chromosome 19. The disease is not exclusive to the Finnish population. Nephrotic syndrome manifests at birth or by age three months, and usually results in death from complications secondary to nephrotic syndrome by age one unless treated with renal transplantation. Microscopic hematuria is often present.

Glomeruli may be immature, more so than expected for term birth, but this may in part reflect the usual premature birth of affected infants. Mature glomeruli have variable mesangial increase and non-specific sclerosis and occasional proliferation (Fig. 1.51). Occasional crescents may be present, but without necrosis. Glomeruli may also be unremarkable by light microscopy. The proximal tubules are dilated (Figs 1.52, 1.53). Tubules may show atrophy and Bowman's capsule may be dilated in some cases, although collecting ducts are not typically dilated. Of note, these typical tubular lesions may be absent in early biopsies.

Fig. 1.51 Congenital nephrotic syndrome of Finnish type. Glomeruli do not show specific lesions, but may have varying mesangial hypercellularity. There is microcystic dilatation of proximal tubules, here associated with global glomerulosclerosis and interstitial fibrosis (hematoxylin and eosin (H&E), ×100).

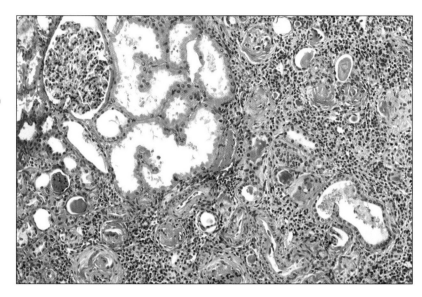

Fig. 1.52 Congenital nephrotic syndrome of Finnish type. Glomeruli are unremarkable and microcystic dilatation of proximal tubules is widespread (Jones' silver stain, ×100).

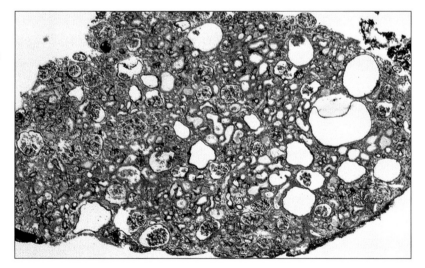

There are no deposits by immunofluorescence. By electron microscopy, there is widespread effacement of foot processes. The glomerular basement membrane may be focally attenuated.

Etiology/pathogenesis

The nephrin gene is mutated in CNF. The nephrin gene is a prominent component of the slit diaphragm of the foot processes of the podocyte. Studies in knock-out mice reveal that intact nephrin is

Fig. 1.53 Congenital nephrotic syndrome of Finnish type. Proximal tubules are microcystically dilated. Glomeruli show normal maturity for age in this newborn (Jones' silver stain, ×200).

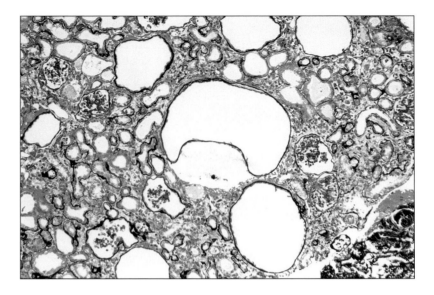

required for maintaining normal capillary permselectivity. Mutations of a protein tightly associated with nephrin, CD2-associated protein (CD2AP) in mice has demon-strated that mutation of other components of the slit diaphragm or its anchoring proteins also lead to nephrotic syndrome with clinical characteristics mirroring many of those of congenital nephrotic syndrome of Finnish type. It is puzzling, based on this elucidation of the genetic abnormality, that approximately one-quarter of patients transplanted develop recurrent nephrotic syndrome. Renal biopsies of the transplant performed from 3 days to 2 weeks after onset of recurrent nephrotic syndrome showed glomerular capillary endo-thelial cell swelling, but without attendant GBM abnormalities to specifically suggest chronic transplant nephropathy. In two patients with recurrent nephrotic syndrome in the transplant, the renal biopsy lesions suggested minimal change disease type morphology, and the patients responded to steroids or cyclophosphamide. The etiology of the recurrent nephrotic syndrome remains unclear. However, recent data show that all recurrences developed in patients with the Fin-major/Fin-major genotype, resulting in completely absent nephrin. Some patients developed anti-nephrin antibodies after transplant, although usual immune complexes were not observed.

Selected reading

Rapola J 1987 Congenital nephrotic syndrome. Pediatric Nephrology 1:441–446.

Huttunen N-P, Rapola J, Wilska J, et al 1980 Renal pathology in congenital nephrotic syndrome of Finnish type: A quantitative light microscopic study on 50 patients. International Journal of Pediatric Nephrology 1:10.

Ruotsalainen V, Ljungberg P, Wartiovaara J, et al 1999 Nephrin is specifically located at the slit diaphragm of glomerular podocytes. Proceedings of the National Academy of Science, USA. 96(14):7962–7967.

Patrakka J, Ruotsalainen V, Reponen P, et al 2002 Recurrence of nephrotic syndrome in kidney grafts of patients with congenital nephrotic syndrome of the Finnish type: role of nephrin. Transplantation 73(3):394–403.

Glomerular diseases that cause nephrotic syndrome: immune complex

Membranous glomerulopathy

Membranous glomerulopathy was until recently the most common cause of nephrotic syndrome in adults in the USA, recently surpassed by focal segmental glomerulosclerosis. The peak incidence is in the fourth and fifth decades, with men affected more commonly than women. Approximately one-third of patients may develop slowly progressive renal disease.

Membranous glomerulopathy is due to diffuse, global subepithelial deposits (Fig. 1.54). At an early time point, these may be only evident by light microscopy by a more rigid-appearing capillary wall without visible deposits (Fig. 1.55). In favorable tangential sections, small areas of lucency seen on Jones' silver stain may be detected, representing the lack of silver staining of the deposits (Fig. 1.56). These so-called 'holes' are the earliest manifestation of membranous glomerulopathy by light microscopy. As deposits persist, the glomerular basement membrane matrix reaction produces small spike-like protrusions visualized by silver stain (Figs 1.57–1.59). With progressive basement membrane reaction, the matrix encircles the deposits resulting in a lace-like splitting or laddering appearance of the GBM on silver stain (Fig. 1.60). The morphologic findings related to these subepithelial deposits have been divided into stages (see below).

Additional lesions may be present, ranging from crescents to sclerosis. Segmental sclerosis, interstitial fibrosis and tubular atrophy are associated with worse prognosis (Figs 1.61, 1.62). Rarely, crescents may be found in cases of apparent idiopathic membranous glomerulopathy, but are more common with lupus-associated lesions (Fig. 1.63).

Fig. 1.54 Membranous glomerulopathy. There is no evident proliferation by light microscopy, with global subepithelial deposits, which may be visualized by light microscopy by the glomerular basement membrane spike reaction on silver stain. At earlier stages, the deposits that do not stain with silver may be seen in tangential sections as holes, producing a corkboard appearance. In advanced stages, the basement membrane reaction may encircle the deposits, with ensuing splitting.

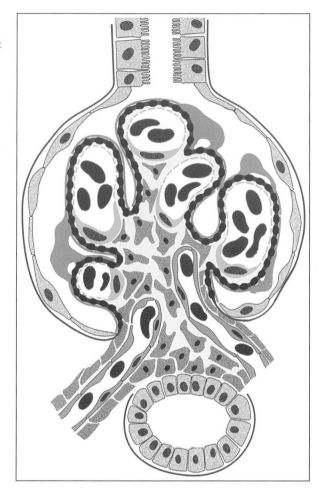

Fig. 1.55 Membranous glomerulopathy. Stage 1 membranous glomerulopathy does not show evident spikes by light microscopy. Only rare holes are evident, with a slightly more rigid appearance of the GBM (Jones' silver stain, ×400).

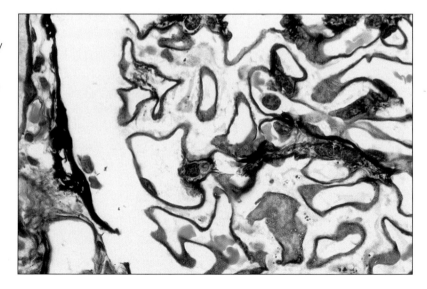

Fig. 1.56 Membranous glomerulopathy. In some cases of stage 1 membranous glomerulopathy, holes may be seen in tangential sections, since the deposits do not stain with Jones' stain. This gives a corkboard, bubbly-type appearance (Jones' silver stain, ×1000).

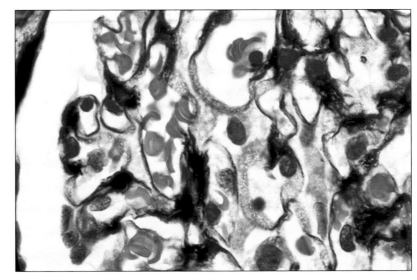

Fig. 1.57 Membranous glomerulopathy. In early stage 2 membranous glomerulopathy, small, stubby spike-like projections are seen, representing the basement membrane reaction to the subepithelial deposits. This gives a thick, 'fuzzy rope' appearance to the GBM (Jones' silver stain, ×400).

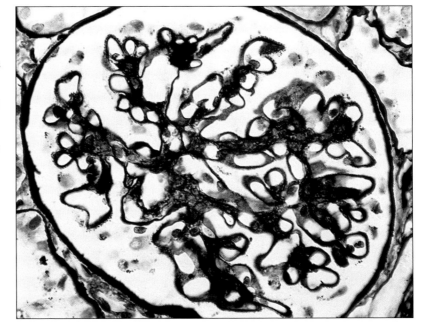

By immunofluorescence, the subepithelial deposits are visualized as diffuse, global granular positivity along the capillary wall (Figs 1.64–1.66). Immunofluorescence microscopy is more sensitive than either light microscopy or electron microscopy for detection of deposits and is very finely granular in Stage 1, and coarsely

Fig. 1.58 Membranous glomerulopathy. There are well-developed spikes and holes in tangential sections in stage 2 membranous glomerulopathy (Jones' silver stain, ×1000).

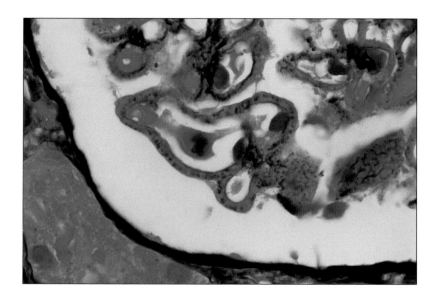

Fig. 1.59 Membranous glomerulopathy. In late stage 2 membranous glomerulopathy, the glomerular basement membrane is markedly thickened, due to extensive basement membrane spike reaction around the deposits (Jones' silver stain, ×1000).

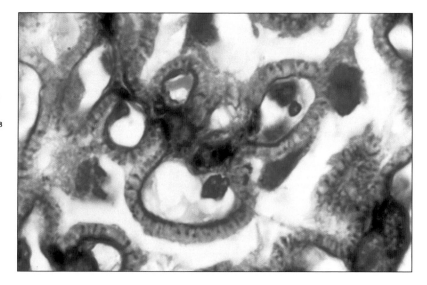

granular with more advanced stages. IgG is typically the predominant immunoglobulin, and C3 is most often also present. In addition, mesangial deposits are typically present in secondary membranous glomerulopathy, and are absent in most cases of idiopathic membranous glomerulopathy. When IgA, IgM and C1q are also present, the possibility of secondary membranous glomerulopathy due to systemic lupus erythematosus should be considered.

Fig. 1.60 Membranous glomerulopathy. In stage 3 membranous glomerulopathy, the basement membrane reaction encircles the deposits, giving rise to a bubbly, split appearance of the GBM. This can readily be distinguished from membranoproliferative glomerulonephritis, due to the lack of associated endocapillary proliferation. Further, the subepithelial/trans/intramembranous location of the deposits is resolved by immunofluorescence and electron microscopy (Jones' silver stain, ×400).

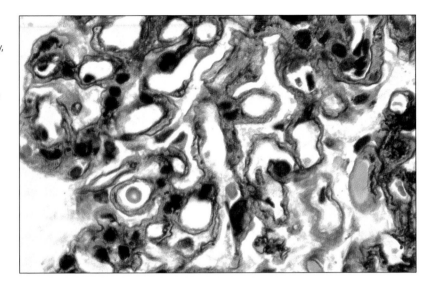

Fig. 1.61 Membranous glomerulopathy. There may be associated sclerosis with tubulointerstitial fibrosis in more advanced membranous glomerulopathy, as shown here (Jones' silver stain, ×100).

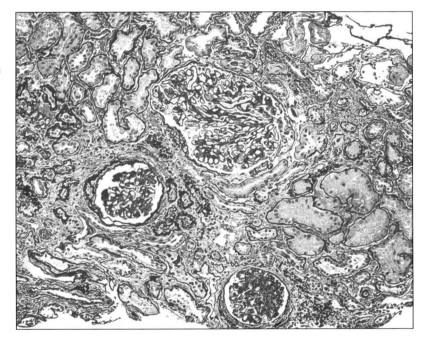

By electron microscopy, deposits corresponding to the stage of membranous glomerulopathy are visualized, with varying surrounding glomerular basement membrane reaction. In early stage 1, membranous glomerulopathy, deposits may be extremely small and inconspicuous with no surrounding glomerular basement mem-

Fig. 1.62 Membranous glomerulopathy. Membranous glomerulopathy may also have associated segmental sclerosis as it becomes more chronic. This is not indicative of a second idiopathic sclerosing process, but rather is thought to reflect the ongoing chronic injury, and is associated with worse prognosis. By light microscopy, the small spikes and thickened glomerular basement membrane are evident, with the diagnosis of membranous glomerulopathy confirmed by IF and EM (Jones' silver stain, ×400).

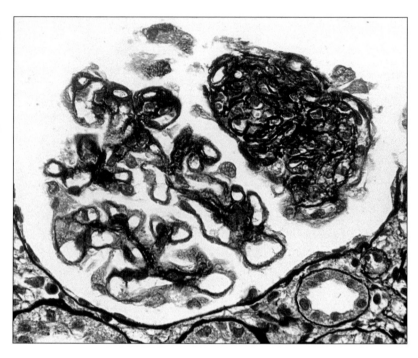

Fig. 1.63 Membranous glomerulopathy. Idiopathic membranous glomerulopathy may rarely be associated with crescents. Crescents are more commonly seen with secondary causes of membranous glomerulopathy, particularly due to systemic lupus erythematosus. The thickened glomerular basement membrane was shown to contain subepithelial deposits by immunofluorescence and electron microscopy (Jones' silver stain, ×400).

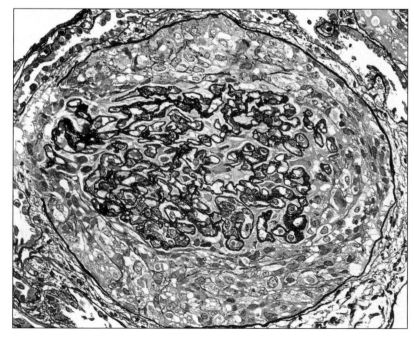

Fig. 1.64 Membranous glomerulopathy. There is an evenly distributed granular capillary loop pattern of positivity in membranous glomerulopathy, corresponding to the evenly distributed subepithelial deposits. Deposits in idiopathic membranous glomerulopathy stain predominately with IgG, with lesser amounts of C3 (anti-IgG immunofluorescence, ×400).

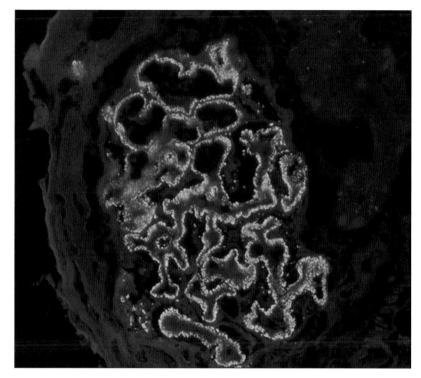

Fig. 1.65 Membranous glomerulopathy. In secondary membranous glomerulopathy, there is often associated mesangial staining, along with a granular capillary loop staining (anti-IgG immunofluorescence, ×200).

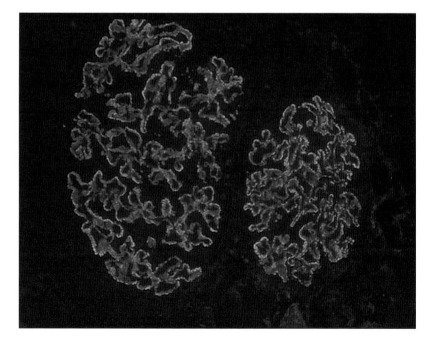

Fig. 1.66 Membranous glomerulopathy. The granularity of the capillary loop deposits characteristic of membranous glomerulopathy is evident (anti-IgG immunofluorescence, ×400).

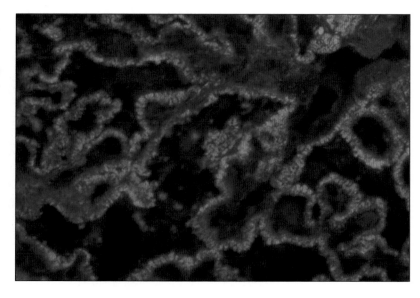

Fig. 1.67 Membranous glomerulopathy. The deposits are inconspicuous by EM in stage 1 membranous glomerulopathy, with blunting and partial effacement of overlying foot processes. There is no surrounding basement reaction (TEM, ×8000).

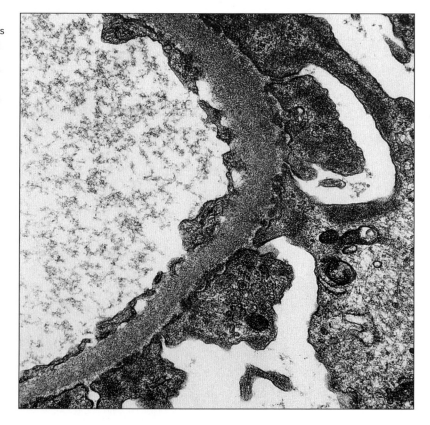

Fig. 1.68 Membranous glomerulopathy. There are slightly larger deposits underneath the podocyte, without surrounding spike reaction in this stage 1 membranous glomerulopathy (TEM, ×9000).

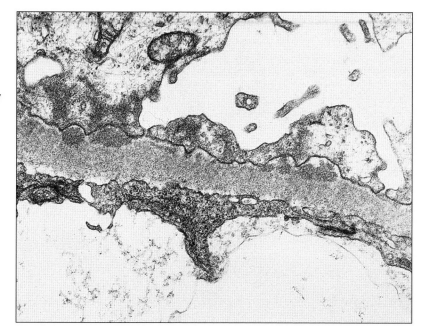

brane reaction, corresponding to the lack of spikes evident by light microscopy (Figs 1.67, 1.68). In stage 2 membranous glomerulopathy, well-formed spike reaction is present (Figs 1.69, 1.70). In stage 3 membranous glomerulopathy, the deposits are encircled by the glomerular basement membrane reaction (Figs 1.71, 1.72). In stage 4 membranous glomerulopathy, the deposits are resorbed, leaving behind rarefied, lucent areas (Figs 1.73, 1.74).

The visceral epithelial cells show diffuse effacement of foot processes. When mesangial deposits are present, the possibility of a secondary etiology of membranous glomerulopathy should be considered (Figs 1.75, 1.76). If reticular aggregates are present in endothelial cell cytoplasm, the possibility of lupus-associated membranous glomerulopathy (WHO Vb, RPS/ISN V) should be considered.

Etiology/pathogenesis

Most cases of membranous glomerulopathy are idiopathic. The subepithelial deposits are thought to arise from *in situ* immune complex formation. The antigen in idiopathic cases remains undefined but is postulated to be a component of the glomerular visceral epithelial cell. Infectious agents, including bacterial, viral or parasitic drugs or thyroglobulin may also be the antigen. Numerous

Fig. 1.69 Membranous glomerulopathy. In stage 2 membranous glomerulopathy, there are well-developed basement membrane reactions surrounding the evenly distributed sub-epithelial deposits (TEM, ×1200).

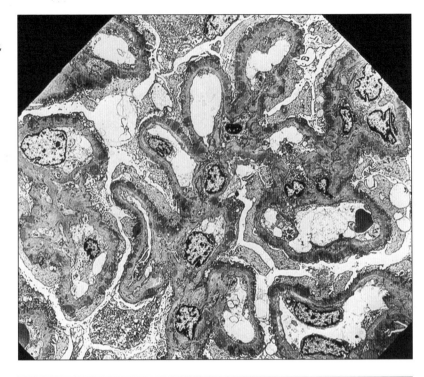

Fig. 1.70 Membranous glomerulopathy. The well-developed basement mem-brane reaction surrounding the deposits is evident in stage 2 membranous glomerulopathy, with over-lying foot process efface-ment (TEM, ×8000).

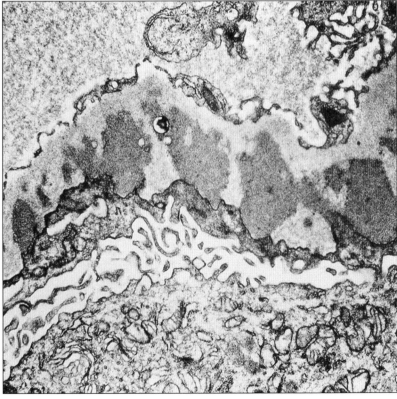

Fig. 1.71 Membranous glomerulopathy. In early stage 3 membranous glomerulopathy, the basement membrane reaction encircles the deposits, and there is early resorption. Overlying foot processes are largely effaced (TEM, ×8000).

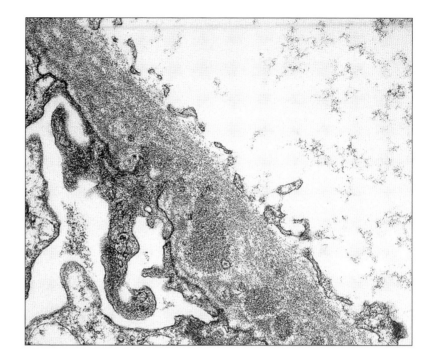

entities have been associated with membranous glomerulopathy, but causality has only been established for some, including hepatitis B, Hashimoto's thyroiditis, systemic lupus erythematosus, syphilis, penicillamine, gold (Fig. 1.77), mercuric chloride and Sjögren syndrome. Malignancies, in particular some carcinomas, sarcomas and leukemias, have been linked to membranous glomerulopathy, but definitive proof of causal linkage, i.e. circulating antibody–antigen immune complexes and tumor antigen within the deposits, is lacking.

Selected reading

Couser W G, Baker P J, Adler S 1985 Complement and the direct mediation of immune glomerular injury: a new perspective. Kidney International 28:879–890.

Dumoulin A, Hill G S, Montseny J J et al 2003 Clinical and morphological prognostic factors in membranous nephropathy: significance of focal segmental glomerulosclerosis. American Journal of Kidney Disease 41:38–48.

Fig. 1.72 Membranous glomerulopathy. Stage 3 membranous glomerulopathy is illustrated, with early resorption and basement membrane reaction overlying the deposits. The tangential section of basement membrane corresponds to the holes seen by light microscopy, since the electron-dense deposits do not stain by Jones' stain, whereas the surrounding basement membrane does (TEM, ×8000).

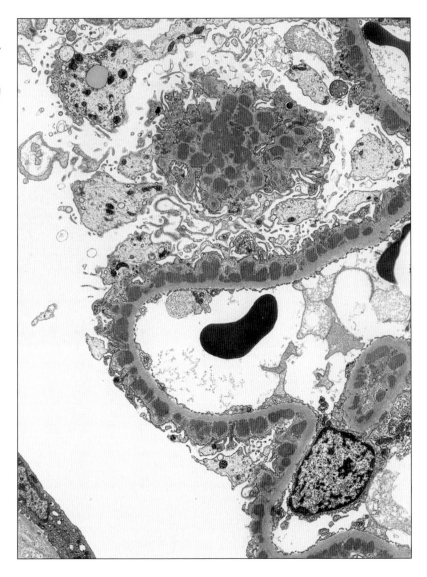

Ehrenreich T, Churg J 1968 Pathology of membranous nephropathy. In: Sommers S C (ed.) Pathology Annual. Appleton-Century-Crofts, New York, 3:145–154.

Gonzalo A, Mampaso F, Barcena R et al 1999 Membranous nephropathy associated with hepatitis B virus infection: long-term clinical and histological outcome. Nephrology, Dialysis and Transplantation 14:416–418.

Jennette J C, Iskandar S S, Dalldorf F G 1983 Pathologic differentiation between lupus and nonlupus membranous glomerulopathy. Kidney International 24:377–385.

Fig. 1.73 Membranous glomerulopathy. In stage 4 membranous glomerulopathy, there is resorption of deposits. Some deposits still remain with surrounding halo or resorption, and the basement membrane reaction encircles the deposits in this largely sclerosed segment (TEM, ×20 250).

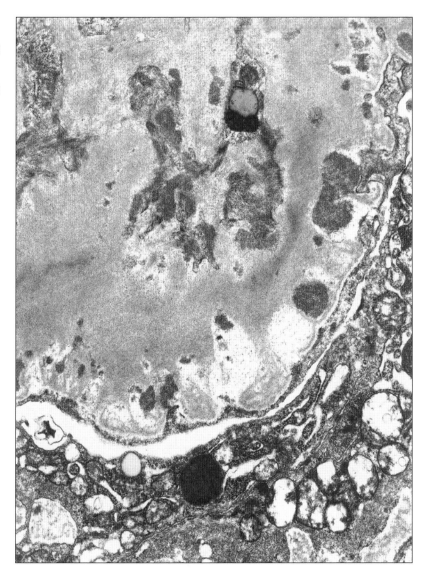

Kerjaschki D 1990 The pathogenesis of membranous glomerulonephritis: From morphology to molecules. Virchows Archiv [B] 58:253–271.

Lee, H S, Koh H I 1993 Nature of progressive glomerulosclerosis in human membranous nephropathy. Clinical Nephrology 39:7–16.

Toth T, Takebayashi S 1992 Idiopathic membranous glomerulonephritis: a clinicopathologic and quantitative morphometric study. Clinical Nephrology 38:14–19.

Fig. 1.74 Membranous glomerulopathy. In stage 4 membranous glomerulopathy, deposits are largely resorbed, with small electron-dense subepithelial deposits overlying the resorbed areas, indicating ongoing active immune complex deposition (TEM, ×4400).

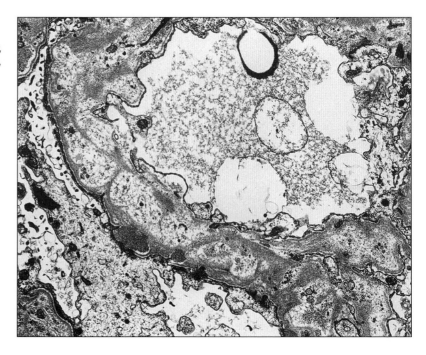

Fig. 1.75 Membranous glomerulopathy. In secondary membranous glomerulopathy, there is mesangial expansion, associated with mesangial deposits, in addition to the peripheral loop subepithelial deposits. This patient's disease was related to hepatitis B infection (Jones' silver stain, ×400).

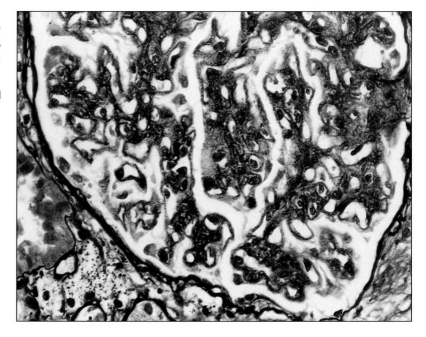

Fig. 1.76 Membranous glomerulopathy. In this case of secondary membranous glomerulopathy, advanced stage 2, there are also associated mesangial deposits, indicating a secondary etiology (TEM, ×8000).

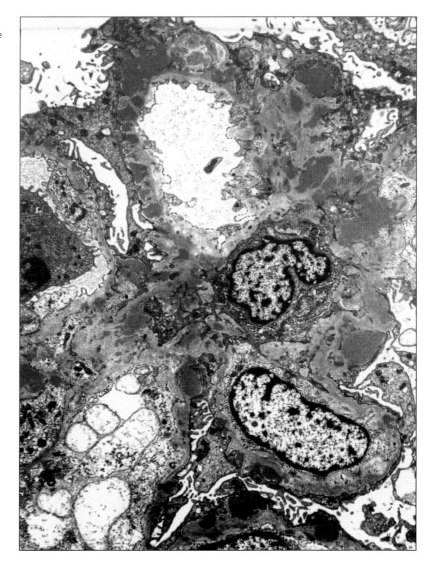

Van Damme B, Tardanico R, Vanrenterghem Y, et al 1990 Adhesions, focal sclerosis, protein crescents, and capsular lesions in membranous nephropathy. Journal of Pathology 161:47–56.

Wakai S, Magil A B 1992 Focal glomerulosclerosis in idiopathic membranous glomerulonephritis. Kidney International 41:428–434.

Wasserstein A G 1997 Membranous glomerulonephritis. Journal of the American Society of Nephrology 8:664–674.

Fig. 1.77 Membranous glomerulopathy. In rare cases of secondary membranous glomerulopathy, the etiology may be definitively determined. In this case, rare gold particles were found within lysosomes in tubules, providing a causal etiology for this patient's secondary membranous glomerulopathy (TEM, ×14 000).

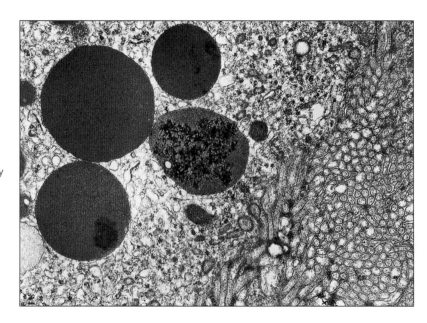

Membranoproliferative glomerulonephritis

Membranoproliferative glomerulonephritis (MPGN) type I typically presents as combined nephritic/nephrotic syndrome with hypocomplementemia. It occurs mostly in children and young adults, and as a lesion secondary to for instance chronic infections in adults. The incidence of MPGN type I appears to have decreased in children in the last decade, for unknown reasons. Children with MPGN type I tend to be older than children with dense deposit disease (also called MPGN type II by some, see 'Dense Deposit Disease'). The presence of the C3 nephritic factor (C3NeF) is more rare and concurrent partial lipodystrophy is very rare in MPGN type I compared to DDD. Patients typically have progressive renal disease, with about 50% renal survival at 10 years in children, and similar rates of progression in adults. Many of the patients reaching end stage died of complications of their kidney disease. Clinical indicators of poor prognosis are hypertension, impaired renal function and nephrotic syndrome. MPGN type I recurs in the transplant in about one-third of patients, and may lead to graft loss, particularly if crescents are present. MPGN can also occur *de novo* in the transplant, related to hepatitis C infection and cryoglobulinemia (see 'Cryoglobulinemia').

The term MPGN describes a light microscopic pattern of injury characterized by diffuse mesangial expansion due to endocapillary proliferation and increased mesangial matrix and thickened capillary walls, often with a split 'tram-track' appearance (Fig. 1.78). The term MPGN is preferably used only when this pattern is caused by immune complex glomerulonephritides. Of note, basement membrane splitting may be seen in other non-immune complex injuries, such as the organizing phase of thrombotic microangiopathy, radiation nephritis, chronic transplant glomerulopathy or in sickle cell disease. Although light microscopy may appear similar to MPGN, immunofluorescence findings and electron microscopy readily allow recognition of the immune complexes in MPGN.

MPGN has been divided into three types, all with similar light microscopic appearance. The term 'mesangiocapillary' glomerulonephritis has also been used for MPGN type I. There is global, diffuse endocapillary proliferation with increased mesangial cellularity and matrix, and lobular simplification (Figs 1.79–83). Increased

Fig. 1.78 There is endocapillary proliferation and glomerular basement membrane splitting, due to mesangial and subendothelial deposits, with resultant interposition and new basement membrane being laid down, causing the split appearance.

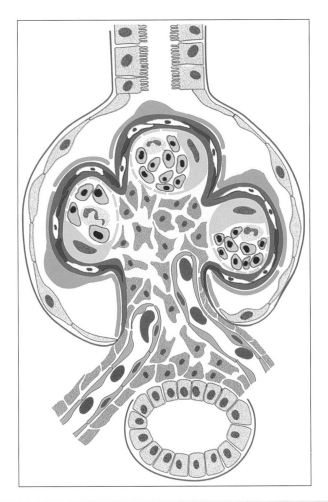

mononuclear cells and occasional neutrophils may be present. The proliferation is typically uniform and diffuse in idiopathic MPGN, contrasting the irregular involvement with proliferative lupus nephritis. In some cases, the glomeruli may appear more solid and

Fig. 1.79 MPGN type I. MPGN is characterized by diffuse endocapillary proliferation, which results in a lobular, uniform appearance of glomeruli (PAS, ×100).

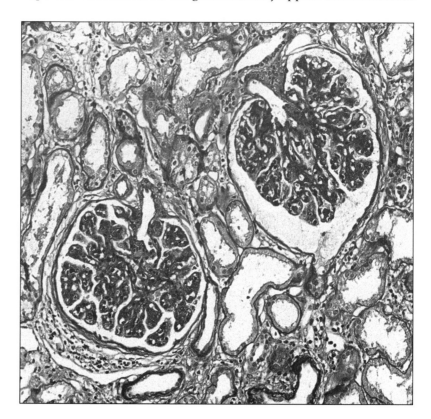

Fig. 1.80 MPGN type I. There is diffuse endocapillary proliferation with extensive duplication of the glomerular basement membrane, with frequent eosinophilic deposits within the split capillary wall. There is marked mesangial prolifera-tion, and endocapillary proliferation with a lobular appearance (Jones' silver stain, ×200).

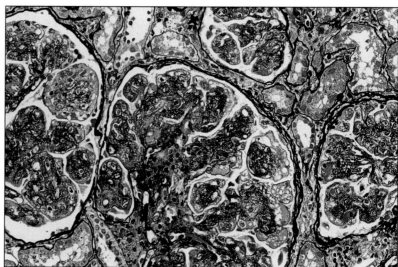

Fig. 1.81 MPGN type I. There is less marked endocapillary proliferation, but still widespread splitting of the glomerular basement membrane, so-called 'tram tracking' (Jones' silver stain, ×400).

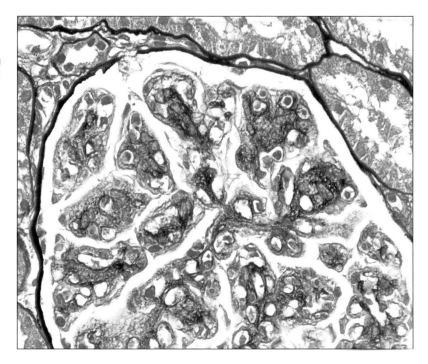

Fig. 1.82 MPGN type I. There is abundant mesangial hypercellularity with proliferation extending to peripheral capillary lumens (endocapillary proliferation), with only segmental glomerular basement membrane splitting in this case. In idiopathic MPGN, the endocapillary proliferation is typically global and diffuse, while in secondary cases, the lesions may be more focal and segmental (Jones' silver stain, ×400).

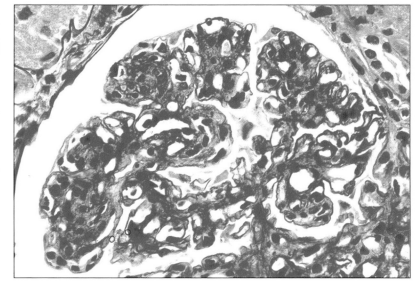

nodular (Fig. 1.84). The capillary wall is thickened with a double contour by silver stains (Figs 1.83, 1.85). This appearance results from the presence of subendothelial deposits and so-called circumferential mesangial interposition, whereby mesangial cells, infiltrating mononuclear cells or even portions of endothelial cells interpose themselves between the endothelium and the basement

Fig. 1.83 MPGN type I. There is segmental inter-position of cells with splitting of peripheral capillary GBM along with subendothelial deposits (Jones' silver stain, ×1000).

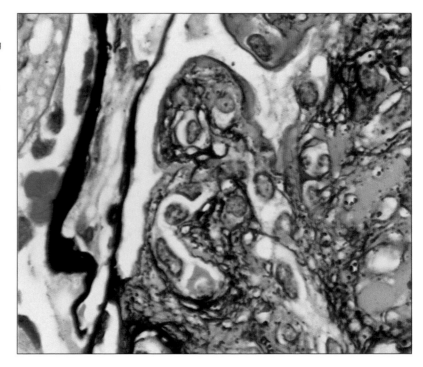

Fig. 1.84 MPGN type I. In some cases of MPGN, there may be nodular glomerulosclerosis and massive deposits. Occasional PMNs are also present, in addition to the mesangial and endocapillary prolifera-tion. A small incipient cellular crescent is present. These morphological features suggest the possibility of a secondary etiology of the MPGN lesion (Jones' silver stain, ×400).

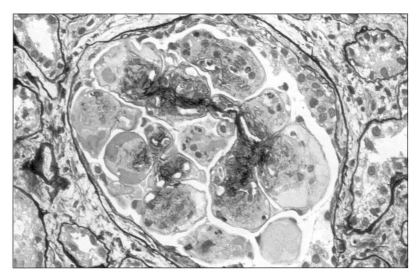

membrane, with new, inner basement membrane being laid down. A circumferential, or partial, double contour basement membrane results. In secondary forms of MPGN, the injury may be more irregular. Crescents may occur in both idiopathic and secondary forms (Fig. 1.84). Greater than 20% crescents has been associated with worse prognosis. Deposits do not involve extraglomerular sites.

Fig. 1.85 MPGN type I. Large subendothelial deposits and interposed cells are evident, along with endocapillary proliferation. A smaller subendothelial deposit is present at the far left, with small nodular expansion in the middle and right capillary loops (same case as in Fig. 1.84) (Jones' silver stain, ×1000).

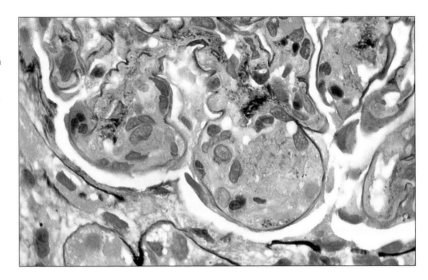

Lesions progress with less cellularity and more pronounced matrix accumulation and sclerosis over time. Tubulointerstitial fibrosis and vascular sclerosis proportional to glomerular scarring are seen late in the course. Tubular atrophy and interstitial fibrosis indicate worse prognosis.

The immunofluorescence findings are variable in MPGN type I. Typically, IgG and IgM and C3 are present in an irregular, chunky capillary and mesangial distribution (Figs 1.86–1.89). IgA is present in only a small proportion of cases. C3 staining may be dominant and staining for immunoglobulin may even be lost, especially in secondary MPGN. The peripheral loop deposits typically are sausage-shaped and have a smooth outer edge because they are subendothelial and molded under the GBM (Fig. 1.89).

By electron microscopy, MPGN type I shows numerous deposits in subendothelial and mesangial areas (Figs 1.90–1.93). The 'subendothelial' deposits actually more commonly lie within the GBM, immediately under the original lamina densa, and thus might more precisely be described as 'intramembranous' (Fig. 1.93). Vague wormy or microtubular substructure suggests a possible cryoglobulin component (Fig. 1.92). So-called mesangial interposition is present. This term refers to the interposition of cytoplasmic processes of mesangial or mononuclear cells between the endothelial cell and the basement membrane (Fig. 1.94). Monocyte interposition is particularly common when the MPGN lesion is related to cryoglobulinemia. Reduplication of new basement material is present

Fig. 1.86 MPGN type I. There is irregular, chunky capillary loop and mesangial staining in MPGN, with coarse, subendothelial deposits with a molded, smooth outer contour (anti-IgG immunofluorescence, ×100).

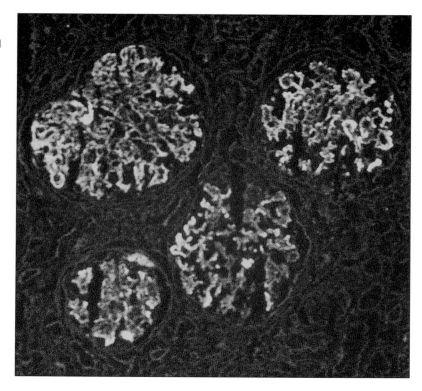

Fig. 1.87 MPGN type I. In addition to IgG, there is often very prominent complement deposition in MPGN, with prominent mesangial and coarse, chunky peripheral loop deposits, corresponding to the subendothelial deposits (anti-C3 immunofluorescence, ×100).

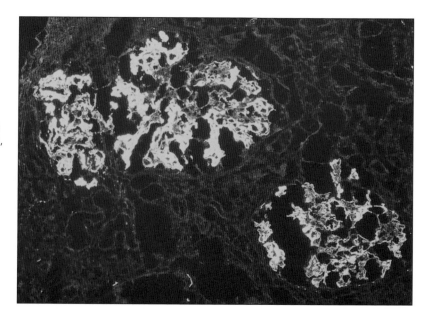

Fig. 1.88 MPGN type I. The smooth outline of the sausage shaped, chunky peripheral loop deposits is evident along with the scattered mesangial deposits. The smooth outer contour of the peripheral loop deposits reflects their subendothelial location, with molding under the GBM (anti-C3 immuno-fluorescence, ×200).

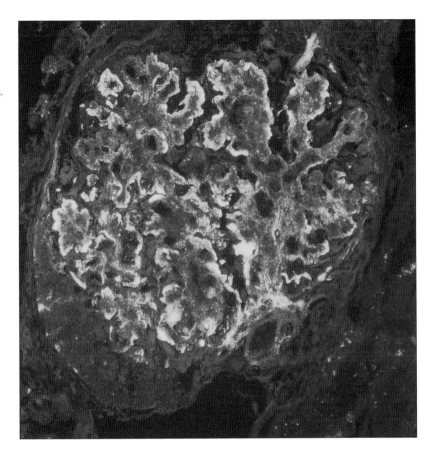

Fig. 1.89 MPGN type I. Both complement pathways are typically activated in MPGN, with frequent C1q positivity in addition to C3. The subendothelial location of the peripheral deposits is evident by their smooth outer contour (anti-C1q immunofluorescence, ×400).

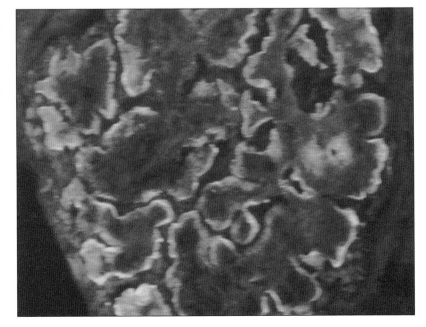

Fig. 1.90   MPGN type I. There are massive subendothelial deposits in the right loop, with minimal endocapillary proliferation, and small, sliver-like deposits on the left and top loops, with associated proliferation. Scattered mesangial deposits are also present. There is subtotal effacement of overlying foot processes. The smooth outer contour of the deposits is also evident by immunofluorescence (see Figs 1.88, 1.89) (TEM, ×8000).

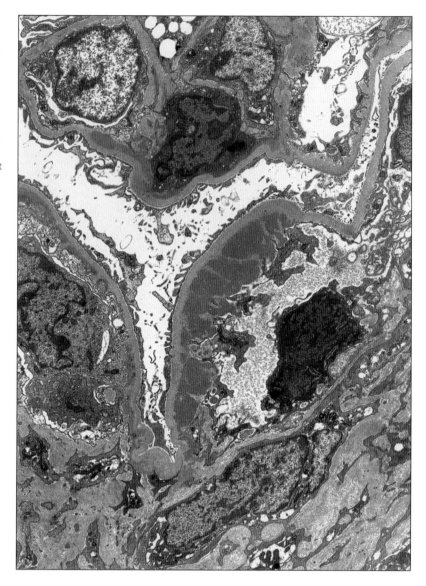

immediately under the swollen endothelial cells. The overlying visceral epithelial cells are effaced. MPGN type III shows in addition to the subendothelial and mesangial deposits, numerous sub-epithelial deposits (Fig. 1.95). It may not, however, represent an entity separate from MPGN type I. Although C3 nephritic factor is rarely found in these patients, clinical distinction of this morphology has not been apparent.

Fig. 1.91   MPGN type I. There is marked endocapillary proliferation, with small subendothelial deposits and a transmembranous deposit (lower right). The endocapillary proliferation is due to a mixture of endothelial cells, mesangial cells and infiltrating mononuclear cells/macrophages (TEM, ×8000).

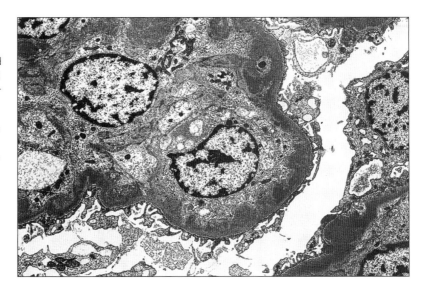

Fig. 1.92   MPGN type I. Subendothelial deposits are present, without attendant proliferation. The mottled, vaguely wormy substructure of the deposits suggests the possibility of a secondary etiology, such as cryoglobulin deposits. Correlation with light microscopy, immunofluorescence and clinical findings can further support or refute this possibility (TEM, ×11 250).

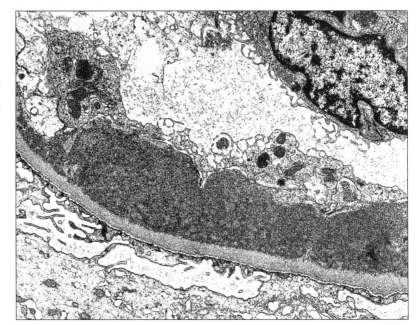

Of note, in non-immune complex diseases with GBM splitting seen by light microscopy (e.g. transplant glomerulopathy, chronic thrombotic microangiopathy), electron microscopy shows that the double contour results from widening of the GBM due to increased lucency of the lamina rara interna with new basement membrane formed underneath the endothelium.

Fig. 1.93 MPGN type I. An intramembranous deposit, molded under the original lamina densa, is associated with an interposed cell and new underlying glomerular basement membrane. Some of the deposit material is subendothelial (far right) (TEM, ×25 625).

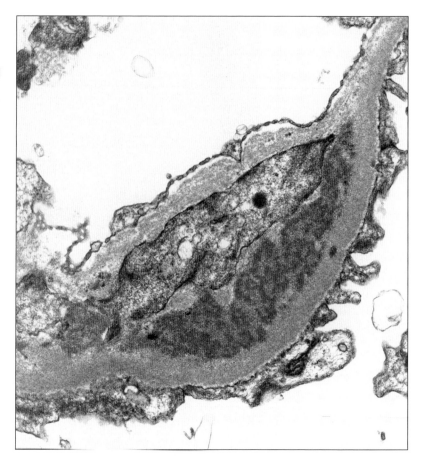

Etiology/pathogenesis

MPGN-like lesions can occur secondary to a number of chronic infectious processes, including hepatitis B, hepatitis C, subacute bacterial endocarditis, cryoglobulin, syphilis, etc., which are discussed separately. Morphologic features do not allow precise classification of the underlying agent in most cases of MPGN. MPGN may rarely occur due to inherited deficiency of complement, or partial lipodystrophy. In adults in the USA, many patients with MPGN have associated hepatitis C infection. This association has not been seen in children with MPGN. These hepatitis C positive cases often show vague substructure of deposits, with short, curved, vaguely fibrillar deposits suggestive of mixed cryoglobulinemia (see 'Cryoglobulinemic glomerulonephritis'). Features suggestive or even diagnostic of cryoglobulin as an underlying cause of MPGN include strongly PAS-positive cryo-'plugs' in capillary lumina,

Fig. 1.94 MPGN type I. This capillary loop shows a complex combination of lesions, with interposed cells and intramembranous and subendothelial deposits. Adjacent areas of the glomerulus show mesangial deposits (far right) and mesangial proliferation (TEM, ×14 000).

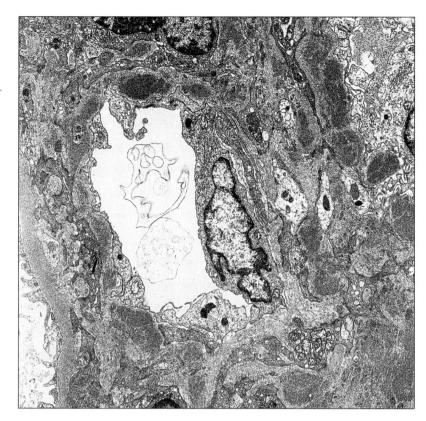

vasculitis, predominant IgM deposits, sometimes with clonality, and vague substructure of deposits by EM. Morphologic clues of an underlying chronic bacterial infection causing MPGN-type lesions are the presence of hump-type subepithelial deposits (see 'Postinfectious glomerulonephritis').

Selected reading

Anders D, Agricola B, Sippel M et al 1997 Basement membrane changes in membranoproliferative glomerulonephritis. II. Characterization of a third type by silver impregnation of ultra thin sections. Virchows Archiv (Pathology and Anatomy) 376:1–19.

Berger J, Galle P 1963 Dépôts denses au sein des membranes basales du rein: étude en microscopies optique et électronique. Presse Medicale 71:2351–2354.

Cameron J S, Turner D R, Heaton J et al 1983 Idiopathic mesangiocapillary glomerulonephritis. Comparison of types I and II in children and adults and long-term prognosis. American Journal of Medicine 74:175–192.

D'Amico G, Ferrario F 1992 Mesangiocapillary glomerulonephritis. Journal of the American Society of Nephrology 2(10 Suppl):S159–166.

Fig. 1.95   MPGN type I. There may be occasional subepithelial or more frequently transmembranous deposits in cases that otherwise appear as MPGN. These lesions may meet morphologic criteria for MPGN III, which commonly has presence of C3 nephritic factor. Occasional transmembranous deposits may, however, be found in any type of MPGN lesion (TEM, ×17 125).

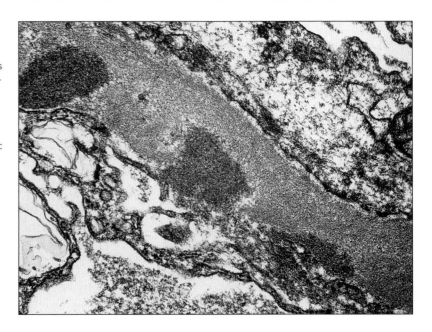

Donadio J V Jr, Slack T K, Holley K E et al 1979 Idiopathic membranoproliferative (mesangiocapillary) glomerulonephritis: a clinicopathologic study. Mayo Clinic Proceedings 54(3):141–150.

Habib R, Kleinknecht C, Gubler M C et al 1973 Idiopathic membranoproliferative glomerulonephritis in children: report of 105 cases. Clinical Nephrology 1:194–214.

Johnson R J, Gretch D R, Yamabe H et al 1993 Membranoproliferative glomerulonephritis associated with hepatitis C virus infection. New England Journal of Medicine 328:465–470.

Katz S M 1981 Reduplication of the glomerular basement membrane: a study of 110 cases. Archives of Pathology and Laboratory Medicine 105:67–70.

Nowicki M J, Welch T R, Ahmad N et al 1995 Absence of hepatitis B and C viruses in pediatric idiopathic membranoproliferative glomerulonephritis. Pediatric Nephrology 9(1):16–18.

Rennke H G 1995 Nephrology forum: Secondary membranoproliferative glomerulonephritis. Kidney International 47:643–656.

Strife C F, Jackson E C, McAdams A J 1984 Type III membranoproliferative glomerulonephritis: long-term clinical and morphological evaluation. Clinical Nephrology 21:323–334.

Strife C F, McEnery P T, McAdams A J et al 1977 Membranoproliferative glomerulonephritis with disruption of the glomerular basement membrane. Clinical Nephrology 7:65–72.

Taguchi T, Bohle A 1989 Evaluation of change with time of glomerular morphology in membranoproliferative glomerulonephritis: a serial biopsy study of 33 cases. Clinical Nephrology 31(6):297–306.

Dense deposit disease (DDD)

DDD is a separate disease entity from membranoproliferative glomerulonephritis (MPGN) type I, but due to its similar light microscopic appearance, it has also been called MPGN type II (Fig. 1.96). DDD is much more rare than type I MPGN, accounting for 15–35% of total MPGN I and DDD cases. Patients with dense deposit disease (DDD) typically present with features of nephritic/ nephrotic syndrome and decreased complements, particularly C3, hypertension and elevated serum creatinine. Early components of the classic pathway, i.e. C1q and C4, usually show normal serum levels. Some patients have partial lipodystrophy associated with DDD. Most patients are children or young adults; girls and boys are affected equally. Progressive renal failure is common, occurring in

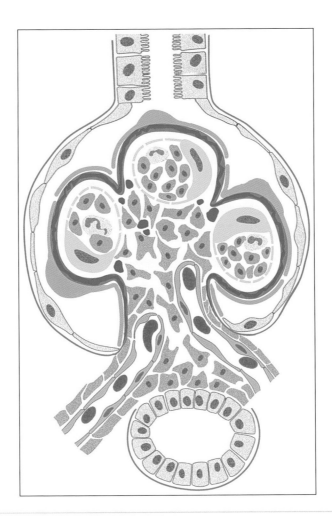

Fig. 1.96 DDD. The glomerulus shows a membranoproliferative pattern, with endocapillary proliferation and GBM splitting. The GBM is altered by dense deposits in a ribbon-like pattern, with mesangial dense material as well.

Fig. 1.97   DDD. Dense deposit disease has membranoproliferative features by light microscopy, with diffuse, global mesangial and often endocapillary proliferation, and frequent glomerular basement membrane splitting. The glomerular basement membrane may in some cases appear more refractile than in idiopathic type I MPGN (H&E, ×400).

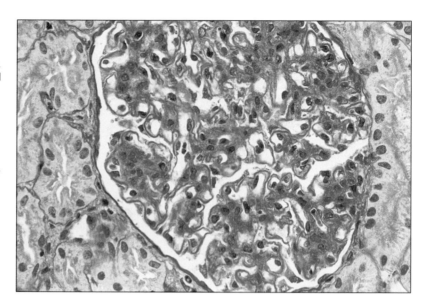

the majority of patients, usually developing over years. Rare cases of spontaneous improvement of the disease have been reported. More rapid progression is associated with crescents. Clinical features alone did not predict progression.

By light microscopy, endocapillary proliferation is present, often with PMN infiltrate (Figs 1.97, 1.98). There may be focal segmental necrotizing proliferative lesions. The glomerular basement membranes are thickened and highly refractile and eosinophilic. The involved areas of the GBM resemble a 'string of sausages'. The deposits are PAS positive and stain brown with silver stain (Figs 1.99, 1.100). The thioflavin T stain also highlights the deposits, as does the toluidine blue stain (Fig. 1.101). Thickening also affects tubular basement membranes and Bowman's capsule. Crescents may be present.

Immunofluorescence in DDD shows C3 staining irregularly along the capillary wall, in a smooth, granular or discontinuous pattern (Fig. 1.102). Mesangial bright granular staining can be present. Immunoglobulin is usually not detected, indicating the dense deposits are not classic antigen–antibody immune complexes. However, segmental IgM or less often IgG and very rarely IgA have been reported.

Fig. 1.98 DDD. There is moderate mesangial proliferation and endocapillary proliferation and segmental glomerular basement membrane splitting with interposition. There are no large eosinophilic sub-endothelial deposits as typically seen in MPGN I (Jones' silver stain, ×200).

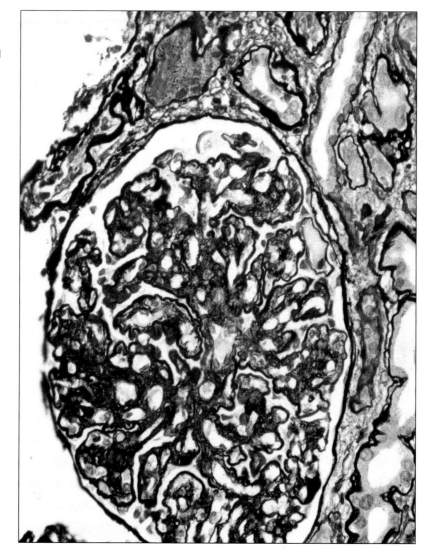

By electron microscopy, the lamina densa of the basement membrane in DDD shows a very dense transformation without discrete immune complex-type deposits (Figs 1.103, 1.104). Similar dense material is often found in the mesangial areas in addition to increased matrix. Increased mesangial cellularity or mesangial interposition are far less common than in type I MPGN. Visceral epithelial cells show varying degrees of reactive changes, from vacuolization, microvillous transformation to foot process effacement. Tubular basement membranes and Bowman's capsule may show similar densities as in the GBM.

Fig. 1.99 DDD. The refractile, dense appearance of the glomerular basement membrane is evident, along with mesangial and endocapillary proliferation. Note that the density is within the basement membrane itself, and not in a subendothelial location (PAS, ×1000).

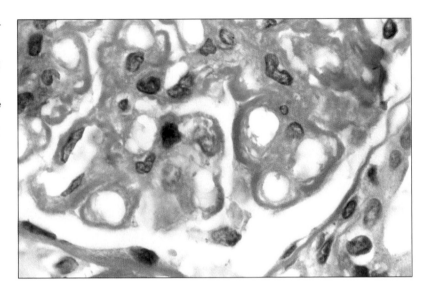

Fig. 1.100 DDD. The refractile, dense GBM of dense deposit disease is apparent. The basement membrane appears ribbon-like. There is associated mesangial and segmental endocapillary proliferation with occasional, segmental interposition (Jones' silver stain, ×1000).

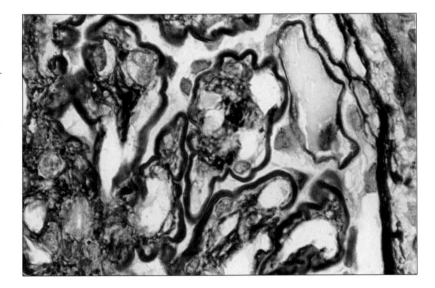

Etiology/pathogenesis

The precise nature of the dense material is not established. However, studies support that these densities represent a biochemical modification of the glycoprotein components of the normal basement membrane.

Fig. 1.101 DDD. On plastic-embedded sections, the ribbon-like dense transformation of the entire glomerular basement membrane is often apparent. There is associated mesangial and endocapillary proliferation (toluidine blue stain, ×1000).

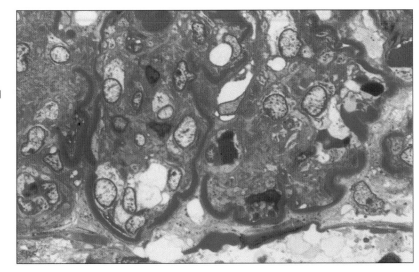

Fig. 1.102 DDD. There is typically only complement positivity in dense deposit disease, with chunky mesangial and coarse, irregular capillary loop positivity. Immunoglobulin staining is typically absent, indicating that there are no true immune complex-type (i.e. antibody–antigen) deposits (anti-C3 immunofluorescence, ×400).

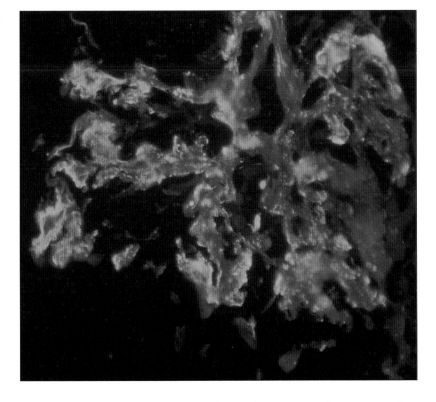

The pathogenesis of DDD is also unknown. Much attention has focused on C3 nephritic factor, C3NeF, which stabilizes the C3 convertase C3bBb, resulting in alternate pathway-mediated C3 breakdown. DDD sometimes occurs in association with partial lipodystrophy, a condition with loss of adipose tissue, decreased

Fig. 1.103 DDD. There is dense transformation of the glomerular basement membrane, with associated endocapillary and mesangial proliferation and occasional large, globular mesangial densities (TEM, ×8000).

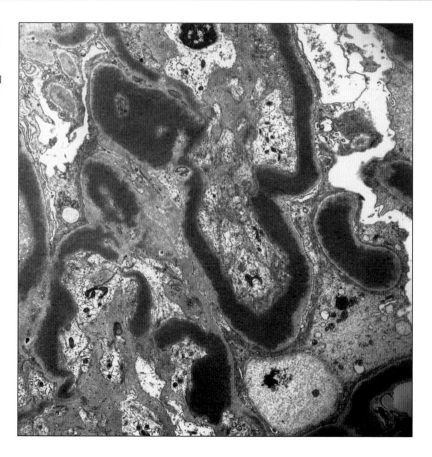

complement and presence of C3NeF. Further, a porcine model of factor H deficiency has similarities to DDD. Factor H inactivates factor C3bBb. These associations have suggested that abnormal complement regulation predisposes to DDD. However, clinical measures of complement, C3NeF, or presence of partial lipodystrophy did not predict clinical outcome amongst patients with DDD, and some patients with MPGN type I also have C3NeF. Some patients with partial lipodystrophy and C3NeF do not have DDD, further indication that complement abnormalities alone are insufficient to produce the disease.

Crescents or PMNs in capillary loops were associated with worse prognosis, whereas focal segmental glomerulonephritic lesions were less frequently associated with progressive renal disease. DDD invariably recurs morphologically in the transplant, although it does not usually cause graft loss.

Fig. 1.104   DDD. There is dense transformation of nearly the entire thickness of the glomerular basement membrane, with associated endocapillary proliferation. Overlying foot processes are extensively effaced. The nature of the transformed material has not been proven (TEM, ×20 250).

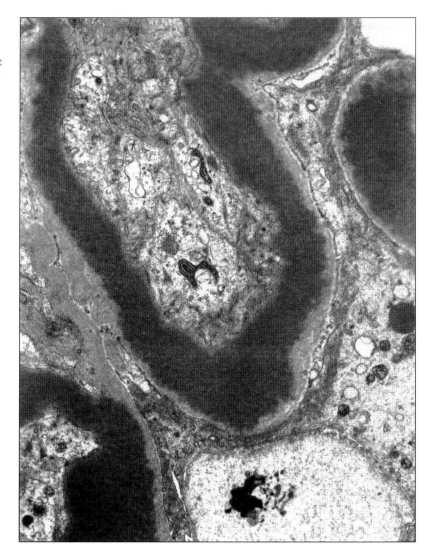

Selected reading

Anders D, Agricola B, Sippel M et al 1977 Basement membrane changes in membranoproliferative glomerulonephritis. II. Characterization of a third type by silver impregnation of ultra thin sections. Virchows Archiv (Pathology and Anatomy) 376:1–19.

Andresdottir M B, Assmann K J, Hoitsma A J et al 1999 Renal transplantation in patients with dense deposit disease: morphological characteristics of recurrent disease and clinical outcome. Nephrology, Dialysis and Transplantation 14(7):1723–1731.

Bennett W M, Fassett R G, Walker R G et al 1989 Mesangiocapillary glomerulonephritis type II (dense-deposit disease): clinical features of progressive disease. American Journal of Kidney Disease 13(6):469–476.

Berger J, Galle P 1963 Dépots denses au sein des membranes basales du rein: étude en microscopies optique et électronique. Presse Medicale 71:2351–2354.

Cameron J S, Turner D R, Heaton J et al 1983 Idiopathic mesangiocapillary glomerulonephritis. Comparison of types I and II in children and adults and long-term prognosis. American Journal of Medicine 74:175–192.

Churg J, Duffy J L, Bernstein J 1979 Identification of dense deposit disease. Archives of Pathology 103:67–72.

Habib R, Gubler M C, Loirat C et al 1975 Dense deposit disease: a variant of membranoproliferative glomerulonephritis. Kidney International 7:204–215.

McEnery P T, McAdams A J 1988 Regression of membranoproliferative glomerulonephritis type II (dense deposit disease): observations in six children. American Journal of Kidney Disease 12(2):138–146.

Fibrillary glomerulonephritis

Fibrillary glomerulonephritis was first reported by Rosenmann and Eliakim as a glomerulopathy with material very similar to amyloid that did not stain with Congo Red. A distinctly different morphologic form of glomerulopathy with larger, microtubular organized structures has been termed immunotactoid glomerulopathy. The classification of these lesions has been controversial. Some investigators have chosen to use the term immunotactoid glomerulopathy to refer to this entire group of disorders. We prefer to use the term fibrillary glomerulonephritis only for the amyloid-like, Congo Red-negative form, as this may have implications for prognosis and pathogenesis.

Fibrillary glomerulonephritis is a disease of adults, with average age of onset ~50 years. Patients are most often Caucasian, with a slight female predominance. This entity comprises about 1% of diagnoses amongst adults undergoing native kidney biopsy. Most patients present with nephrotic syndrome and frequently have associated hematuria. Rapidly progressive glomerulonephritis clinically was present in approximately one-third of patients. The prognosis is one of progression to renal loss in approximately 40% of cases over 5 years, with a median renal survival time of only 24 months from time of biopsy in one large series. Better prognosis was seen in patients younger than 40 years at presentation. No specific treatment has been described. Patients who progress to end stage renal disease generally did so rapidly, reaching end stage within 10 months on average after diagnosis. Elevated serum creatinine at presentation was a clinical sign of poor prognosis. Recurrence in the transplant

Fig. 1.105 Fibrillary glomerulonephritis. The light microscopic pattern varies from mesangial to membranoproliferative. This case shows moderate mesangial proliferation and occasional basement membrane splitting (Jones' silver stain, ×400).

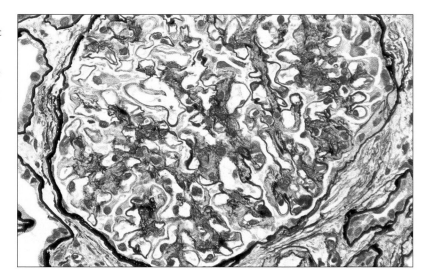

Fig. 1.106 Fibrillary glomerulonephritis. In some cases of fibrillary glomerulonephritis, there may be a lobular or nodular proliferative pattern, which may resemble diabetic nephropathy, as in this case (PAS, ×100).

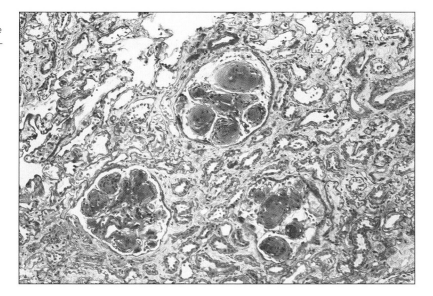

has been described for fibrillary glomerulonephritis cases, with a slower course of loss of GFR in the graft than in the native kidney.

The light microscopic appearance in fibrillary glomerulonephritis most frequently is that of a membranoproliferative, typically lobular, glomerulonephritis, with GBM splitting (Figs 1.105–1.107). Less frequently there is a mesangial proliferative or diffuse endocapillary proliferative pattern. Some cases may even appear similar to diabetic nephropathy, with large nodular expansion of mesangial matrix

Fig. 1.107 Fibrillary glomerulonephritis. A membranoproliferative pattern is evident with mesangial and endocapillary proliferation and basement membrane reduplication and interposition (Jones' silver stain, ×400).

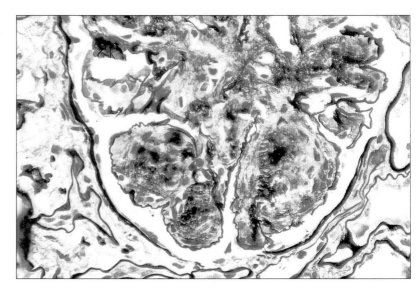

Fig. 1.108 Fibrillary glomerulonephritis. In our series, approximately one-third of cases showed crescents. In this case, there is associated moderate mesangial proliferation, an important feature indicating by LM that this crescentic lesion is likely not pauci-immune crescentic glomerulonephritis or anti-GBM antibody-mediated glomerulonephritis. Periglomerular fibrosis and early adhesions are also evident (Jones' silver stain, ×400).

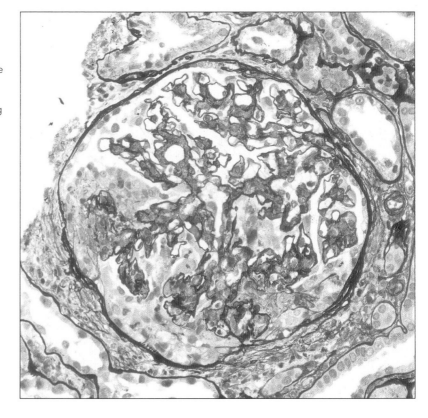

Fig. 1.109 Fibrillary glomerulonephritis. Immunofluorescence patterns in fibrillary glomerulonephritis mirror the light microscopic changes, ranging from mesangial to membranoproliferative or even membranous patterns. There is typically a smudgy positivity with particularly predominant mesangial staining. This case illustrates chunky mesangial staining and irregular, coarsely granular peripheral loop staining, corresponding to a light microscopic membranoproliferative pattern. Deposits typically stain for IgG and C3 and are polyclonal, but restricted to IgG4 subclass (anti-IgG, ×400).

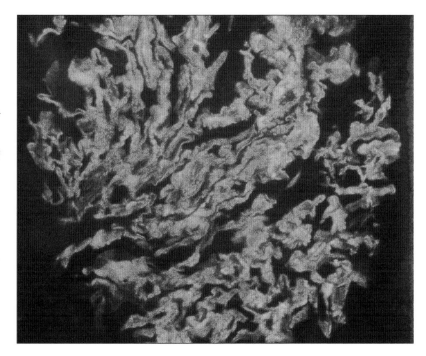

(Fig. 1.106). In rare cases there are GBM spikes in a membranous pattern, reflecting GBM reaction to the fibrillary deposits in a subepithelial location. Areas of deposits stain weakly PAS and silver positive. Crescents, either cellular or fibrocellular, were present in one-third of cases in one series (Fig. 1.108). Crescents more commonly are associated with diffuse endocapillary proliferation, and may be associated with worse outcome. Sclerosis is associated with more severe disease (Fig. 1.108). By definition, Congo red stains are negative. The interstitium shows interstitial fibrosis and tubular atrophy, proportional to glomerular changes. Vessels do not show any specific lesions.

Immunofluorescence demonstrates prominent, but smudgy IgG and lesser amounts of C3 in mesangial areas, and segmental, usually chunky, staining along glomerular basement membranes, occasionally in a membranous pattern (Figs 1.109, 1.110). IgG4 is the dominant or exclusive subclass. In about half of cases, weaker IgA and IgM and C1q may also be detected. Rare cases of other patterns have been reported; with predominant IgA deposits, or distinct fibrillar deposits by EM but no immunoglobulin staining. Not infrequently, the deposits are so diffuse as to provide an apparent linear staining by immunofluorescence (Fig. 1.110). This

Fig. 1.110 Fibrillary glomerulonephritis may also show a membranous pattern of deposits in some cases, with corresponding coarsely granular peripheral loop deposits, along with coarse mesangial deposits as shown here (anti-IgG immuno-fluorescence, ×400).

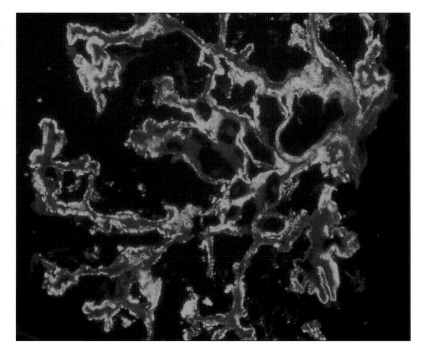

Fig. 1.111 Fibrillary glomerulonephritis. The deposits in fibrillary glomerulonephritis may be localized anywhere in the glomerulus. Randomly arranged fibrillar deposits, approximately 15 nm in diameter, permeate the thickened glomerular basement membrane, with overlying foot process effacement (TEM, ×4400).

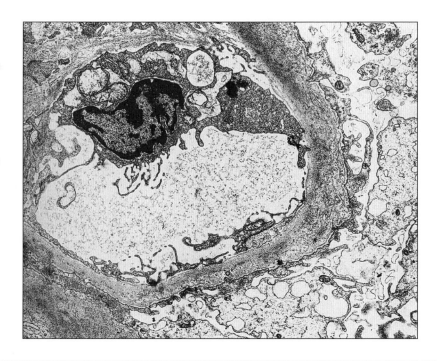

Fig. 1.112 Fibrillary glomerulonephritis. Randomly arranged fibrils of fibrillary glomerulonephritis permeate the glomerular basement membrane with blunting of overlying foot processes. The fibrils are slightly thicker than those seen in amyloid, but there may be overlap in fibril size in individual cases (TEM, ×7000).

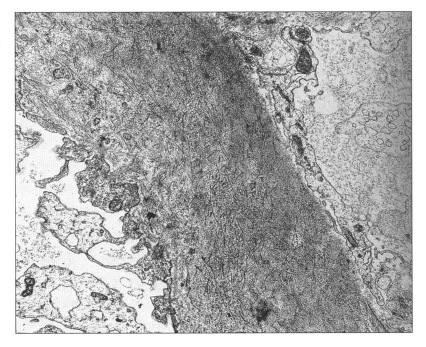

may, especially in cases with crescents, lead to an initial erroneous impression of possible anti-GBM antibody-mediated glomerulonephritis. The smudgy, predominantly mesangial staining suggests the specific diagnosis, confirmed by electron microscopy and negative Congo red stain.

The electron microscopic findings are then confirmatory of the diagnosis of fibrillary glomerulonephritis, showing the presence of randomly aligned fibrils that resemble amyloid fibrils but are larger (Figs 1.112–1.114). However, a precise distinction from amyloid cannot, in our experience, be made on fibril diameter alone. Fibril diameters in some series were 20–22 nm, with a range of 13–39 nm, contrasting amyloid cases with a mean of approximately 10 nm. However, in our series of fibrillary glomerulonephritis, there was some overlap, with average fibril diameter in fibrillary glomerulonephritis cases of 14 nm (range 10.4–18.4 nm). Therefore, it is critical to also use Congo Red-negative staining and typical immunofluorescence staining, as described above, as diagnostic criteria.

Fig. 1.113   Fibrillary glomerulonephritis. Large chunky deposits composed of randomly arranged fibrils are seen in this case of fibrillary glomerulonephritis, with interspersed more amorphous deposits. The overlying foot processes are completely effaced (TEM, ×8000).

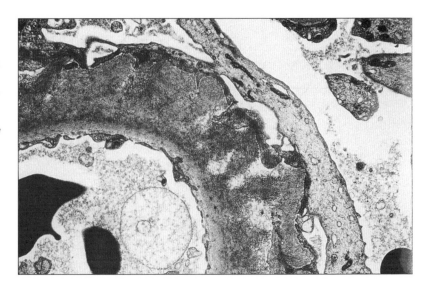

Fig. 1.114   Fibrillary glomerulonephritis. Randomly arranged fibrils, approximately 15 nm in diameter, in fibrillary glomerulonephritis, localized to the mesangium (TEM, ×15 000).

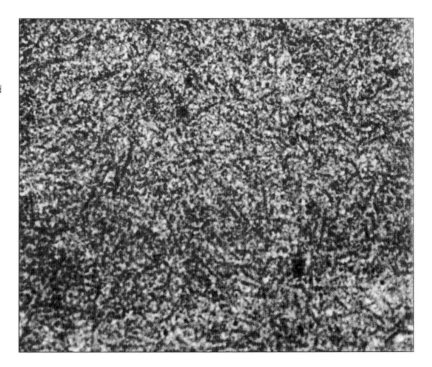

Electron microscopy may show fibrils in all glomerular compartments, including mesangium and basement membrane in intramembranous, subepithelial and subendothelial locations. Additional dense deposits without distinct fibrillary composition have been observed in some cases (Fig. 1.113). Rare tubular basement membrane fibrillary deposits may occur (Fig.1.115).

Fig. 1.115 Fibrillary glomerulonephritis. Rarely, there may be fibrillary deposits in tubular basement membranes in cases of fibrillary glomerulonephritis, (TEM, ×7000). Case shared by Dr Robert G. Horn.

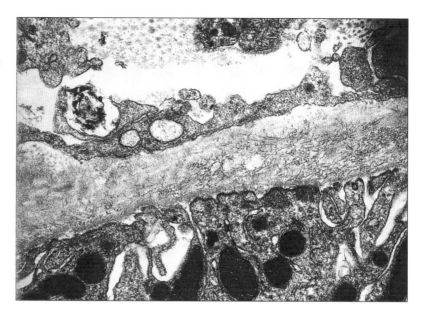

Etiology/pathogenesis

The etiology of fibrillary glomerulonephritis is unknown. Amyloid P has been found to be bound to the fibrils. Cryoprecipitated mixed immunoglobulin–fibronectin complexes were detected in the serum of a patient with fibrillary glomerulonephritis who had no evidence of a systemic disease process. The immunoglobulin component was polyclonal and consisted of IgG, IgM, heavy and light chains. These exciting findings indicate that serum precursors can lead to formation of fibrillary deposits. Occasional association with hepatitis C infection has been reported, but causality has not been proven. Importantly, fibrillary glomerulonephritis is not associated with lymphoproliferative disorders or monoclonality of deposits, in contrast to immunotactoid glomerulopathy.

Selected reading

Alpers C E 1992 Immunotactoid (microtubular) glomerulopathy: An entity distinct from fibrillary glomerulonephritis? American Journal of Kidney Disease 19:185–191.

Alpers C E, Rennke H G, Hopper J J et al 1987 Fibrillary glomerulonephritis: An entity with unusual immunofluorescence features. Kidney International 31:781–789.

Bridoux F, Hugue V, Coldefy O et al 2002 Fibrillary glomerulonephritis and immunotactoid (microtubular) glomerulopathy are associated with distinct immunologic features. Kidney International 62(5):1764–1775.

Churg J, Venkataseshan V S 1993 Fibrillary glomerulonephritis without immunoglobulin deposits in the kidney. Kidney International 44:837–842.

Fogo A, Quereshi N, Horn R G 1993 Morphologic and clinical features of fibrillary glomerulonephritis versus immunotactoid glomerulopathy. American Journal of Kidney Disease 22:367–377.

Iskandar S S, Falk R J, Jennette J C 1992 Clinical and pathological features of fibrillary glomerulonephritis. Kidney International 42:1401–1407.

Korbet S M, Schwartz M M, Rosenberg B F et al 1985 Immunotactoid glomerulopathy. Medicine 64:228–243.

Pronovost P H, Brady H R, Gunning M E et al 1996 Clinical features, predictors of disease progression and results of renal transplantation in fibrillary/immunotactoid glomerulopathy. Nephrology, Dialysis and Transplantation 11:837–842.

Rosenmann E, Eliakim M 1977 Nephrotic syndrome associated with amyloid-like glomerular deposits. Nephron 18:301–308.

Rosenstock J L, Markowitz G S, Valeri A M et al 2003 Fibrillary and immunotactoid glomerulonephritis: Distinct entities with different clinical and pathologic features. Kidney International 63(4):1450–1461.

Schwartz M M, Lewis E J 1980 The quarterly case: Nephrotic syndrome in a middle aged man. Ultrastructural Pathology 1:575–582.

Immunotactoid glomerulopathy

The classification of lesions with organized non-amyloid fibrillar or microtubular deposits has been controversial. Some investigators have chosen to use the term immunotactoid glomerulopathy to refer to this entire group of disorders. We prefer to use the term fibrillary glomerulonephritis only for the amyloid-like, Congo Red-negative form, as this may have implications for prognosis and pathogenesis. We will here discuss immunotactoid glomerulopathy, defined as large microtubular deposits typically >30 nm in diameter, often arranged in parallel arrays. This entity is very rare, less than 0.06% of adult native kidney biopsies. Patients are typically older than those with fibrillary glomerulonephritis, around 60–70 years vs. around 50 years on average and are mostly Caucasian. Patients present with nephrotic syndrome, hematuria, and some have hypocomplementemia. Importantly, there is associated monoclonal gammopathy and hematologic malignancy in about two-thirds of patients and deposits may stain in a monoclonal pattern. Patients do not generally have definable cryoglobulins, which may also give rise to organized deposits (see 'Cryoglobulinemic glomerulo-nephritis'). Renal survival appears better than in fibrillary glomerulonephritis, but published series have been too small and/

Fig. 1.116 Immunotactoid glomerulopathy. Light microscopic changes typically are those of a mesangial or membranoproliferative process, without crescents. Extensive glomerular basement membrane splitting and segmental adhesions are present in this case (Jones' silver stain, ×200).

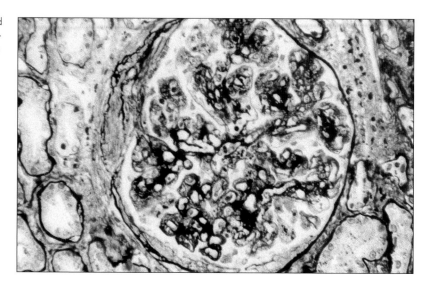

Fig. 1.117 Immunotactoid glomerulopathy. There is extensive glomerular basement membrane reduplication and interposition with mild mesangial and endocapillary proliferation (Jones' silver stain, ×400).

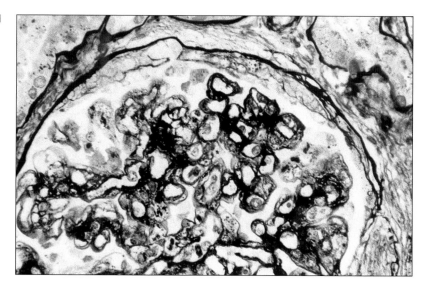

or had too short follow-up for definitive analysis. In our six patients, renal function remained stable, while one patient in a series of patients reported by the Columbia group reached end stage in 2 months. Chemotherapy directed at the underlying lymphoproliferative disease led to remission of nephrotic syndrome in some patents with immunotactoid glomerulopathy. Recurrence in the transplant has been described for immunotactoid glomerulopathy, with a slower course of loss of GFR in the graft than in the native kidney.

Light microscopy shows a mesangioproliferative or membrano-proliferative pattern (Figs 1.116, 1.117). The glomerular basement

Fig. 1.118 Immunotactoid glomerulopathy. Immuno-fluorescence shows coarse positivity in a mesangial and membranoproliferative pattern, typically with IgG and C3. The subendothelial location of these deposits is evident by the smooth outer border of peripheral loop deposits. There are also chunky mesangial deposits (anti-IgG, immuno-fluorescence ×400).

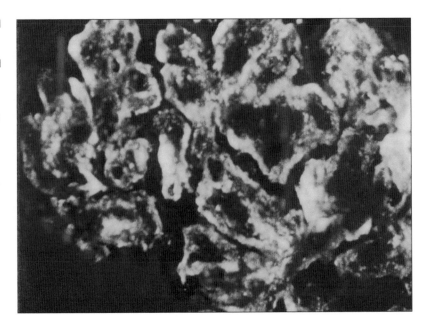

membrane may show only splitting, or occasionally spikes. Tubules and interstitium show atrophy and fibrosis proportional to glomerular injury. Vessels do not show specific lesions. Crescents are rare. Congo red stains are by definition negative.

Immunofluorescence shows predominant IgG with lesser IgA and IgM in occasional cases (Fig. 1.118). C3 is also usually positive, with less frequent C1q. The staining is chunky, irregular along capillary loops and in the mesangium. It does not appear smudgy as does fibrillary glomerulonephritis deposits by IF. The staining is usually stronger in capillary loops rather than in the mesangium, the converse of the pattern in fibrillary glomerulonephritis. Some cases may show monoclonal staining.

Electron microscopy shows large microtubular deposits, usually >30 nm in diameter and sometimes >50 nm. The microtubules have a hollow core and are frequently arranged in parallel arrays, and may have a 'stacked wood' arrangement (Figs 1.119, 1.20). The distribution mirrors that seen by IF, with predominant subendo-thelial and mesangial deposits. Some cases also have subepithelial or intramembranous deposits.

Fig. 1.119 Immunotactoid glomerulopathy. The specific diagnosis of immunotactoid glomerulopathy is made by electron microscopy. The deposits are microtubular and/or organized in parallel arrays, appearing like 'kindling wood stacked up for the winter'. The tubules are frequently 30–50 nm in diameter, and are here seen both in longitudinal and cross section, revealing their tubular nature. A similar appearance may be seen in some cases of cryoglobulinemic glomerulonephritis (TEM, ×12 000).

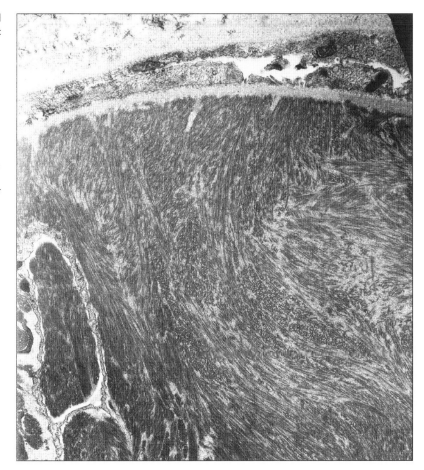

Etiology/pathogenesis

Immunotactoid glomerulopathy, defined by microtubular deposits, often in organized arrays, is significantly more frequently associated with monoclonal protein and hematopoietic malignancy than is fibrillary glomerulonephritis. Further, these immunotactoid deposits stain monoclonally in about two-thirds of cases. The clinical improvement of proteinuria when treatment was directed at the hematopoietic disorder, with parallel improvement of hematological parameters, further supports a role for monoclonal proteins in some of these patients.

Fig. 1.120 Immunotactoid glomerulopathy. The microtubular nature of the deposits in immunotactoid glomerulopathy is illustrated, with microtubules cut in cross and longitudinal orientation. The deposits are intramembranous and subendothelial, with associated foot process effacement and interposition (TEM, ×26 000).

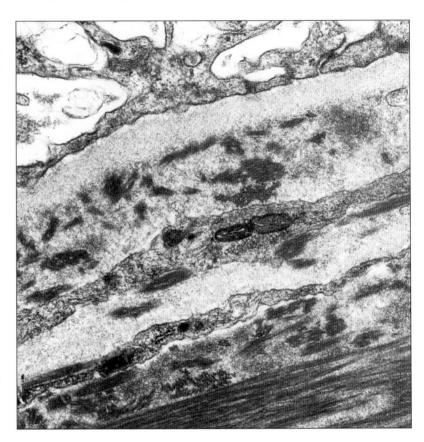

Selected reading

Alpers C E 1992 Immunotactoid (microtubular) glomerulopathy: An entity distinct from fibrillary glomerulonephritis? American Journal of Kidney Disease 19:185–191.

Bridoux F, Hugue V, Coldefy O et al 2002 Fibrillary glomerulonephritis and immunotactoid (microtubular) glomerulopathy are associated with distinct immunologic features. Kidney International 62(5):1764–1775.

Fogo A, Quereshi N, Horn R G 1993 Morphologic and clinical features of fibrillary glomerulonephritis versus immunotactoid glomerulopathy. American Journal of Kidney Disease 22:367–377.

Korbet S M, Schwartz M M, Rosenberg B F et al 1985 Immunotactoid glomerulopathy. Medicine 64:228–243.

Pronovost P H, Brady H R, Gunning M E et al 1996 Clinical features, predictors of disease progression and results of renal transplantation in fibrillary/immunotactoid glomerulopathy. Nephrology, Dialysis and Transplantation 11:837–842.

Rosenstock J L, Markowitz G S, Valeri A M et al 2003 Fibrillary and immunotactoid glomerulonephritis: Distinct entities with different clinical and pathologic features. Kidney International 63(4):1450–1461.

Glomerular diseases that cause hematuria or nephritic syndrome: immune complex

Acute postinfectious glomerulonephritis

Postinfectious glomerulonephritis presents as acute nephritic syndrome. Classically, this condition follows streptococcal infection. Other bacterial, viral, mycotic or even protozoan infections may give rise to the same type of glomerulonephritis. In tropical climates, skin infection rather than throat infection may lead to acute glomerulonephritis. Acute poststreptococcal glomerulonephritis is more common in children and young adults, with boys affected more than girls. Patients with typical poststreptococcal glomerulonephritis following a pharyngitic infection usually have a rapid course with rapid resolution, and thus are not biopsied. Biopsies therefore may over-represent more severe lesions. A small subset of patients has persistent renal dysfunction long-term after the acute nephritis subsides. Unrecognized subclinical disease related to postinfectious glomerulonephritis may also contribute to chronic renal disease. In a large series of predominantly adult patients, the majority of patients had glomerulosclerosis on re-biopsy 3–15 years from onset.

The light microscopic characteristic features in the acute phase are diffuse, exudative proliferative glomerulonephritis, with prominent endocapillary proliferation (Fig. 1.121) and numerous neutrophils (Figs 1.122–1.129). The proliferative lesions are diffuse and global. Small hump-shaped deposits may occasionally be visualized even by light microscopy with silver, trichrome or toluidine blue stains (Fig. 1.129). Crescents are present in severe cases, and may portend worse prognosis (Fig. 1.125). When biopsy is performed later in the course, the neutrophilic infiltrate is less prominent with remaining diffuse mesangial hypercellularity (Figs 1.126–1.128).

By immunofluorescence, scattered fine or large chunky deposits are present along the glomerular basement membrane, along with scattered mesangial deposits. The deposits typically stain with IgG with even more prominent C3 staining after the first few weeks. IgM and IgA staining is absent or minimal. Three immunofluorescence patterns have been described: starry sky, garland and mesangial patterns (Figs 1.130–1.133). The starry sky or garland patterns are seen early in the course of the disease, with garland-type deposits

Fig. 1.121 Acute post-infectious glomerulonephritis. There is an exudative proliferation with numerous PMNs and endocapillary proliferation, with scattered mesangial and large hump-shaped subepithelial deposits.

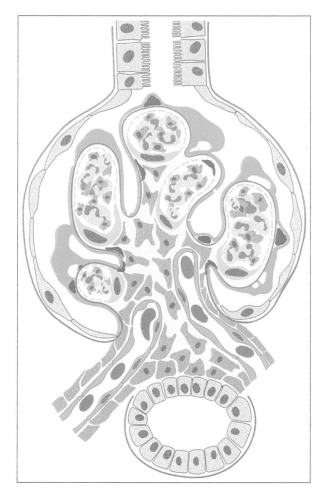

Fig. 1.122 Acute post-infectious glomerulo-nephritis. There is diffuse, global exudative proliferation with prominent endocapillary proliferation and numerous neutrophils. There is also surrounding inflammation in the tubulointerstitium (PAS, ×400).

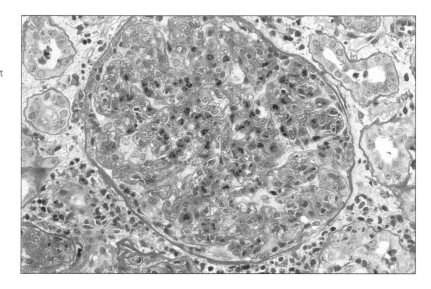

Fig. 1.123 Acute postinfectious glomerulonephritis. The numerous PMNs filling capillary lumens are clearly demonstrated, along with endocapillary proliferation and segmental interposition (Jones' silver stain, ×400).

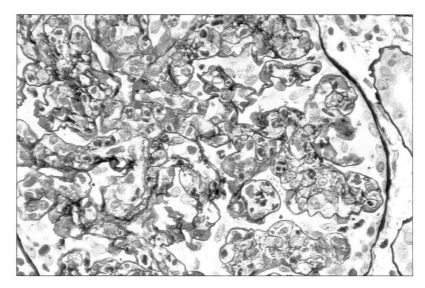

Fig. 1.124 Acute postinfectious glomerulonephritis. Endocapillary proliferation and numerous PMNs both within capillary loops and within the mesangial area are present. Deposits are not visualized here, although they may occasionally be seen by light microscopy (see Fig. 1.129) (H&E, ×1000).

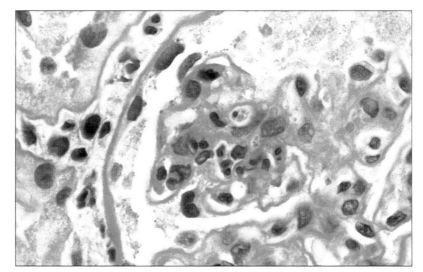

extending to the peripheral loops, associated with an exudative hypercellular glomerular lesion. Starry sky refers to the irregularly distributed coarse fluorescence positivity along the glomerular basement membrane. The garland pattern shows thicker, more elongated deposits along the capillary wall, is more commonly present in adults and has been associated with worse prognosis (Fig. 1.132).

Fig. 1.125 Acute post-infectious glomerulonephritis. In biopsied patients, there may frequently be crescents as these patients typically have an unusual clinical course with more severe injury. The cellular crescents are associated with endo-capillary proliferation and abundant PMNs. There is also associated extensive edema and tubulointerstitial inflammation (Jones' silver stain, ×100).

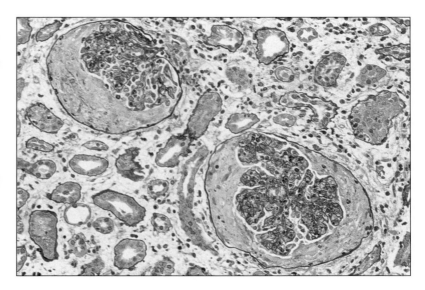

Fig. 1.126 Acute postin-fectious glomerulonephritis. In the latter stages follow-ing onset of the disease, there may be less promi-nent neutrophilic infiltrate with focal segmental mesangial and/or endo-capillary proliferation. Immunofluorescence and electron microscopy studies are then key in pointing to a postinfectious etiology (PAS, ×200).

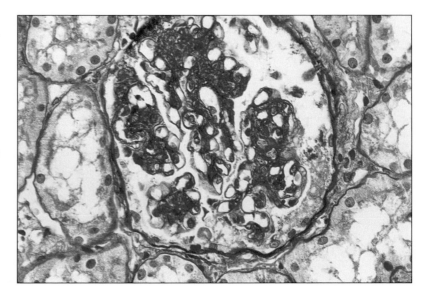

By EM, there are scattered subepithelial, hump-shaped deposits overlying the glomerular basement membrane without surrounding basement membrane reaction (Figs 1.134–1.136). These hump deposits are particularly numerous in the acute phase and may be variegated. Occasional mesangial and subendothelial deposits are present. When biopsies are performed at a later stage, peripheral hump-type deposits are more rare. Hump-shaped deposits may then only be present in the subepithelial area overlying the mesangium (the 'notch' or 'waist' area) (Fig. 1.136). In the more chronic phase

Fig. 1.127 Acute postinfectious glomerulonephritis. In this case of postinfectious glomerulonephritis, there is only segmental mesangial proliferation with very segmental endocapillary extension of the proliferation. No PMNs remain at this late state where deposits are visualized in the mesangial area and at '9 o'clock', confirmed by immunofluorescence and electron microscopy studies (Jones' silver stain, ×200).

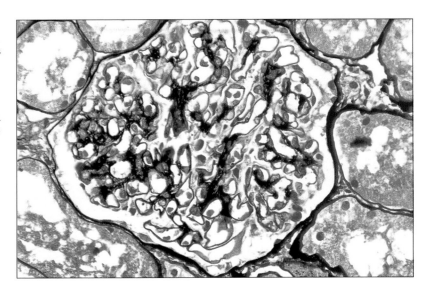

Fig. 1.128 Acute postinfectious glomerulonephritis. In later stages, there may be also diffuse, global endocapillary proliferation. In this case, there is extensive glomerular basement membrane reduplication, and PMNs still remain. The postinfectious etiology was strongly suggested by immunofluorescence findings with predominant C3 and hump-shaped, rare deposits by electron microscopy (Jones' silver stain, ×400).

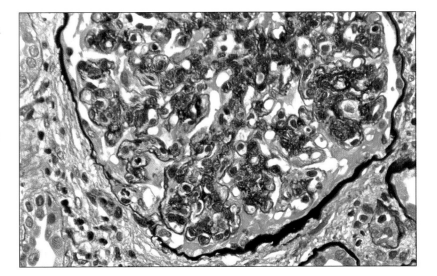

of the disease, mesangial deposits predominate, usually with less endocapillary proliferation and exudation. The finding of even rare hump-type subepithelial deposits strongly points to an infectious etiology of an immune complex glomerulonephritis, and is quite helpful in determining etiology when biopsy is done in the more chronic phase where only mesangial proliferation or focal membranoproliferative changes are present by light microscopy. A recent study by Haas also suggests that clinically silent post-infectious glomerulonephritis resulted in healed 'incidental' post-infectious

Fig. 1.129 Acute postinfectious glomerulonephritis. Large, hump-shaped deposits may occasionally be seen by light microscopy (Jones' silver stain, ×1000).

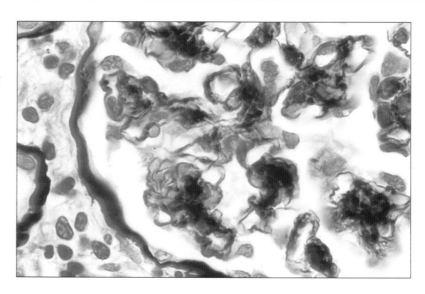

Fig. 1.130 Acute postinfectious glomerulonephritis. Starry sky pattern of immunofluorescence positivity is shown, with coarse, irregularly distributed fluorescence along the glomerular basement membrane, along with some mesangial staining (anti-IgG immunofluorescence, ×400).

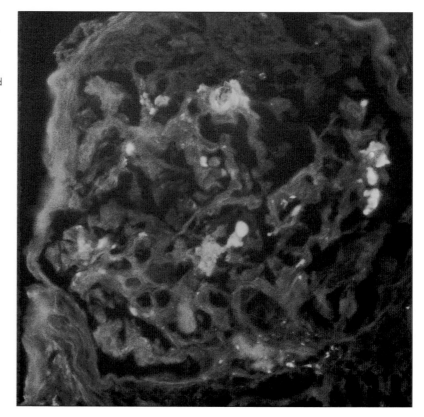

Fig. 1.131 Acute postinfectious glomerulonephritis.
C3 positivity is often even
stronger than IgG in postinfectious glomerulonephritis.
This is the same case as in
Figure 1.129, with predominant starry sky pattern, with
occasional segments with
thicker, more elongated
deposits, so-called 'garland
pattern' (bottom) (anti-C3
immunofluorescence, ×400).

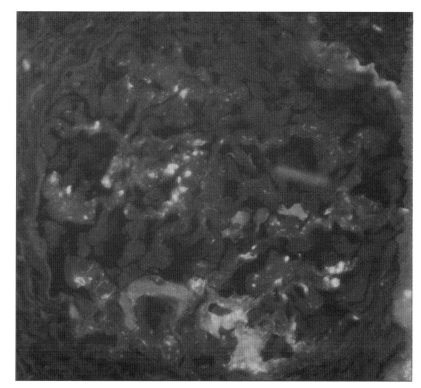

Fig. 1.132 Acute postinfectious glomerulonephritis.
A more extensive garland
pattern with elongated
peripheral loop deposits is
illustrated, along with occasional small mesangial
deposits (anti-C3 immuno-
fluorescence, ×400).

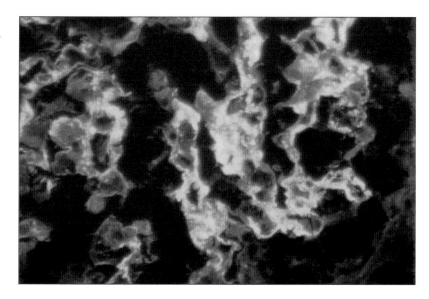

Fig. 1.133 Acute postinfectious glomerulonephritis. In the more chronic phase of the disease, mesangial deposits may be predominant, usually with less endocapillary proliferation and exudation, as illustrated here. There are very few, scattered subepithelial deposits, corresponding to rare hump-type deposits by EM (anti-C3 immunofluorescence, ×400).

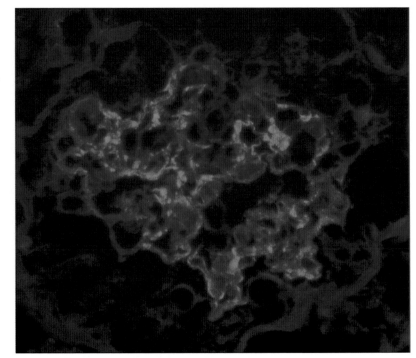

Fig. 1.134 Acute postinfectious glomerulonephritis. There is an intraluminal PMN, a platelet and endocapillary proliferation, with scattered intramembranous and large hump-shaped deposits without surrounding basement membrane reaction (TEM, ×3000).

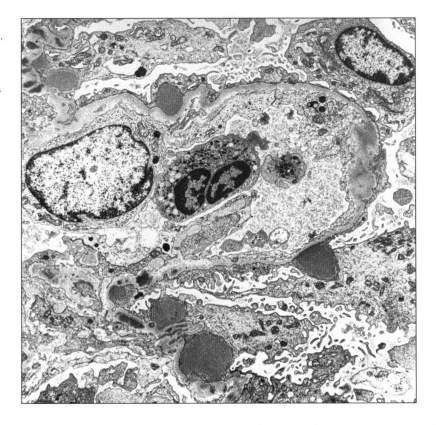

Fig. 1.135 Acute postinfectious glomerulonephritis. More continuous areas of hump-shaped subepithelial deposits are present, corresponding to the garland pattern by immunofluorescence. Rare small intramembranous and subendothelial deposits (bottom) are also present, along with endocapillary proliferation (TEM, ×3000).

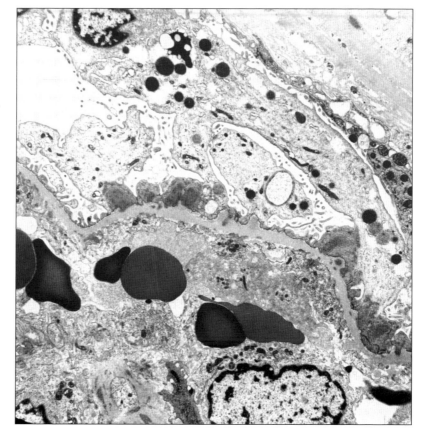

lesions, deduced by presence of these subepithelial deposits by EM. These deposits were associated with a variety of other renal lesions, and may be additional contributors to progressive renal damage.

Etiology/pathogenesis

The immunopathogenesis of poststreptococcal glomerulonephritis has been studied extensively. Numerous streptococcal antigens have been proposed as the target antigen. Erythrogenic toxin type B (ETB) produced by Streptococci may be a key part of the immune complexes in post-infectious glomerulonephritis. The antigens from other pathogens such as Staphylococcus and Pneumococcus that can induce an identical glomerulonephritis are not known. Whether circulating immune complexes deposit in the glomeruli, or the antigens traverse the GBM and bind to sites within the glomerulus and stimulate antibody and subsequent complement activation, is

Fig. 1.136 Acute postinfectious glomerulonephritis. Small mesangial deposits and a large, variegated, hump-shaped deposit located subepithelially in the waist region are present. This area is the last place where hump-shaped deposits persist. The presence of even rare hump-shaped deposits is a useful indicator of an underlying infectious etiology for an immune complex glomerulonephritis (TEM, ×25 625).

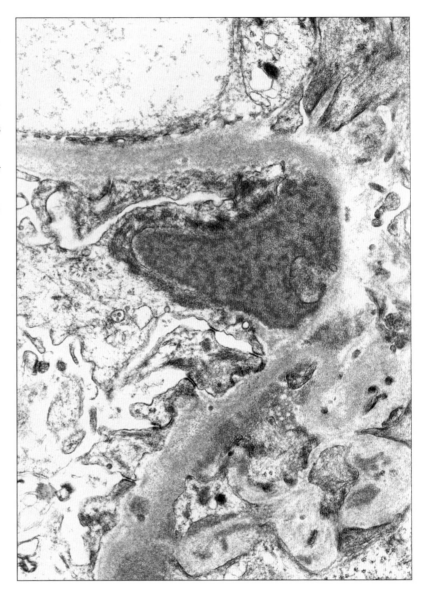

not determined. Individual variability in susceptibility to glomerulonephritis after infection with 'nephritogenic' strains of bacteria is linked to HLA class II allelic variation, with resistance to disease in those patients with reduced immune responsiveness.

Selected reading

Baldwin D S, Gluck M C, Schacht R G et al 1974 The long-term course of poststreptococcal glomerulonephritis. Annals of Internal Medicine 80:342–358.

Edelstein C L, Bates W D 1992 Subtypes of acute postinfectious glomerulonephritis: A clinico-pathological correlation. Clinical Nephrology 38:311–317.

Haas M 2003 Incidental healed postinfectious glomerulonephritis: a study of 1012 renal biopsy specimens examined by electron microscopy. Human Pathology 34:3–10.

Kotb M, Norrby-Teglund A, McGeer A et al 2002 An immunogenetic and molecular basis for differences in outcomes of invasive group A streptococcal infections. Nature Medicine 8(12):1398–1404.

Lewy J E, Salinas-Madrigal L, Herdson P B et al 1971 Clinico-pathologic correlations in acute poststreptococcal glomerulonephritis. A correlation between renal functions, morphologic damage and clinical course of 46 children with acute poststreptococcal glomerulonephritis. Medicine (Baltimore) 50:453–501.

Sagel I, Treser G, Ty A et al 1973 Occurrence and nature of glomerular lesions after group A streptococci infections in children. Annals of Internal Medicine 79(4):492–499.

Sorger K, Balun J, Hubner F K et al 1983 The garland type of acute postinfectious glomerulonephritis: morphological characteristics and follow-up studies. Clinical Nephrology 20:17–26.

Sorger K, Gessler M, Hubner F K et al 1987 Follow-up studies of three subtypes of acute postinfectious glomerulonephritis ascertained by renal biopsy. Clinical Nephrology 27:111–124.

Sorger K, Gessler U, Hubner F K et al 1982 Subtypes of acute postinfectious glomerulonephritis. Synopsis of clinical and pathological features. Clinical Nephrology 17:114–128.

IgA nephropathy

IgA nephropathy (IgAN) is the most common glomerulonephritis in renal biopsies worldwide. Patients with IgAN present with hematuria, either microscopic or macroscopic, and varying proteinuria. Occasionally proteinuria may reach nephrotic range. The disease occurs in all age groups. The incidence of IgAN in African-Americans and Africans is much lower than in other populations. The apparent higher incidence of IgA nephropathy in biopsy series from Japan likely reflects the practice of widespread screening urinalysis and frequent renal biopsy for isolated microscopic hematuria. The clinical presentation gives useful prognostic information in patients with IgA nephropathy, with worse prognosis in older male patients with hypertension, marked proteinuria and increased creatinine at presentation and persistent microscopic hematuria. Prognosis is quite variable, with some patients showing rapid progression and approximately one-third developing chronic renal failure over long-term, 30-year, follow-up. Recurrence in the transplant occurs in up to 60% of patients, but morphologic recurrence does not equate to graft loss.

The light microscopic appearance in IgA nephropathy varies from minimal mesangial expansion (Fig. 1.137) to diffuse proliferative lesions with crescents or widespread sclerosis. There is often mesangial area increase due to increase in both mesangial cells, matrix and deposits (Figs 1.139–1.141). In some cases, deposits can be outlined on the silver stain as they are silver negative (Fig. 1.142). Endocapillary proliferation may be present, in either focal segmental or diffuse distribution, and is typically associated with extension of deposits to peripheral loops (Fig. 1.143). These deposits can result in mesangial interposition and GBM splitting. With severe injury, there may be segmental necrosis and crescents (Fig. 1.144, 1.145). In chronic cases, there is often segmental sclerosis, with proportional tubular atrophy and interstitial fibrosis (Figs 1.146–1.148).

Fig. 1.137   IgA nephropathy. There is mesangial cell and matrix increase, with mesangial deposits.

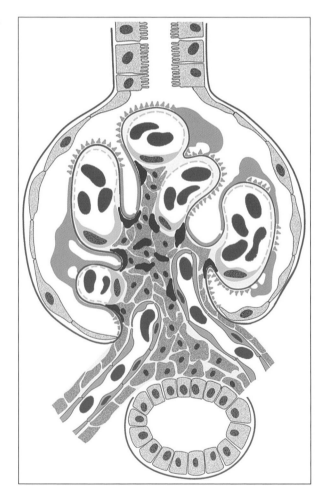

Fig. 1.138 IgA nephropathy. There may be inconspicuous changes by light microscopy with only minimal or no apparent increase in matrix. In these cases, the diagnosis rests on immunofluorescence and electron microscopy for a specific diagnosis of IgA nephropathy (Jones' silver stain, ×200).

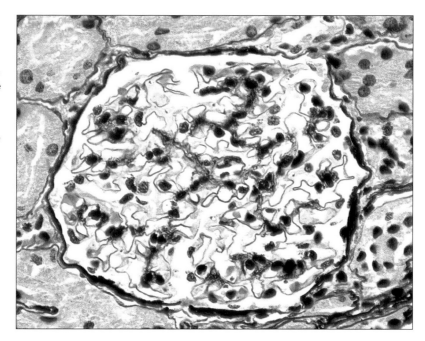

Fig. 1.139 IgA nephropathy. There is mild mesangial matrix expansion and a mild increase in mesangial cellularity, with three or more nuclei in most mesangial areas in this early case of IgA nephropathy (PAS, ×200).

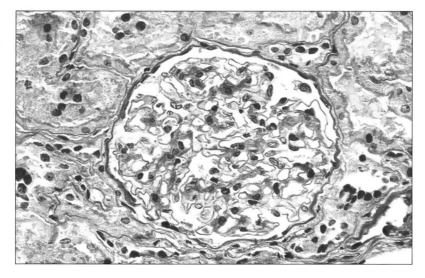

The relative frequency of proliferative lesions versus sclerosing lesions and minimal light microscopic findings likely reflect biopsy practices. In a large series, 13% of biopsies showed only minimal mesangial expansion, 6% showed diffuse mesangial hypercellularity, 80% showed focal segmental glomerulosclerosis and/or focal segmental proliferative lesions with crescents, and 1% showed an end-stage kidney. Classifications based on light microscopic appearance

Fig. 1.140 IgA nephropathy. The expanded mesangial matrix is evident, with more lucent, weakly PAS positive areas representing the immune deposits, verified by immunofluorescence and electron microscopy (Jones' silver stain, ×1000).

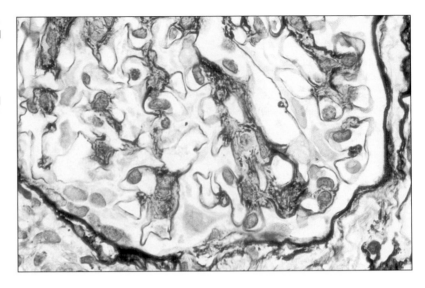

Fig. 1.141 IgA nephropathy. There is marked mesangial expansion, with segmental proliferation extending out to peripheral capillary loops, and early focal proliferative lesion (Masson trichrome stain, ×200).

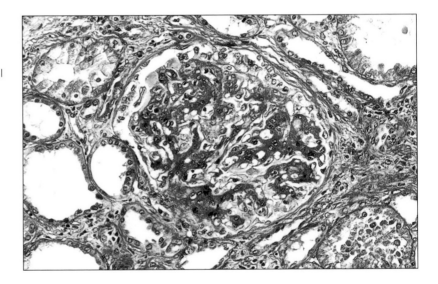

have been proposed, with parallels to the commonly used WHO classification for SLE nephritis (Tables 1.3, 1.4).

Henoch-Schönlein purpura may be thought of as the systemic counterpart of IgA nephropathy. The lesions in the kidney are indistinguishable, and differentiation is made based on clinical pathological features. The International Study of Kidney Disease in Children used a classification for renal disease in patients with Henoch-Schönlein purpura with many similarities to the IgAN classification (see section on 'Henoch-Schönlein purpura').

Fig. 1.142 IgA nephropathy. Massive deposits are visualized as PAS positive areas within the mesangium in this case of advanced IgA nephropathy with mesangial proliferation and segmental sclerosis (top upper right) (Jones' silver stain, ×400).

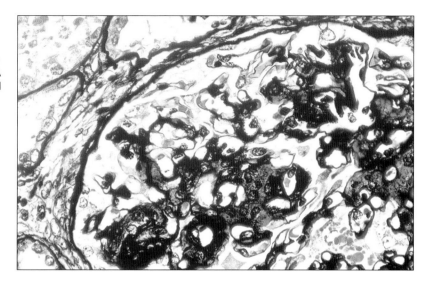

Fig. 1.143 IgA nephropathy. There is diffuse mesangial proliferation with segmental endocapillary proliferation and occasional peripheral basement membrane splitting, evidence of deposits extending to peripheral loops (Jones' silver stain, ×200).

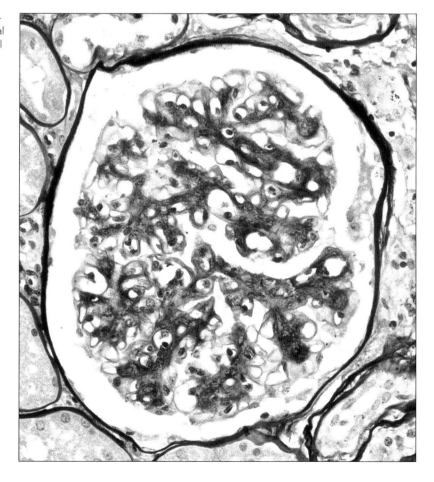

Fig. 1.144 IgA nephropathy. Mild mesangial proliferation is associated with segmental peripheral capillary loop splitting and endocapillary proliferation, and a small area of segmental fibrinoid necrosis (Jones' silver stain, ×400).

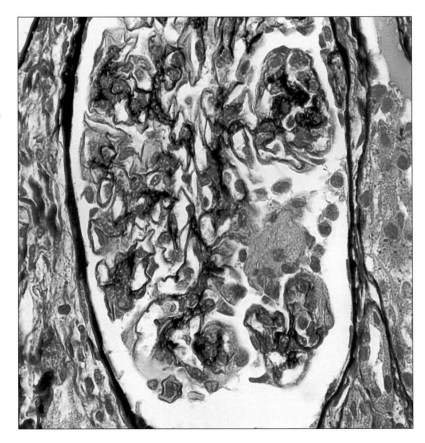

Fig. 1.145 IgA nephropathy. The underlying IgA nephropathy giving rise to the crescentic injury is evident by moderate mesangial proliferation with segmental peripheral capillary loop alteration (right). In addition, characteristic IgA positivity by IF and EM demonstration of well-defined deposits were present (Jones' silver stain, ×200).

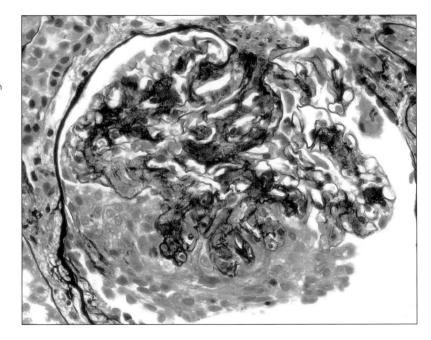

Fig. 1.146 IgA nephropathy. With ongoing injury, there may be extensive glomerulosclerosis, both segmental and global, often with associated more active lesions of endocapillary proliferation and cellular or fibrocellular crescents. Numerous adhesions with thickened areas of Bowman's capsule, indicative of past healed proliferative lesions, are present, in addition to the extensive global sclerosis and segmental sclerosis. There is associated tubulointerstitial atrophy and fibrosis (Jones' silver stain, ×100).

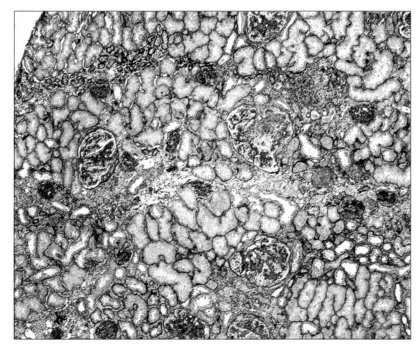

Fig. 1.147 IgA nephropathy. Mild to moderate mesangial proliferation, segmental endocapillary proliferation, early cellular crescent formation (left and top) with numerous adhesions, indicative of organization of past active lesions are present. There is early tubulointerstitial fibrosis, and active tubulointerstitial infiltrate surrounds the glomeruli with early crescentic injury and disruption of Bowman's capsule (Jones' silver stain, ×200).

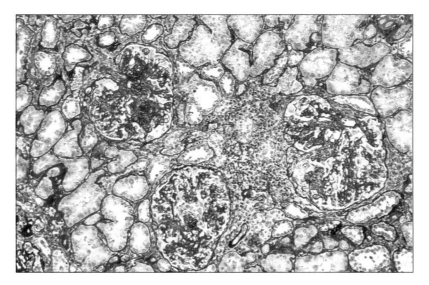

Immunofluorescence microscopy reveals the definitive characteristic dominant or co-dominant deposits of IgA. These deposits may be confined to the mesangium (Fig. 1.149), or extend to peripheral capillary loops, typically associated with proliferative lesions (Fig. 1.150). C3 is almost invariably present, but C1q is

Fig. 1.148 IgA nephropathy. Lesions may be quite complex, with combination of adhesions, small cellular crescents, mesangial and endocapillary proliferation with peripheral basement membrane splitting. There is also early surrounding tubulointerstitial fibrosis and inflammation (Jones' silver stain, ×200).

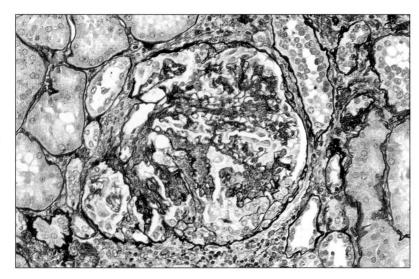

TABLE 1.3   Haas classification of IgAN

I.   Minimal or no mesangial hypercellularity.

II.   Focal and segmental glomerulosclerosis without cellular proliferation

III. Focal proliferative glomerulonephritis

IV.   Diffuse proliferative glomerulonephritis

V.   ≥40% global glomerulosclerosis, and/or ≥40% cortical tubular atrophy

Focal refers to <50% of glomeruli with the lesion

TABLE 1.4   WHO classification of IgAN

I.   Minimal lesion

II.   Minor changes with small segmental proliferation

III. Focal and segmental glomerulonephritis (<50% involved)

IV.   Diffuse mesangial lesions with proliferation and sclerosis

V.   Diffuse sclerosing glomerulonephritis affecting >80% of glomeruli

Fig. 1.149 IgA nephropathy. Definitive diagnosis is made by dominant or codominant staining with IgA in a predominantly mesangial pattern, as shown here. The mesangial location results in a 'pruned shrub' appearance (anti-IgA immunofluorescence, ×400).

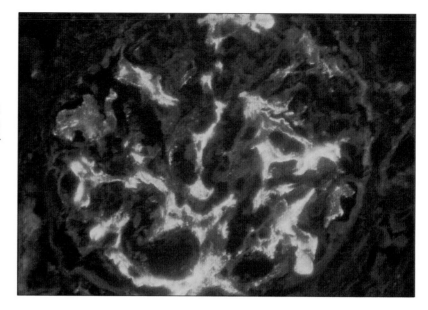

Fig. 1.150 IgA nephropathy. Definitive diagnosis is made by immunofluorescence, showing dominant or codominant IgA staining in the mesangium. In cases with more active lesions, there is frequent extension to peripheral capillary loops, as seen segmentally in this case (left) (anti-IgA immunofluorescence, ×400).

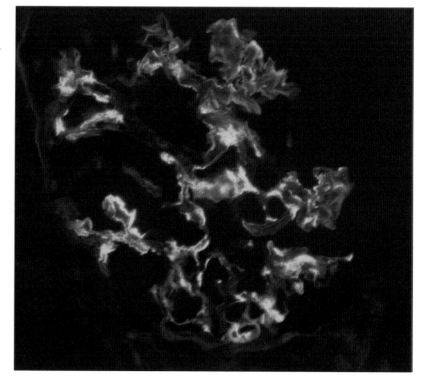

Fig. 1.151   IgA nephropathy. The deposits are in the mesangial area, underneath the paramesangial basement membrane. In this case, there is no extension of deposits to peripheral loops, and there was only mesangial proliferation by light microscopy (TEM, ×3000).

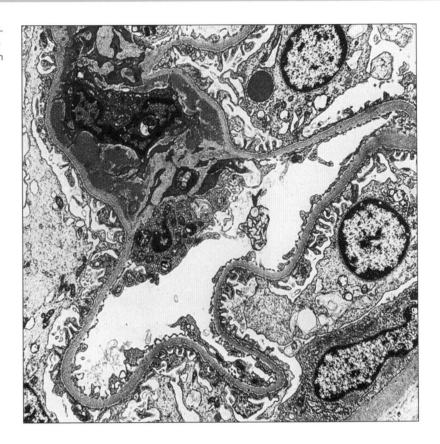

rarely positive. The immunofluorescence positivity for IgA is diffuse and global, although the light microscopic lesions may be focal and segmental. Of note, lambda staining is typically more predominant than kappa staining, in contrast to predominance of kappa in other polyclonal immune complex diseases. IgG and/or IgM may also be present, but by definition, are not present in greater intensity than IgA.

By electron microscopy, deposits are found in the mesangial areas, underlying the paramesangial glomerular basement membrane (Figs 1.151, 1.152). There is increased mesangial matrix and mesangial cellularity may also be increased. Subendothelial deposits are typically present in cases with endocapillary proliferation, and extend out from the mesangial area (Fig. 1.153). Occasionally there may be subepithelial or intramembranous deposits. Foot processes are effaced over areas with sclerosis. The distribution of deposits mirrors the IF pattern (Fig. 1.154).

Fig. 1.152 IgA nephropathy. There are mesangial deposits, but with extension towards the peripheral loop basement membranes (TEM, ×17 125).

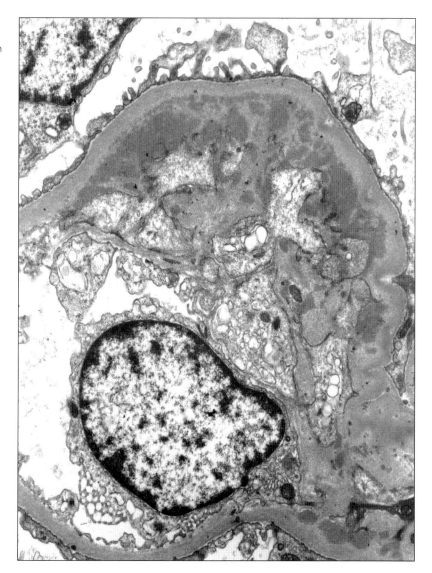

Etiology/pathogenesis

The pathogenesis of progressive injury in IgAN is unknown. Morphological features provide additional prognostic information over the clinical findings. The extent of global and/or segmental sclerosis or adhesions, tubular atrophy and interstitial fibrosis, interstitial cellular infiltrate, and peripheral capillary wall alterations (including splitting, deposits or endocapillary proliferation) are all associated with worse outcome. Efforts to develop quantitative scoring systems to predict outcomes have been tested with varying

Fig. 1.153 IgA nephropathy. Extension of deposits to peripheral loop is often associated with mesangial interposition. Overlying foot processes show diffuse effacement, and there is associated endocapillary proliferation (TEM, ×17 125).

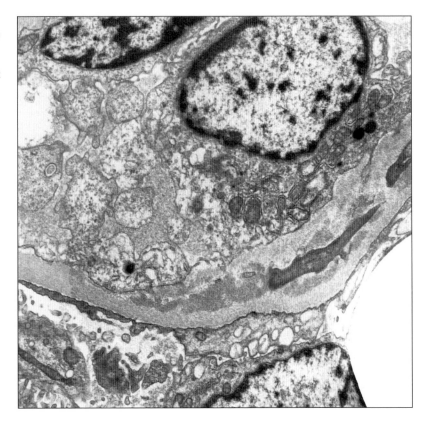

results. Mesangial cellularity and matrix increase, capillary lumen narrowing, sclerosis, crescents and adhesions were scored and combined in a severity index that gave more prognostic information than individual lesions.

Interestingly, IgAN recurs in the transplant, and conversely, IgAN regressed when transplantation of kidneys with mild IgAN into patients with end stage renal disease from other causes was inadvertently performed. These observations strongly indicate that IgAN has a systemic basis. The etiology of IgA nephropathy remains unknown. Current research has focused on abnormal mucosal immune reactivity, production of IgA with an abnormal hinge region resistant to proteolysis, and genetic factors. The hinge region of IgA1 usually has bound oligosaccharides that are O-linked to serine or threonine residues. Abnormal oligosaccharides are postulated to be causal in resistance to proteolysis of the IgA deposits. In support of this hypothesis, the deposits in IgAN are predominantly IgA1 subclass, which accounts for 90% of serum IgA, while IgA2 comprises 60% of

Fig. 1.154 IgA nephro-pathy. Deposits may be quite massive (same case as Fig. 1.142) (TEM, ×3000).

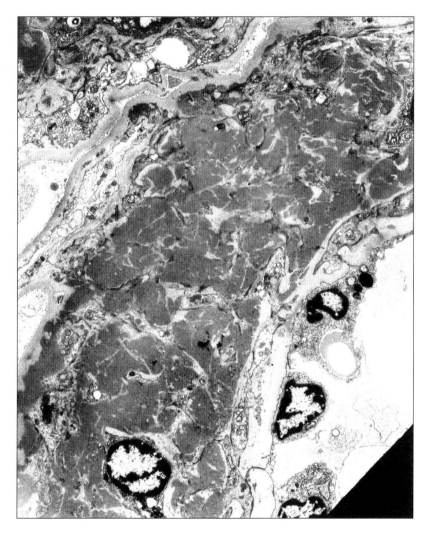

IgA in secretions. African Americans commonly have a form of IgA1 with deletion of these hinge region amino acids, which could explain the rarity of IgAN in this population. Abnormal mucosal plasma cell production of J chain, required for transport of IgA into mucosal secretions may also contribute to IgAN. Studies in familial IgA nephropathy have identified linkage to a region of chromosome 6. Whether this gene plays a role in sporadic IgAN is not known.

Selected reading

Berger J 1969 IgA glomerular deposits in renal disease. Transplantation Proceedings 1:939–944.

Berger J, Hinglais N 1968 Les depots intercapillaires d'IgA-IgG. Journal of Urology 74:694–695.

D'Amico G, Imbasciati E, Di Belgioso G B et al 1985 Idiopathic IgA mesangial nephropathy. Clinical and histological study of 374 patients. Medicine 64:49–60.

D'Amico, Imbasciati E, Barbiano Di Belgioso G et al 1985 Idiopathic IgA mesangial nephropathy. Clinical and histological study of 374 patients. Medicine 64:49–60.

Donadio J V, Grande J P 1997 Predicting renal outcome in IgA nephropathy. Journal of the American Society of Nephrology 8:1324–1332.

Emancipator S N 1994 IgA nephropathy: morphologic expression and pathogenesis. American Journal of Kidney Disease 23(3):451–462.

Floege J, Burg M, Kliem V 1998 Recurrent IgA nephropathy after transplantation not a benign condition. Nephrology, Dialysis and Transplantation 13:1933–1935.

Frohnert P P, Donadio J V, Velosa J A et al 1997 The fate of renal transplants in patients with IgA nephropathy. Clinical Transplantation 11:127–133.

Gharavi A G, Yan Y, Scolari F et al 2000 IgA nephropathy, the most common cause of glomerulonephritis, is linked to 6q22-23. Nature Genetics 26(3):354–357.

Haas M 1997 Histologic subclassification of IgA nephropathy: A clinicopathologic study of 244 cases. American Journal of Kidney Disease 29:829–842.

Ibels L S, Gyory A Z 1994 IgA nephropathy: analysis of the natural history, important factors in the progression of renal disease, and a review of the literature. Medicine (Baltimore) 73:79–102.

Lee S M K, Rao V M, Franklin W A et al 1982 IgA nephropathy: Morphologic predictors of progressive renal disease. Human Pathology 13:314–322.

Radford M G Jr, Donadio J V Jr, Bergstralh E J, Grande J P 1997 Predicting renal outcome in IgA nephropathy. Journal of the American Society of Nephrology 8(2):199–207.

Secondary glomerular diseases

Diseases associated with nephrotic syndrome

Monoclonal immunoglobulin deposition disease

Monoclonal immunoglobulin production may be seen as a consequence of multiple myeloma, Waldenström's macroglobulinemia, B-cell lymphoma, or represent monoclonal gammopathy of undetermined significance (MGUS). Multiple myeloma is the most common underlying disease in monoclonal immunoglobulin deposition disease (MIDD) and accounts for 40–50% of pure MIDD. The incidence of overt multiple myeloma is even greater in patients with MIDD associated with light chain cast nephropathy (>90%). In patients with multiple myeloma, approximately 5% are found to have MIDD at autopsy. The diagnosis of MIDD by renal biopsy often precedes other clinical evidence of dysproteinemia (70%) and is commonly the presenting disease, which leads to the discovery of multiple myeloma. Some 15–30% of patients with MIDD on renal biopsy may not have a detectable urine or serum monoclonal protein. Conversely, not all patients with monoclonal protein have related renal disease. Of note, about 60% of our biopsied patients with monoclonal protein had unrelated renal disease. Most had MGUS detected by screening tests as part of the workup for their renal disease. The spectrum of diagnoses in these patients reflected the spectrum of diagnoses seen in our general adult renal biopsy population. Thus, diabetic nephropathy and FSGS were the most common diseases in these proteinuric MGUS patients.

The most common monoclonal immunoglobulin-mediated nephropathies include AL-amyloidosis light chain cast nephropathy, cryoglobulinemia (type I and II), light chain cast nephropathy and the monoclonal immunoglobulin deposition diseases (MIDD). The MIDD are characterized by non-Congophilic, nonfibrillar electron dense deposits distributed in various tissues. MIDD predominantly affects the kidneys, but can also commonly involve the heart and liver. Non-amyloid glomerular MIDD is divided into three categories based on the type of immunoglobulin deposits: light chain deposition disease (LCDD), light and heavy chain deposition disease (LHCDD) and heavy chain deposition disease (HCDD). Among these three entities, LCDD is the most common and thus best understood with respect to its clinical and pathological features, and appears to have a slightly better prognosis than LHCDD or HCDD. LHCDD is less frequent, comprising less than 10% of MIDD. HCDD has been reported in only 11 cases to date. MIDD may recur in the transplant.

Amyloidosis

Amyloidosis is defined as the deposition of proteins that have the capacity to form beta-pleated sheets and are therefore resistant to degradation. Amyloid is a systemic disease, and different amyloids have somewhat differing propensities for tissue-specific involvement. The most common presentation of AA amyloidosis (due to active serum amyloid A protein) is that of renal disease, and AL amyloid (due to monoclonal light chain) also frequently involves the kidney. When amyloid involves the kidney, nearly half of patients have nephrotic range proteinuria, regardless of the peptide origin of the amyloid. Occasionally patients present with concentrating defects due to tubulointerstitial amyloid deposition. Additional extrarenal manifestations include carpal tunnel syndrome, peripheral neuropathy, liver dysfunction and congestive heart failure due to cardiac amyloidosis. Cardiac involvement is rare in AA amyloidosis, contrasting the frequent heart abnormalities in AL and transthyretin (ATTR) amyloidosis. In a large USA series of mostly adult native kidney biopsies, amyloidosis was the diagnosis in 2% of renal biopsies, and AL amyloid was the most common type of amyloid. In contrast, in developing and Mediterranean countries, renal amyloid is more commonly AA amyloid. The age of the patients reflects the underlying conditions causing amyloid formation. Patients with amyloid due to light chain are typically older adults. In contrast, familial Mediterranean fever may result in amyloid even in early childhood.

The prognosis of patients with amyloidosis varies according to the type of amyloid and underlying associated condition. With AL amyloidosis, the median survival is only one to two years, contrasting up to 15-year survival with ATTR amyloidosis. For AL amyloidosis, treatment of the underlying plasma cell dyscrasia has been attempted with melphalan with remission in some patients. Vigorous treatment and removal of the underlying inciting inflammation in AA amyloidosis may halt progression. Colchicine has been used in some cases of familial Mediterranean fever-associated

AA amyloidosis, although the efficacy of this approach in other forms of amyloidosis has not been shown.

By light microscopy, there may be only minimal mesangial expansion or segmental areas of amorphous, acellular pale eosinophilic material ('cotton candy' appearance) (Figs 1.155, 1.156). The glomeruli may also have massive amyloid deposits and show a nodular appearance, typically without marked increase in cellularity (Figs 1.157–1.159). The glomerular basement membrane may also

Fig. 1.155 Amyloidosis. Amyloid deposits may be small and inconspicuous by light microscopy. There is only minimal mesangial expansion, and occasional small feathery spikes along the peripheral basement membrane. Amyloid deposition must be verified by Congo red positivity, and can also be verified by electron microscopy (Jones' silver stain, ×400).

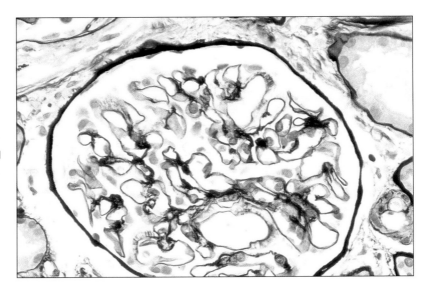

Fig. 1.156 Amyloidosis. There is very segmental amorphous, eosinophilic, fluffy 'cotton candy' appearance material in the mesangium, and very segmentally along the capillary wall (Jones' silver stain, ×400).

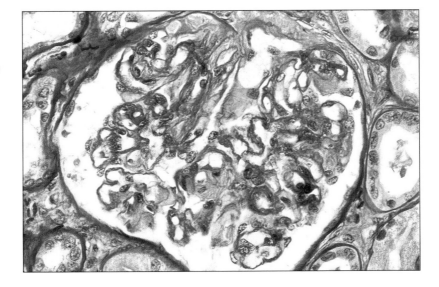

Fig. 1.157 Amyloidosis. Massive amyloid deposits are present in glomeruli and arterioles. There is a nodular appearance due to amorphous, acellular eosinophilic pale material, characteristic of amyloid (H&E, ×100).

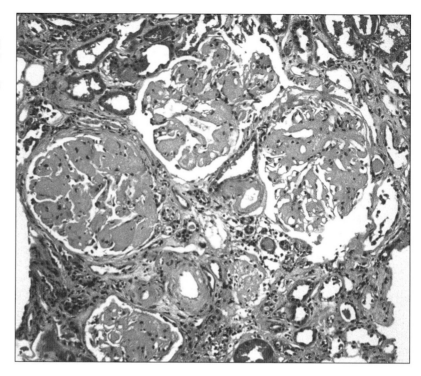

Fig. 1.158 Amyloidosis. The slightly chunky appearance of the amorphous, acellular amyloid deposits expanding the mesangial areas with focal extension to capillary loops is shown (H&E, ×200).

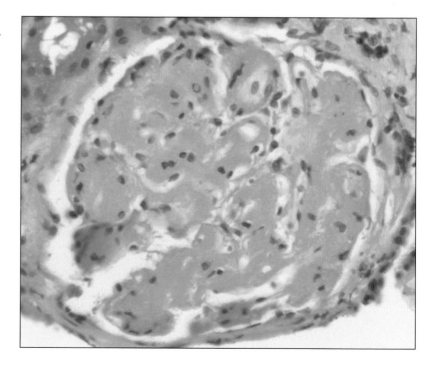

Fig. 1.159 Amyloidosis. There is massive amyloid deposition within the arteriole, and moderate expansion of the mesangium with amorphous, pale, 'cotton candy appearance' material within the mesangium with occasional peripheral loop alteration (Jones' silver stain, ×200).

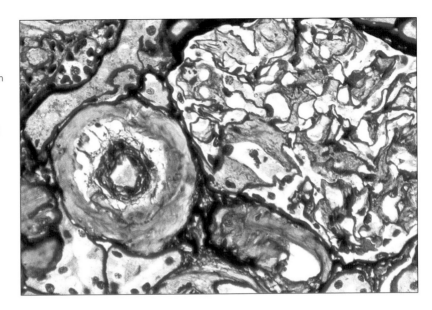

Fig. 1.160 Amyloidosis. Moderate mesangial expansion due to amyloid is shown, along with segmental feathery spikes. These are not as short and well-defined as the spikes due to the glomerular basement membrane reaction in membranous glomerulonephritis, and appear rather like the 'fringe on a rug'. These feathery spikes may be seen with marked peripheral loop amyloid deposit due to the basement membrane reaction (Jones' silver, ×400).

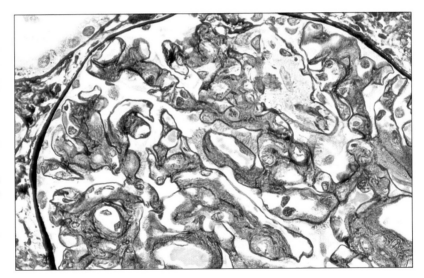

have amyloid deposits, which typically are segmental, giving rise to irregular thickening with a feathery spike appearance on Jones' silver stain (Figs 1.160, 1.161). Amyloid deposits often also involve arterioles and arteries, with acellular chunky, pale material (Fig. 1.159). The interstitium and tubules may also show similar acellular, pale eosinophilic amyloid material (Fig. 1.162). Histologic pattern of renal involvement is not useful in differentiating various forms of amyloid.

Definitive diagnosis is made by Congo red stain detecting apple-green birefringence under polarized light (Figs 1.163–1.165). This

Fig. 1.161 Amyloidosis. Large feathery spike reaction due to amyloid infiltration of the peripheral capillary loop is shown, with a tangential section of such a spike reaction giving a corona appearance (bottom left) (Jones' silver stain, ×400).

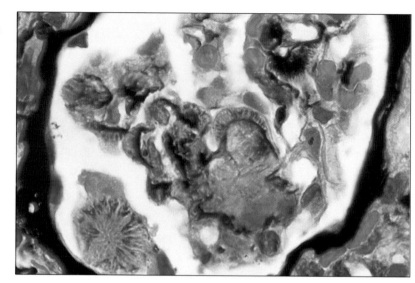

Fig. 1.162 Amyloidosis. Amyloid may also involve the tubulointerstitium, with pale, amorphous acellular areas, which should not be mistaken for areas of necrosis (H&E, ×200).

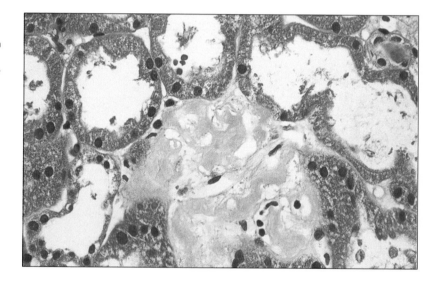

stain should be done on a section cut thicker, 8 μm, than normal to optimize detection of amyloid proteins. Preexposure of slides to potassium permanganate tends to abolish Congo red positivity of AA, but not AL amyloid, although this technique is no longer in common use with the availability of antibodies to AA and light chain proteins.

By immunofluorescence, AL amyloid may show positivity for the corresponding light chain in a smudgy pattern, mirroring the light

Fig. 1.163 Amyloidosis. Congo red positivity gives a specific diagnosis of amyloid. The specific positivity of the Congo red stain must be verified by viewing under polarized light (see Fig. 1.164) (Congo red, ×200).

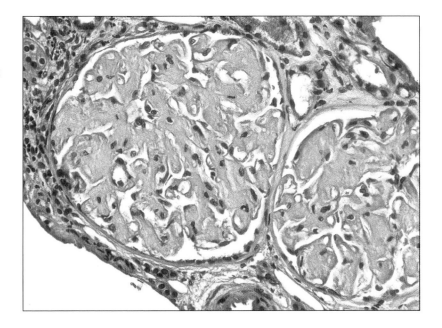

microscopic distribution (Fig. 1.166). In non-light chain amyloid, immunofluorescence shows no specific staining (Fig. 1.167).

Electron microscopy shows non-branching 8–12 nm in diameter fibrils with random orientation (Figs 1.168–1.170). Amyloid fibrils may be present in the mesangium, along the basement membrane where they form the feathery spike appearance by light microscopy, in arterioles and tubulointerstitium. Of note, the fibrils in fibrillary glomerulonephritis tend to be slightly thicker than amyloid fibrils, but there may be overlap in individual cases. Fibrillary glomerulo-nephritis also has distinct immunofluorescence findings, with prominent mesangial, and to lesser degree capillary wall staining with polyclonal IgG and complement, which also differentiates this entity from amyloid. Congo red staining should be used for ulti-mate, specific diagnosis of amyloid.

Etiology/pathogenesis

Amyloid proteins are a group of proteins that share the common characteristic of the ability to form beta-pleated sheets, which are resistant to proteolysis. More than 17 different types of amyloid

Fig. 1.164 Amyloidosis. Amyloid gives a characteristic apple-green birefringence when stained with Congo red and viewed under polarized light. There is amyloid deposition in the mesangial area, capillary loops, and weakly in the interstitium (Congo red under polarized light, ×200).

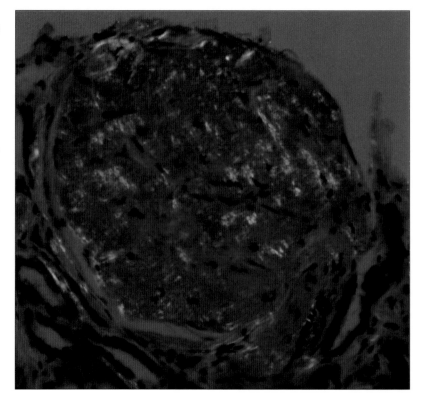

have been identified. Light chain (AL) amyloid is much more commonly lambda than kappa, likely reflecting the propensity of the molecules to form beta-pleated sheets. AA amyloid is due to the acute phase protein formed in response to chronic infection such as tuberculosis, osteomyelitis or chronic inflammatory conditions such as rheumatoid arthritis. Other amyloids are associated with familial conditions (transthyretin), familial Mediterranean fever, or dialysis (β2-microglobulin). Recent evidence has focused interest on amyloid P protein, which associates with the amyloid. Amyloid is resistant to proteolysis due at least in part to its binding to serum amyloid P component (SAP). Recent exciting results have been obtained with targeted pharmacological depletion of SAP. A palindromic compound, abbreviated CPHPC, that acts as a competitive inhibitor of SAP binding to amyloid resulted in crosslinking with

Fig. 1.165 Amyloidosis. Tubular Involvement with amyloid is verified by apple-green birefringence under polarized light. By light microscopy, these deposits were not readily apparent (Congo red under polarized light, ×400).

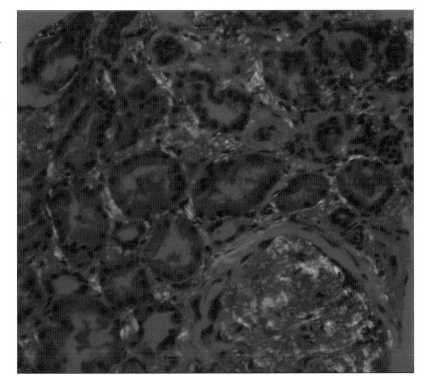

Fig. 1.166 Amyloidosis. Amyloid due to light chain deposition (AL amyloid) will often show preferential staining with the light chain. Lambda light chain more frequently is amyloidogenic than kappa light chain. The positivity is usually smudgy, and follows the distribution of amyloid seen by light microscopy (anti-lambda immunofluorescence, ×400).

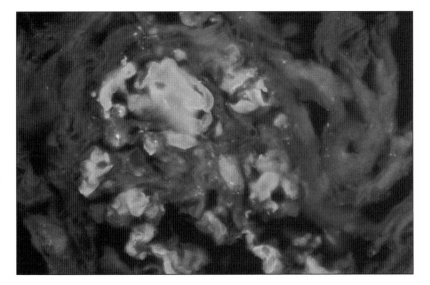

amyloid, dimerization and rapid clearance by the liver with decreased amyloid load in patients by whole body scintigraphy. Inhibition of amyloid fibril formation by small molecules that appear to function by shifting the aggregation equilibrium away from the amyloid state has been successful in treating transthyretin amyloid.

Fig. 1.167 Amyloidosis. Secondary amyloid due to the acute phase reactant protein may be diagnosed by specific immunostaining (AA amyloid). This patient had tuberculosis infection as the presumed underlying etiology of her extensive amyloid deposits (anti-AA immunohistochemistry, ×100).

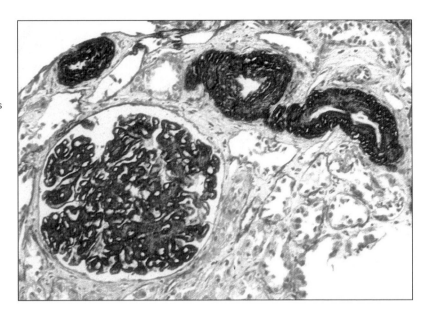

Fig. 1.168 Amyloidosis. Amyloid appears as randomly oriented fibrils, approximately 10 nm in diameter by electron microscopy. Fibrils can be found in the mesangium, the glomerular basement membrane, tubules, inter-stitium and vessels. A specific diagnosis of amyloid should be verified by Congo red positivity, as there may be some overlap in fibril size with fibrillary glomerulo-nephritis. In this case, there is moderate expansion of the mesangium due to amyloid, with segmental capillary loop involvement (TEM, ×3000).

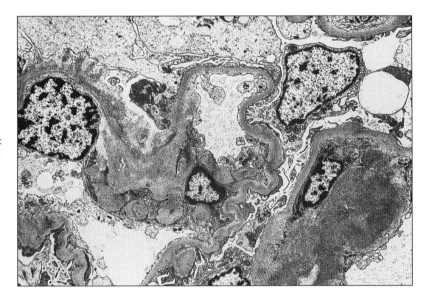

Light chain deposition disease

By light microscopy, glomeruli show varying degrees of mesangial proliferation (Figs 1.171, 1.172). Early lesions consist of mild mesangial increase (Figs 1.173–1.175). Over time, this typically progresses to nodular glomerular lesions. In many cases, lesions may by light

Fig. 1.169 Amyloidosis. Under higher magnification, the random, fibrillary arrangement of amyloid fibrils in the mesangium, underlying the endothelium, is apparent (TEM, ×20 000).

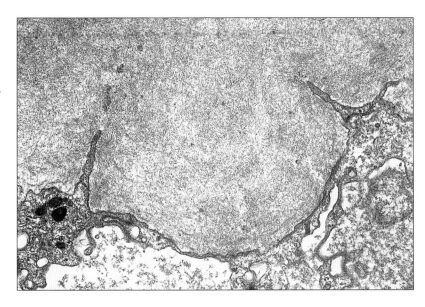

Fig. 1.170 Amyloidosis. Randomly oriented, 8–10 nm fibrils, typical of amyloid within the mesangium (TEM, ×25 000).

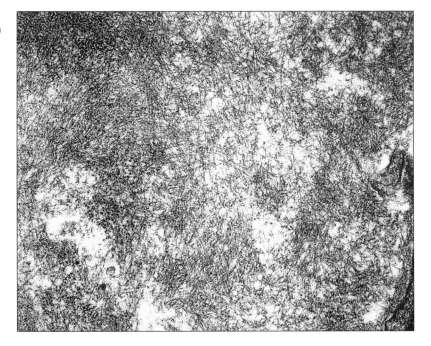

microscopy be nearly indistinguishable from nodular lesions of diabetic nephropathy (Figs 1.175, 1.176). The nodules are PAS-positive, lightly eosinophilic, PAS methenamine silver negative, and Congo-red negative. Capillary microaneurysms may be present.

Rarely, crescents are found. The nodular glomerular lesions of MIDD are similar by light microscopy to those found in other glomerular diseases, including nodular diabetic glomerulosclerosis, amyloidosis, and membranoproliferative glomerulonephritis. There are several characteristics that have been proposed to distinguish MIDD from diabetic glomerulosclerosis. In MIDD there tends to be multiple nodules within the glomerulus which generally stain PAS-positive but methenamine silver PAS-negative, and the efferent arterioles do not exhibit extensive hyalinosis. Conversely, diabetic glomerulosclerosis is characterized by solitary nodules within the glomerulus which stain PAS-positive and methenamine silver PAS-positive in the presence of extensive hyalinosis in the afferent and efferent arterioles. However, some patients with MIDD have silver positive nodules, and LM alone does not allow definitive distinction from

Fig. 1.171   LCDD. LCDD is characterized by nodular glomerulosclerosis, although GBMs are not as thick as in diabetic nephropathy. By EM and IF, deposits of monoclonal light chain are visualized on the inner aspect of the GBM and outer aspect of the TBM.

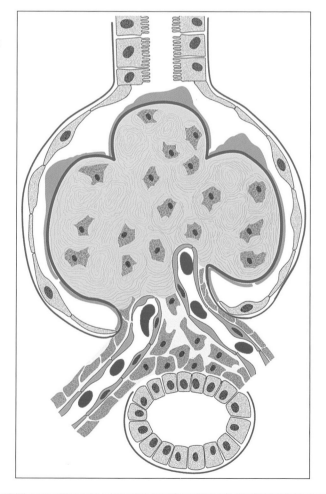

Fig. 1.172 LCDD. There may be only minimal mesangial expansion by light microscopy, with mild increase in mesangial cellularity and matrix. Specific diagnosis is made by immunofluorescence and confirmed by electron microscopy (Jones' silver stain, ×200).

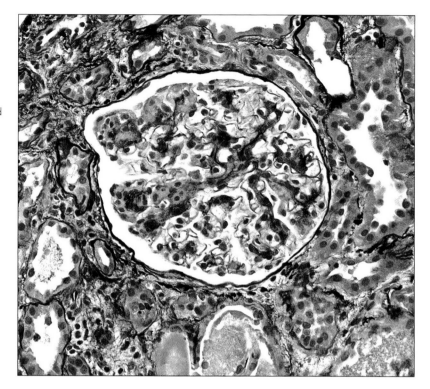

diabetic nephropathy in our experience (Figs 1.175, 1.176). Other causes of nodular glomerulosclerosis may more readily be excluded by light microscopy: Amyloidosis is excluded from the differential diagnosis of MIDD by negative Congo-red staining, and also the absence of fibrils on electron microscopy. Membranoproliferative glomerulonephritis is distinguished from MIDD by the presence of double-contours of the glomerular basement membrane and dominant cellular proliferation. In addition, immunopathology and ultrastructural evaluation will differentiate the other glomerular diseases from MIDD.

The renal tubular basement membranes in light chain deposition disease (LCDD) demonstrate 'ribbon-like' thickening (Fig. 1.177). Tubular atrophy and interstitial fibrosis are typical findings with refractile, PAS-positive deposits found in both the tubular basement membranes and interstitium (occurring in 50% of cases of MIDD). PAS-positive deposits can also be found in the vascular basement membranes of arterioles and small interlobular arteries.

Fig. 1.173 LCDD. Small nodular areas of mesangial increase are present in this glomerulus (same case as Fig. 1.155) (H&E, ×400).

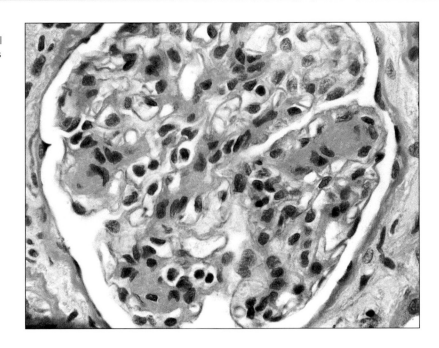

Fig. 1.174 LCDD. The characteristic nodular appearance of LCDD is illustrated. This may be difficult to distinguish from diabetes, although peripheral glomerular basement membranes are not quite as prominent as in diabetic nephropathy. Morphology of the nodules has been suggested to allow distinction between diabetic nephropathy and LCDD. However, in our experience, there is substantial overlap, and immunofluorescence and/or EM is necessary for diagnosis (PAS, ×200).

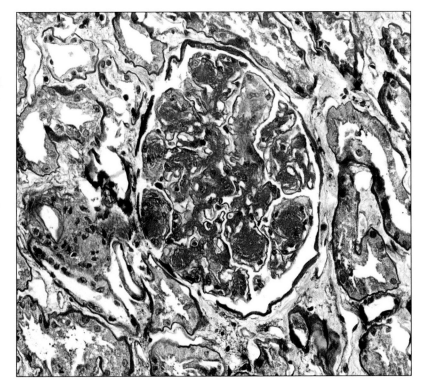

Fig. 1.175 LCDD. In this case, the nodules are variable from glomerulus to glomerulus, and vary in number and in size, and stain with silver stain, all features postulated to allow distinction between diabetic nephropathy, which shows the aforementioned features, and light chain deposition disease, postulated to not show these features. There is even arteriolar hyalinization. However, IF and EM studies confirmed the diagnosis of LCDD, corresponding to the patient's monoclonal protein (Jones' silver stain, ×200).

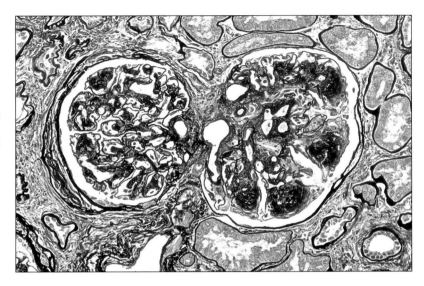

Fig. 1.176 LCDD. The expanded nodules of LCDD are shown. In this case, the GBM also appears slightly prominent by light microscopy, although IF and EM studies confirmed the diagnosis of LCDD (periodic acid Schiff, ×400).

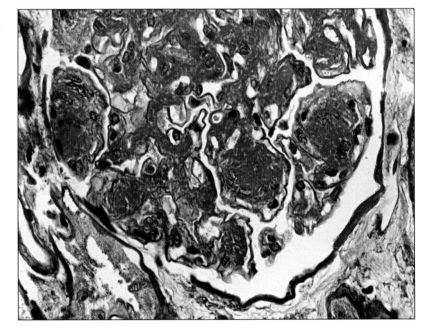

In some patients with MIDD, there is combined LCDD and light chain cast nephropathy, with attendant worse prognosis. Classic findings of cast nephropathy with interstitial nephritis, severe tubular injury and interstitial fibrosis, and brittle, fractured casts with syncytial giant cell reaction are typically present. Of note, casts

Fig. 1.177 LCDD. The tubular basement membranes are also affected by deposits in LCDD, and are commonly thick and refractile. However, this appearance overlaps with the thickening and fibrosis that occur with any tubulointerstitial fibrosis (Jones' silver stain, ×200).

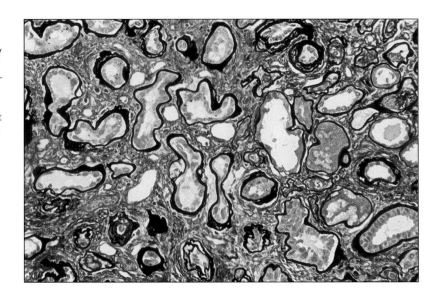

in light chain cast nephropathy may not stain monotypically in all cases, presumably due to nonselective proteinuria and/or abnormal monoclonal protein not recognized by standard commer-cial antibodies (see 'Light Chain Cast Nephropathy').

Definitive diagnosis of LCDD is by immunofluorescence (Figs 1.178, 1.179). The pathognomonic finding of MIDD is the presence of monoclonal immunoglobulin deposits in the GBM and tubular basement membranes. Linear staining is present in the tubular basement membranes, glomerular basement membrane, often in the mesangium, and less often in interstitium and vascular basement membranes. The deposits in LCDD are most frequently kappa light chains with a kappa to lambda case ratio of 9:1 in a recent large series. In contrast, AL amyloid most frequently is due to lambda light chain. Occasionally deposits that appear typical for LCDD by electron microscopy in patients with known mono-clonal protein fail to stain with either kappa or lambda antisera, perhaps reflecting altered antigenicity.

By electron microscopy, granular, amorphous deposits are present along the inner aspect of the glomerular basement membrane and the outer aspect of tubular basement membranes in LCDD (Figs 1.180–1.183). Vascular basement membranes and mesangial nodules may also have deposits. The mesangial deposits are not

Fig. 1.178 LCDD. Specific diagnosis of LCDD is made by immunofluorescence, with monoclonal light chain, more commonly kappa, staining of glomeruli in tubular basement membranes (anti-kappa immunofluorescence, ×100).

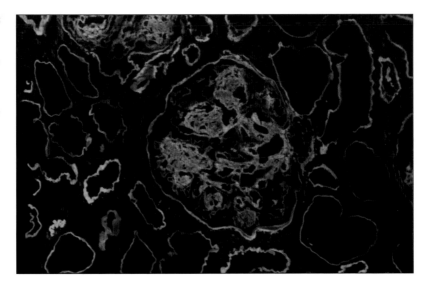

Fig. 1.179 LCDD. The TBM staining in LCDD is illustrated (anti-kappa immunofluorescence, ×400).

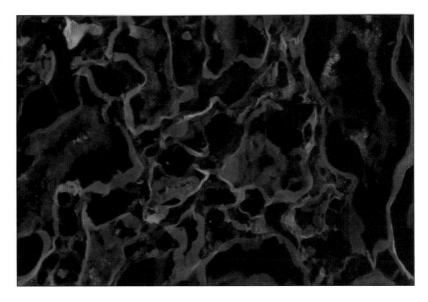

Fig. 1.180   LCDD. The deposits are finely granular and more amorphous than usual immune complexes, and generally are found along the internal aspect of the GBM, filling up the lamina rara interna, sometimes with extension to the lamina densa (TEM, ×11 250).

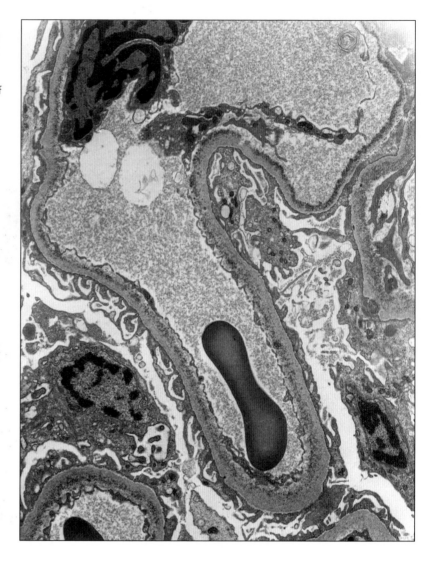

sharply demarcated. Foot process effacement is variable. In general, there is no substructural organization within the deposits. Very rarely, there may be coexistent amyloid fibrils.

Light and heavy chain deposition disease and heavy chain deposition disease

The clinical presentations of light and heavy chain deposition disease and heavy chain deposition disease (LHCDD and HCDD) are usually nephrotic syndrome with hypertension and hematuria. Some

Fig. 1.181   LCDD. The granular, somewhat amorphous deposits of LCDD are shown. There is not a clear border between the deposits and the remaining GBM. Occasional granular deposits permeate into the lamina densa, but the deposits are mostly concentrated along the lamina rara interna (TEM, ×40 000).

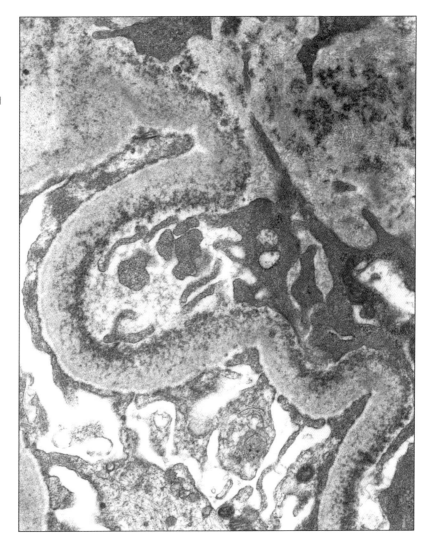

patients with HCDD may have hypocomplementemia. Interestingly, some HCDD and LHCDD patients have falsely positive hepatitis C antibody tests. Monoclonal protein in the blood may be present, but the truncated monoclonal heavy chain in HCDD may be difficult to detect in circulation.

Light microscopy in LHCDD and HCDD is indistinguishable from LCDD. There is mesangial proliferation or membranoproliferative or nodular lesions (Figs 1.184–1.186). As in LCDD, crescents may occasionally be present. Definitive diagnosis and distinction of these MIDD diseases is made by immunofluorescence.

Fig. 1.182 LCDD. A thin granular line of deposits is shown in an early case of LCDD, with specific diagnosis confirmed by IF (TEM, ×12 000).

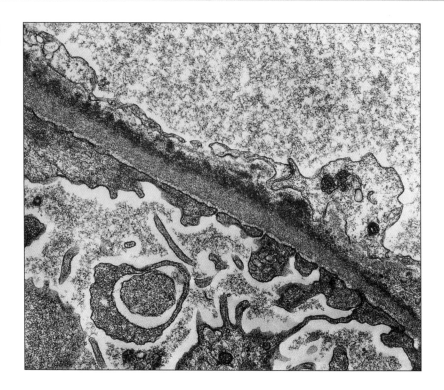

In LHCDD the immunofluorescence studies reveal both a monotypic heavy and light chain within the deposits, whereas in HCDD only a monotypic heavy chain is identified. The deposits are present along the GBM, mesangium and tubular basement membranes (Figs. 1.187, 1.188). The predominant class of heavy chain in HCDD is gamma although rare cases of alpha have also been reported.

By electron microscopy, deposits in LHCDD have been divided into three differing types. These deposits may be punctate as in LCDD, confluent and homogenous as in immune complex disease, or they may lack density and be invisible at the ultrastructural level (Figs 1.189–1.192). We have rarely observed combined subendothelial and subepithelial deposits in LHCDD (Fig. 1.190). In HCDD, the deposits appear finely granular, and ill-defined, permeating the lamina densa of the GBM and the mesangial nodules. Finely granular deposits are also present within the tubular basement membranes and vascular basement membranes (Fig. 1.193).

Fig. 1.183 LCDD. The deposits of the tubular basement membrane are granular, and typically along the outer aspects (TEM, ×4400).

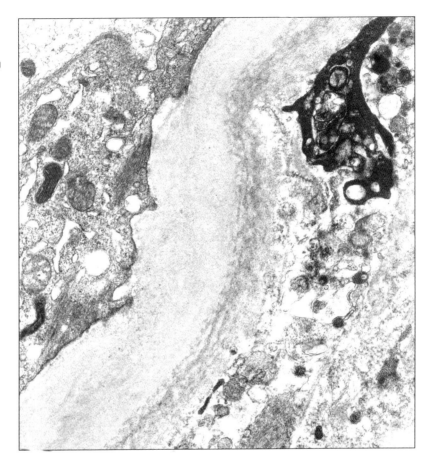

Etiology/pathogenesis of MIDD

The physicochemical properties of the monoclonal protein determine whether it results in light chain deposition disease (or LHCDD, or HCDD), amyloid, light chain cast nephropathy, or rarely, combined lesions. Elegant experiments infusing monoclonal proteins from patients into mice replicated the type of renal lesion caused by the monoclonal protein in patients in the mouse model. The predominance of kappa monoclonal light chain resulting in LCDD whereas lambda monoclonal protein more frequently manifests as amyloid is consistent with the dominant precursor proteins, Vkappa4 and Vlambda6, in LCDD and amyloidosis, respectively. Evidence supports that LHCDD and HCDD result from deletion of one of the heavy chain domains, resulting in truncated heavy chains both in the circulation and in the renal deposits. Gamma heavy chain is the most common Ig resulting in HCDD. The CH1 deletion of the heavy

Fig. 1.184 Light and heavy chain deposition disease. The light microscopic appearance may range from minor mesangial expansion with increased mesangial matrix and cellularity to an overt nodular sclerosis. There is early surrounding tubulointerstitial fibrosis (Jones' silver stain, ×100).

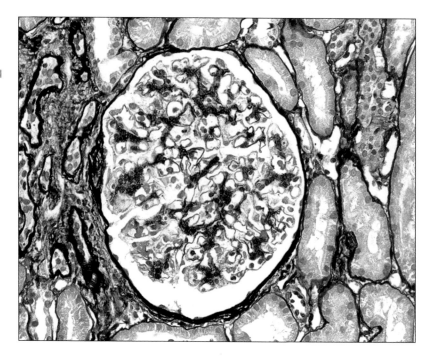

Fig. 1.185 Light and heavy chain deposition disease. A membranoproliferative pattern with increased mesangial cells and matrix is evident in this case of LHCDD, confirmed by IF and EM. There is mesangial interposition, but no overt endocapillary proliferation (Jones' silver stain, ×400).

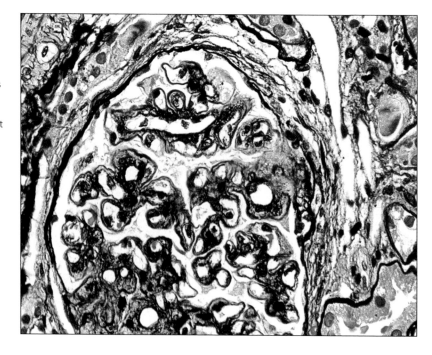

Fig. 1.186 Light and heavy chain deposition disease. This case demonstrated nodular glomerulosclerosis, indistinguishable by light microscopy from LCDD. Specific diagnosis was made by IF and EM (Jones' silver stain, ×200).

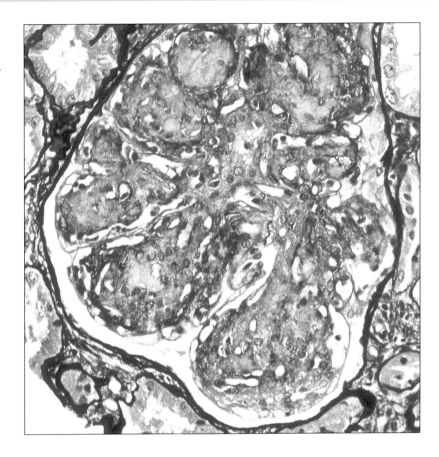

Fig. 1.187 Light and heavy chain deposition disease. There is strong glomerular capillary loop and mesangial staining in a smudgy, continuous pattern along the GBM. There is also TBM staining (left) (anti-IgG immunofluorescence, ×400).

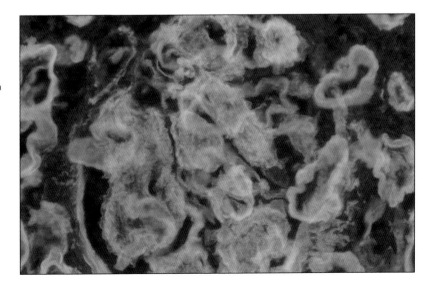

Fig. 1.188 Light and heavy chain deposition disease. The diagnosis of LHCDD was specifically confirmed by monoclonal staining with light chain, in addition to restricted heavy chain staining. Staining for lambda was negative (anti-kappa immunofluorescence, ×400).

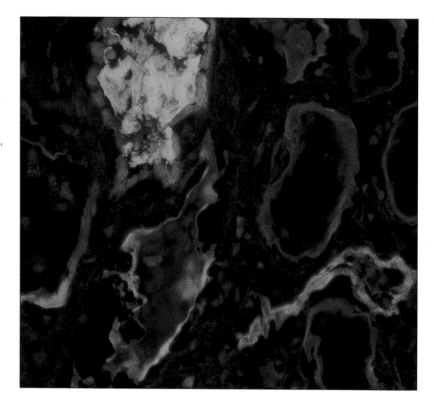

chain appears to play a key pathogenic role in these rare cases of HCDD, preventing binding to heavy chain binding protein in the endoplasmic reticulum and appropriate assembly with light chains.

Selected reading

Amyloidosis

Dikman S H, Churg J, Kahn T 1998 Morphologic and clinical correlates in renal amyloidosis. Human Pathology 12(2):160–169.

Faulk R H, Comenzo R L, Skinner M 1997 The systemic amyloidoses. New England Journal of Medicine 337:898–909.

Glenner G G 1980 Amyloid deposits and amyloidosis. The beta-fibrilloses. New England Journal of Medicine 302(23):1283–1292.

Glenner G G 1980 Amyloid deposits and amyloidosis: the beta-fibrilloses. New England Journal of Medicine 302 (24):1333–1343.

Hammarstrom P, Wiseman R L, Powers E T et al 2003 Prevention of transthyretin amyloid disease by changing protein misfolding energetics. Science 31; 299(5607):713–716.

Kyle R A, Gertz M A 1995 Primary systemic amyloidosis: clinical and laboratory features in 474 cases. Seminars in Hematology 32:45–59.

Looi L-M, Cheah P-L 1997 Histomorphological patterns of renal amyloidosis: a correlation between histology and chemical type of amyloidosis. Human Pathology 28:847–849.

Fig. 1.189 Light and heavy chain deposition disease. Subendothelial deposits are present with a vague, coarsely fibrillar substructure. There is also mesangial interposition (TEM, ×20 250).

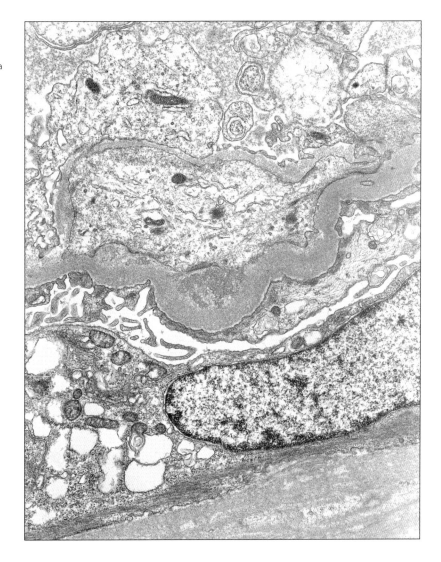

Pepys M B, Herbert J, Hutchinson W L et al 2002 Targeted pharmacological depletion of serum amyloid P component for treatment of human amyloidosis. Nature 417(6886):254–259.

LCDD, LHCDD and HCDD

Gallo G, Picken M, Buxbaum J et al 1989 The spectrum of immunoglobulin deposition disease associated with immunocytic dyscrasias. Seminars in Hematology 26:234–245.

Gallo G R, Feiner H D, Buxbaum J N 1982 The kidney in lymphoplasmacytic disorders. Pathology Annual 17(1):291–317.

Gallo G R, Lazowski P, Kumar A et al 1998 Renal and cardiac manifestations of B-cell dyscrasias with nonamyloidotic monoclonal light chain and light and heavy chain deposition diseases. Advances in Nephrology at Necker Hospital 28:355–382.

Fig. 1.190 Light and heavy chain deposition disease. Subendothelial and subepithelial deposits are present, with a coarsely fibrillar substructure. The specific diagnosis was verified by immunofluorescence (TEM, ×8000).

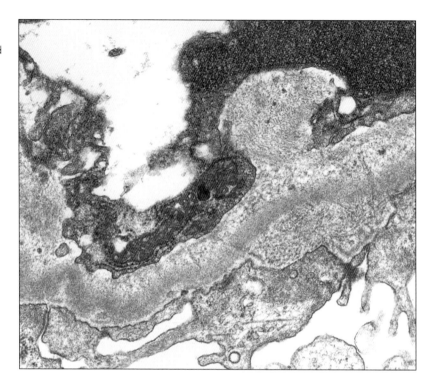

Fig. 1.191 Light and heavy chain deposition disease. In other cases of LHCDD, the deposits may be granular, as in LCDD, or appear as usual immune complex-type deposits, as in areas of this case. There are massive mesangial deposits, which extended into the subendothelial areas (TEM, ×8000).

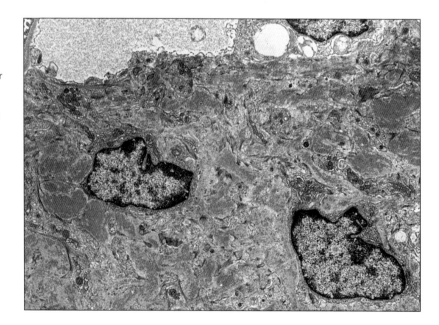

Fig. 1.192 Light and heavy chain deposition disease. On higher power, a vague, short fibrillary substructure is evident in this case of LHCDD (same case as in Fig. 1.191) (TEM, ×40 000).

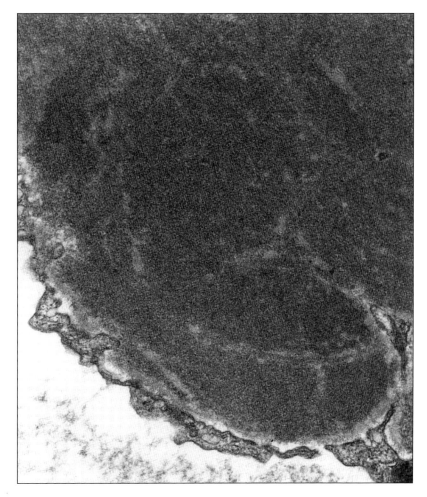

Ganeval D, Mignon F, Preud'homme J L et al 1982 Visceral deposition of monoclonal light chains and immunoglobulins: a study of renal and immunopathologic abnormalities. Advances in Nephrology 11:25–63.

Ganeval D, Noel L H, Preud'homme J L et al 1984 Light-chain deposition disease: its relation with AL-type amyloidosis. Kidney International 26:1–9.

Kambham N, Markowitz G S, Appel G B et al 1999 Heavy chain deposition disease: The disease spectrum. American Journal of Kidney Disease 33:954–962.

Lin J, Markowitz G S, Valeri A M et al 2001 Renal monoclonal immunoglobulin deposition disease: the disease spectrum. Journal of the American Society of Nephrology 12(7):1482–1492.

Pirani C L, Silva F, D'Agati V, Chander P et al 1987 Renal lesions in plasma cell dyscrasias: ultrastructural observations. American Journal of Kidney Disease 10:208–221.

Pirani C L, Silva F, D'Agati V et al 1987 Renal lesions in plasma cell dyscrasias: ultrastructural observations. American Journal of Kidney Disease 10.208–221.

Preud'homme J L, Aucouturier P, Touchard G et al 1994 Monoclonal immunoglobulin deposition disease (Randall type). Relationship with

Fig. 1.193 Light and heavy chain deposition disease. There are frequent tubular basement membrane deposits in LHCDD. They are granular without discrete borders (TEM, ×25 625).

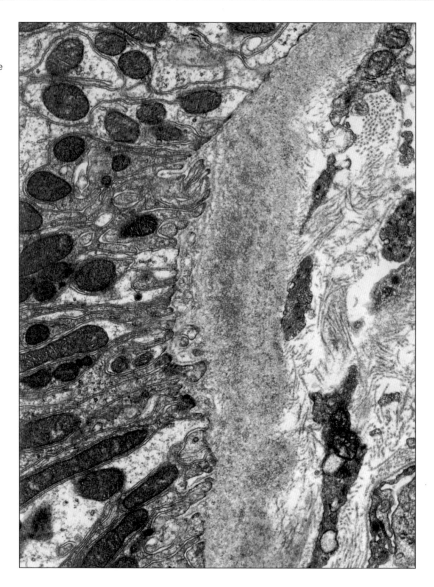

structural abnormalities of immunoglobulin chains. Kidney International 46:965–972.

Randall R E, Williamson W C Jr, Mullinax F et al 1976 Manifestations of systemic light chain deposition. American Journal of Medicine 60:293–299.

Sanders P W, Herrera G A, Kirk K A et al 1991 Spectrum of glomerular and tubulointerstitial renal lesions associated with monotypical immunoglobulin light chain deposition. Laboratory Investigation 64:527–537.

Sanders P W, Herrera G A 1993 Monoclonal immunoglobulin light chain-related renal diseases. Seminars in Nephrology 23:324–341.

Solomon A, Weiss D T, Kattine A A 1991 Nephrotoxic potential of Bence Jones proteins. New England Journal of Medicine 324:1845–1851.

HIV-associated nephropathy

Patients present with nephrotic-range proteinuria, often with rapid downhill course of GFR. Despite marked proteinuria, patients usually do not manifest edema or hypertension. Renal enlargement is common. HIV-associated nephropathy (HIVAN) may precede other manifestations of HIV infection.

By light microscopy, there is a collapsing form of focal segmental glomerulosclerosis with collapse of the glomerular tuft and hyperplasia and hypertrophy of overlying podocytes with prominent protein droplets (Figs 1.194–1.199). This proliferation should not be mistaken for a crescent. The entire tuft or just segments of the glomerulus are collapsed with wrinkling of the GBM. Bowman's space may therefore appear dilated. With progressive disease, there may be

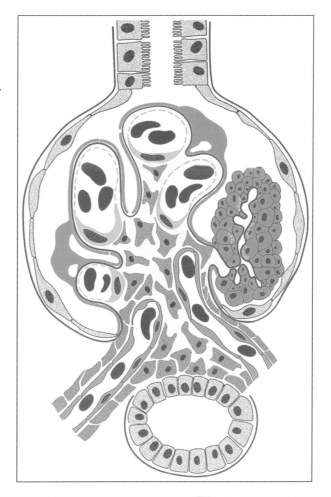

Fig. 1.194   HIVAN. There is segmental or global collapse of the capillary tuft with over-lying visceral epithelial cell hyperplasia, without deposits. In addition, frequent reticular aggregates are present in the endothelial cell cytoplasm, seen by EM.

Fig. 1.195 HIVAN. There is disproportionately severe microcystic tubular injury with tubulointerstitial inflammation, and extensive glomerulosclerosis. Some of the glomeruli have retracted and collapsed, with apparent dilatation of Bowman's space (top left), in this autopsy specimen from a patient who died with HIVAN (Jones' silver stain, ×100).

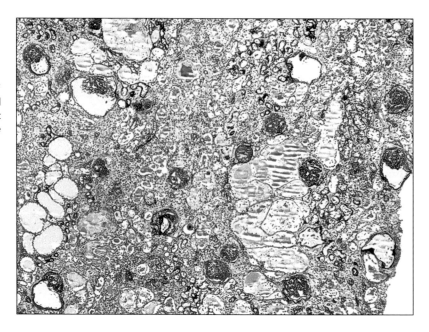

Fig. 1.196 HIVAN. The microcystic tubular injury with proteinaceous casts is shown, along with interstitial edema and early fibrosis, with a lymphoplasmacytic infiltrate (H&E, ×200).

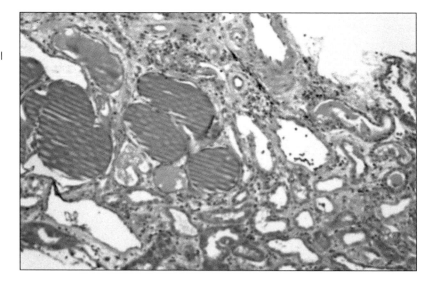

solidification and segmental sclerosis and adhesions (Fig. 1.195). There are associated disproportionately severe tubulointerstitial lesions with cystic dilatation of tubules, and tubular degeneration affecting all tubule segments (Fig. 1.196). Tubular epithelial cells often contain prominent protein droplets. The interstitium shows edema and a variable infiltrate with mainly lymphocytes and occasional monocytes and plasma cells (Fig. 1.196). With progression,

Fig. 1.197 HIVAN. There is microcystic tubular injury and collapse of the glomerular tuft with overlying visceral epithelial cell proliferation (Jones' silver stain, ×200).

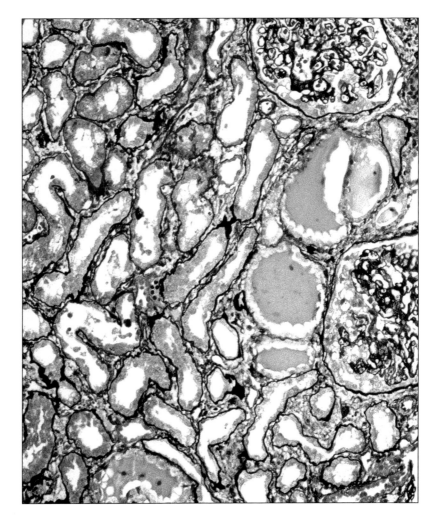

there is interstitial fibrosis and tubular atrophy. Vessels do not show any specific changes.

Immunofluorescence studies do not show immune complex deposits, but may show nonspecific IgM and C3 in mesangial areas. The protein droplets in the podocytes may stain for any Ig, including IgG and IgA. The specific location and round, globular pattern of this staining allows distinction from immune complexes.

Electron microscopy demonstrates collapse and proliferation of the podocytes with foot process effacement (Fig. 1.200). Reticular aggregates, also known as tubuloreticular inclusions, are present in endothelial cell cytoplasm (Fig. 1.201) in HIV-infected patients, whether they have nephropathy or not. These ~25 nm diameter structures are related to elevated levels of interferon-alpha, and are

Fig. 1.198 HIVAN. The glomeruli show a collapsing form of injury, where the lobule is retracted and collapsed with overlying glomerular visceral epithelial cell hyperplasia, often with prominent protein droplets (Jones' silver stain, ×200).

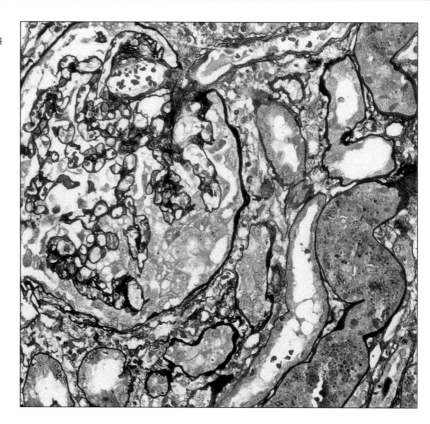

Fig. 1.199 HIVAN. The segmental collapse of the lobule of the glomerulus is shown with prominent overlying visceral epithelial cell proliferation, with protein droplets (Jones' silver stain, ×400).

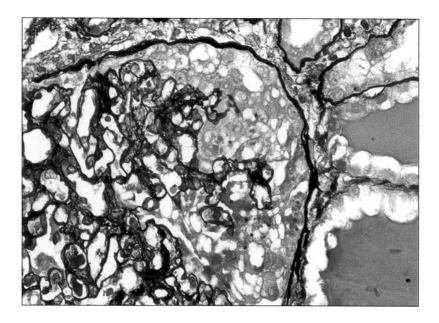

Fig. 1.200   HIVAN. There are no immune deposits, but affected glomeruli show extensive corrugation and collapse of the basement membrane, with overlying visceral epithelial cell hyperplasia and extensive foot process effacement.
In distinction to idiopathic collapsing glomerulopathy, there frequently are numerous reticular aggregates in endothelial cell cytoplasm (TEM, ×8000).

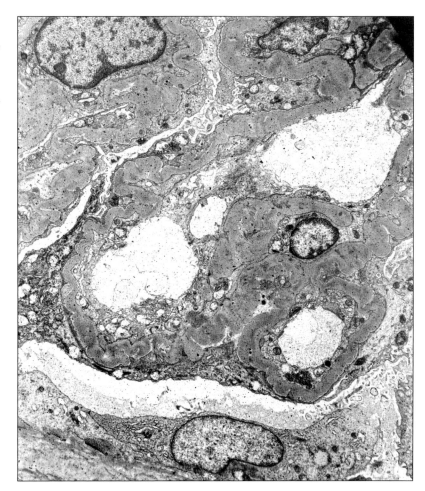

Fig. 1.201   HIVAN. In HIVAN, there typically are numerous reticular aggregates in endothelial cell cytoplasm throughout the body, a marker of HIV infection and high interferon levels. (TEM, ×25 625).

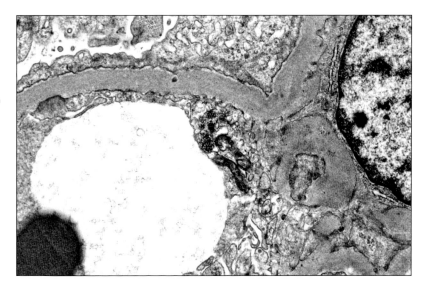

present systemically in the endoplasmic reticulum, particularly in endothelial cells. Reticular aggregates are particularly numerous in patients with HIV infection or with SLE, and are markers of the underlying systemic condition, not specifically of nephropathy.

Etiology/pathogenesis

The specific pathogenesis of HIVAN has not been determined. Some investigators have found HIV antigens in tubular epithelium, but this finding has not been widely confirmed. Whether HIV directly infects resident glomerular cells, and thereby causes the lesions, or whether injury is due to secondary cytokine effects, has not been definitively proven. HIV transgenic mice and primates with simian AIDS have been extensively studied to elucidate the role of specific viral genes and systemic vs. renal parenchymal factors in injury.

The podocyte is a major target of injury in HIVAN. There is dedifferentiation of podocytes with loss of differentiation markers, such as the Wilms' tumor antigen WT-1, and loss of cyclin-dependent kinase inhibitors, allowing proliferation of podocytes. Other factors must contribute to pathogenesis, in that HIVAN occurs much more commonly in African Americans with HIV infection than in Caucasians; 80%–85% of HIVAN patients are African American. In contrast, Caucasian HIV-infected individuals with renal disease studied in Europe had various immune complex and nonimmune glomerular diseases rather than HIVAN.

Selected reading

Alpers C E, Tsai C C, Hudkins K L et al 1997 Focal segmental glomerulosclerosis in primates infected with a simian immunodeficiency virus. AIDS Research in Human Retroviruses 13(5):413–424.

Cohen A H, Nast C C 1988 HIV-associated nephropathy. A unique combined glomerular, tubular, and interstitial lesion. Modern Pathology 1:87–97.

Cohen A H, Sun N C, Shapshak P et al 1989 Demonstration of human immunodeficiency virus in renal epithelium in HIV-associated nephropathy. Modern Pathology 2(2):125–128.

D'Agati V, Suh J I, Carbone L et al 1988 Pathology of HIV-associated nephropathy: a detailed morphologic and comparative study. Kidney International 35:1358–1370.

Kimmel P L, Phillips T M, Ferreira-Centeno A et al 1993 HIV-associated immune-mediated renal disease. Kidney International 44:1327–1340.

Nochy D, Glotz D, Dosquet P et al 1993 Renal disease associated with HIV infection: a multicentric study of 60 patients from Paris hospitals. Nephrology, Dialysis and Transplantation 8:11–19.

Ross M J, Klotman P E 2002 Recent progress in HIV-associated nephropathy. Journal of the American Society of Nephrology 13(12):2997–3004.

Winston J A, Bruggeman L A, Ross M D et al 2001 Nephropathy and establishment of a renal reservoir of HIV type 1 during primary infection. New England Journal of Medicine 344(26):1979–1984.

Sickle cell nephropathy

Patients with sickle cell anemia are at risk for developing progressive renal disease, which initially manifests as microalbuminuria in childhood, progressing to overt proteinuria and progressive decrease in renal function after age 20 years. Some 5% to 8% of all sickle cell patients develop renal failure. Patients typically also have hematuria and urinary concentrating defects. The prognosis is poor when patients have nephrotic syndrome and sickle cell nephropathy, with two-thirds developing renal failure and half dying within 2 years.

The most common renal diseases in sickle cell patients can be categorized as acute injury, including cortical infarcts, related to sickle cell crisis; acute or more insidious injury of the medulla resulting in papillary necrosis and/or fibrosis; and chronic glomerular injury manifest as a secondary focal segmental glomerulosclerosis (FSGS). Sickle cell crisis causes sludging of sickled red blood cells in vessels (Fig. 1.202). The medullary vasa recta are particularly

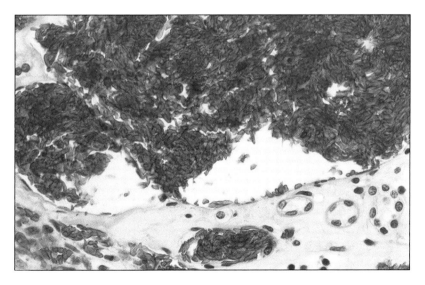

Fig. 1.202 Sickle cell nephropathy. In sickle cell crisis, massive sludging of red blood cells may occur in large vessels due to agglutination of the sickled red blood cells (H&E, ×100).

Fig. 1.203   Sickle cell nephropathy. Even without sickle cell crisis, there may be sickling of red blood cells in peritubular capillaries and in the vasa recta. There is surrounding edema and tubular injury in this patient who had sickle cell trait and died after extreme exertion and dehydration (H&E, ×400).

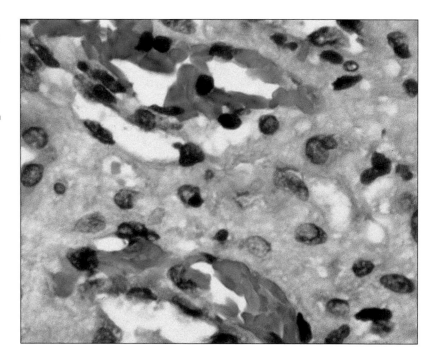

Fig. 1.204   Sickle cell nephropathy. Sickling may cause congestion of glomeruli in addition to peritubular capillaries. There is associated diffuse tubular injury and ATN in this patient who had acute sickle cell crisis (H&E, ×200).

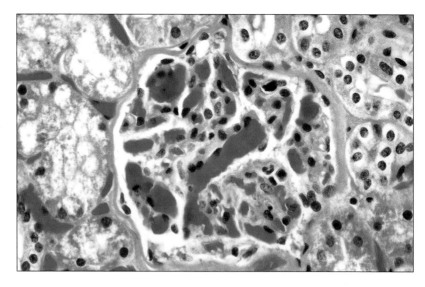

vulnerable (Fig. 1.203). The occlusion of normal blood flow may cause cortical infarcts or occlude glomeruli with surrounding tubular injury (Fig. 1.204). Acute or more insidious injury due to subclinical sickling in the vasa recta can result in papillary necrosis, tubulointerstitial fibrosis and urinary concentrating defects. In the more chronic glomerular injury of sickle cell nephropathy, there is

Fig. 1.205   Sickle cell nephropathy. Chronically, sickle cell patients may have glomerular lesions characterized by extreme glomerulomegaly, and a membranoproliferative and/or focal segmental sclerosis pattern of injury. Most often there are not immune complexes, and glomerular basement reduplication and mesangial proliferation are due to chronic endothelial injury. Rare sickled cells are present (right) (H&E, ×200).

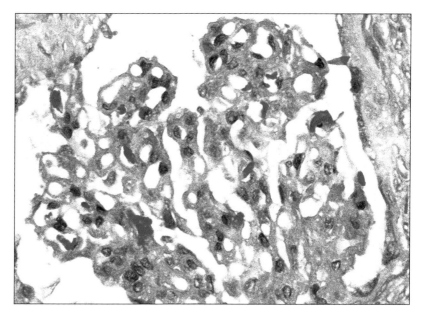

Fig. 1.206   Sickle cell nephropathy. The corrugated, split glomerular basement membrane in chronic sickle cell nephropathy is evident, along with mild congestion. There is segmental sclerosis (left), a secondary process presumed linked to the chronic endothelial injury (Jones' silver stain, ×400).

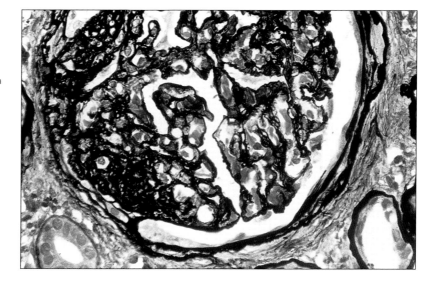

remarkable glomerular enlargement by light microscopy (Fig. 1.205). The mesangium may be expanded, but there is no overt proliferation. Secondary lesions of focal segmental and global glomerulosclerosis can develop later in the course (Fig. 1.206). These lesions are predominantly hilar, and have been associated with hyalinosis, lipid vacuoles and foam cells. The glomerular basement membrane may be thickened and split, but without immune complex-type

Fig. 1.207 Sickle cell nephropathy. There is irregular glomerular basement membrane splitting and corrugation, along with mild mesangial proliferation with rare sickled cells in peripheral loops. This patient had secondary focal segmental glomerulosclerosis and marked proteinuria and no immune deposits (Jones' silver stain, ×1000).

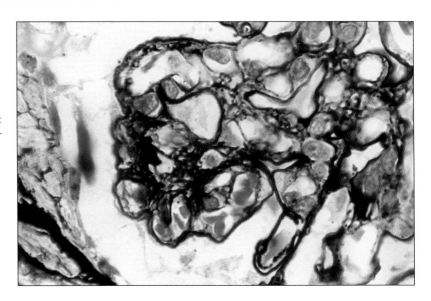

Fig. 1.208 Sickle cell nephropathy. Due to chronic hemolysis, there may be hemosiderin present in tubules and even glomerular cells. The hemosiderin is seen as brown chunky pigment within tubules. There is associated mild tubular atrophy and interstitial fibrosis. The glomerulus is markedly enlarged with mild mesangial expansion (H&E, ×200).

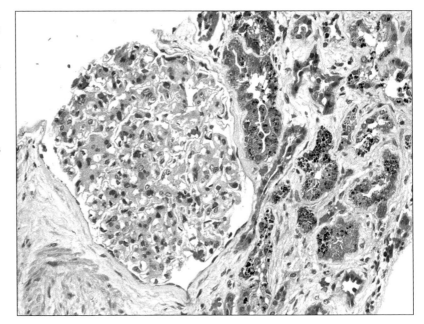

deposits (Figs 1.206, 1.207). Hemosiderin may be present in the glomerulus, including podocytes, and in tubular epithelial cells (Figs 1.208–1.210). There is proportional tubulointerstitial fibrosis in cases. Vessels show no specific lesions. In stable patients not undergoing sickle cell crisis, only rare sickled cells can be detected, even when overt sclerotic lesions are present.

Fig. 1.209   Sickle cell nephropathy. Iron is readily and specifically demonstrated by a Prussian blue stain. There is iron within tubules, occasional interstitial macrophages and rare staining of glomerular resident cells (Prussian blue stain, ×200).

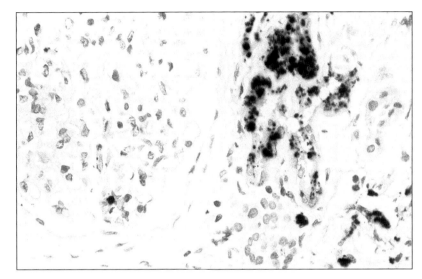

Fig. 1.210   Sickle cell nephropathy. There is apparent mesangial and podocyte localization of iron in this patient with chronic sickle cell nephropathy (Prussian blue stain, ×1000).

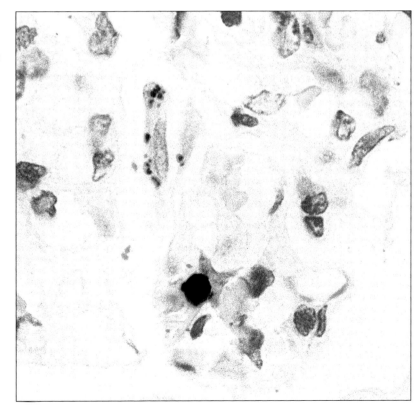

Fig. 1.211 Sickle cell nephropathy. The capillary loop is greatly distorted due to swollen endothelial cells and interposition without well-defined immune complexes. The capillary lumen is obliterated by sickled cells. The overlying foot processes are extensively effaced (TEM, ×19 000).

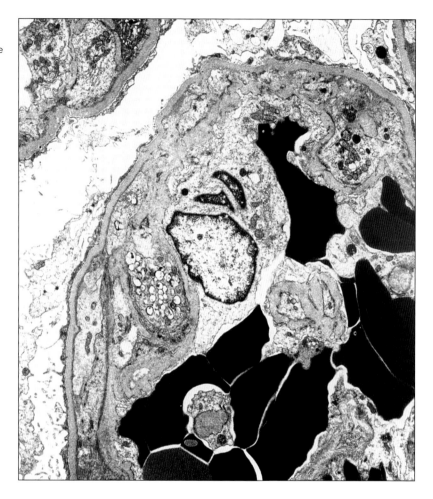

Immunofluorescence microscopy typically shows only IgM, C3 and C1q in the sclerosed areas. Electron microscopy in sickle cell nephropathy with secondary focal segmental glomerulosclerosis shows subtotal foot process effacement overlying areas of sclerosis. Sickled cells may be detected (Fig. 1.211). In cases with glomerular basement membrane splitting by light microscopy, there typically is only mesangial interposition by electron microscopy without well-defined immune complex-type deposits (Fig. 1.211, 1.212). Sickle cell nephropathy can also recur in the transplant.

Etiology/pathogenesis

Patients with either homozygous sickle cell disease or sickle cell-thalassemia or hemoglobinopathy SC may develop any renal

Fig. 1.212 Sickle cell nephropathy. There is marked mesangial matrix expansion and corrugation of the glomerular basement membrane. The capillary lumen is nearly occluded by sickled cells (TEM, ×21 000).

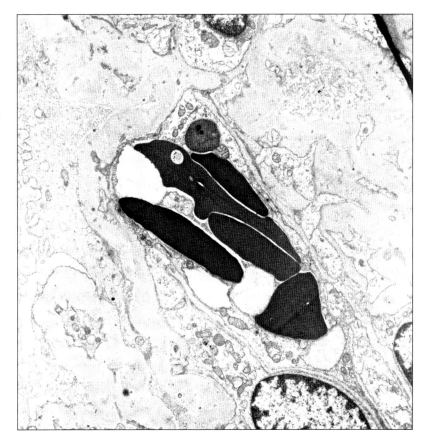

disease related to sickling, including sickle cell nephropathy. Sickle cell trait may also result in significant sickling and even sickle cell crisis, but has only rarely been reported to cause sickle cell nephropathy. The pathogenesis of sickle cell crisis is related to decreased oxygen tension, particularly due to dehydration and exercise, triggering sickling. The vasa recta are particularly vulnerable due to relative hypoxia, low pH and hypertonicity of the medulla, which all promote polymerization of the abnormal hemoglobin and sickling of RBCs. Papillary necrosis occurs secondary to the sickled RBCs occluding blood flow. In patients with gradual development of proteinuria and chronic renal insufficiency, the postulated pathogeneses relate to chronic hypoxia, endothelial injury related to iron/heme components and sickling of RBCs, imbalance in nitric oxide, and secondary mechanisms of marked glomerular hypertrophy/hypertension and hyperfiltration, all culminating in segmental sclerosis. Transgenic sickle cell mice are being studied to further elucidate the pathogenesis of renal disease and efficacy of interventions.

Clinical trials are ongoing to treat sickle cell patients with micro-albuminuria, evidence of early renal injury, with ACE inhibitors.

Selected reading

Bernstein J, Whitten C F 1960 A histological appraisal of the kidney in sickle cell anemia. Archives in Pathology 70:407–417.

Bhathena D B, Sondheimer J H 1991 The glomerulopathy of homozygous sickle hemoglobin (SS) disease: morphology and pathogenesis. Journal of the American Society of Nephrology 1(11):1241–1252.

Buckalew V M Jr, Someren A 1974 Renal manifestations of sickle cell disease. Archives of Internal Medicine 133(4):660–669.

Elfenbein I B, Patchefsky A, Schwartz W et al 1974 Pathology of the glomerulus in sickle cell anemia with and without nephrotic syndrome. American Journal of Pathology 77(3):357–374.

Falk R J, Scheinman J, Phillips G et al 1992 Prevalence and pathologic features of sickle cell nephropathy and response to inhibition of angiotensin-converting enzyme. New England Journal of Medicine 326(14):910–915.

Pham P T, Pham P C, Wilkinson A H et al 2000 Renal abnormalities in sickle cell disease. Kidney International 57(1):1–8.

Scheinman J I 2003 Sickle cell disease and the kidney. Seminars in Nephrology 23(1):66–76.

Fabry's disease

Fabry's disease is an X-linked deficiency of alpha-galactosidase A leading to accumulation of glycosphingolipids. Hemizygous males experience multisystem symptoms starting in infancy or childhood, with painful neuropathies, skin, cardiovascular and renal disease. The early renal manifestations are a concentrating defect, with proteinuria appearing in adulthood, and renal failure developing by age 40–50 years. Patients also develop hemangiomas, conjunctival telangiectasias, corneal and lenticular opacities, and abnormal intestinal mobility. The typical skin lesion is the red nonblanching papular angiokeratoma corporis diffusum. Renal transplantation has obviated death from chronic renal failure, but does not provide sufficient normal enzyme to prevent systemic manifestations of disease. Patients with residual enzyme activity and heterozygous females have milder course of the disease. However, heterozygous females may also be affected, depending on degree of lyonization of the mutated allele.

With standard processing, the accumulated galactosyl ceramide is extracted by xylene. Lectin histochemistry on Epon-embedded material to stain lysosomal sugar residues can be useful for specific

Fig. 1.213 Fabry's disease. The podocytes and parietal epithelial cells show a vacuolated, honey-comb appearance due to accumulation of the abnormal glycosphingolipid in Fabry disease. Endothelial and mesangial cells are less prominently affected in this glomerulus (H&E, ×200).

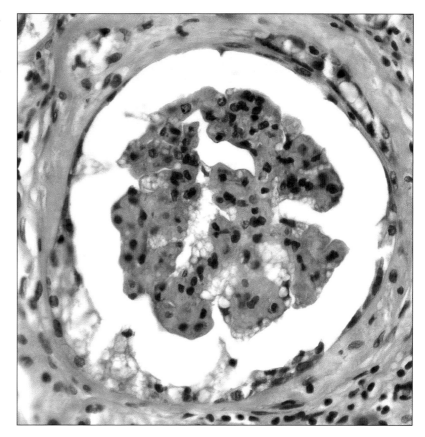

Fig. 1.214 Fabry's disease. There is prominent enlargement of glomerular visceral epithelial cells with a vacuolated, honeycomb appearance. There is also associated mild mononuclear cell infiltrate. Lesser glycosphingolipid accumulation is present in the parietal epithelial cells (H&E, ×200).

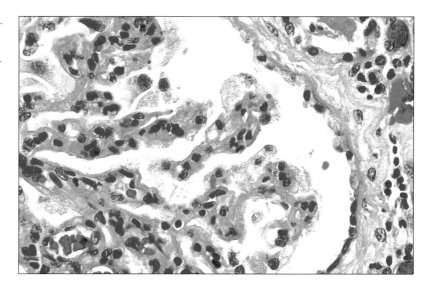

diagnosis. By light microscopy, glomerular visceral epithelial cells and tubular cells are prominently vacuolated (Figs 1.213–1.215). With progressive disease, mesangial expansion and glomerulosclerosis develop, with proportional interstitial fibrosis and tubular atrophy. There may be segmental glomerular basement membrane

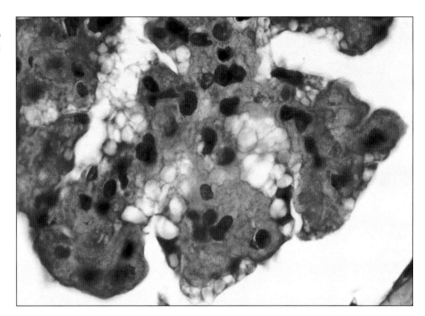

Fig. 1.215 Fabry's disease. The vacuolated, honeycomb appearance of the podocytes is due to the accumulation of glycosphingolipid. Lesser accumulation in mesangial or endothelial cell is seen on the left, along with a mononuclear cell infiltrate (H&E, ×400).

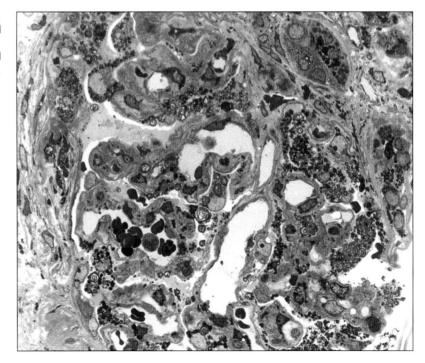

Fig. 1.216 Fabry's disease. On the toluidine blue-stained plastic-embedded sections, the lysosomal inclusions and myelin bodies are numerous, especially in the podocytes. Surrounding tubular epithelium also shows this accumulated glycosphingolipid, with focal accumulation in parietal epithelial cells (toluidine blue, ×400).

Fig. 1.217 Fabry's disease. Massive accumulation of lysosomal inclusions and myelin bodies is present in podocytes with lesser accumulation in parietal epithelium and adjacent tubular epithelium (toluidine blue, ×400).

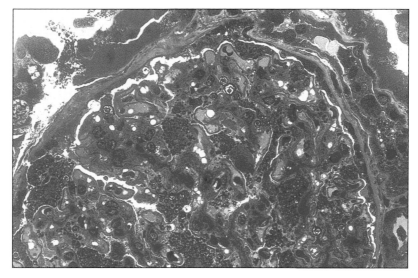

Fig. 1.218 Fabry's disease. The myelin bodies and lysosomal inclusions, some of which are lamellated, are abundant in podocytes with lesser accumulation in mesangial cells and adjacent proximal tubular cells and parietal epithelial cells (toluidine blue, ×1000).

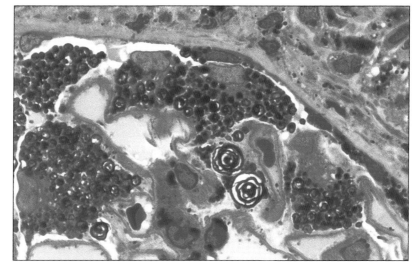

splitting. Inclusions are also present early in Henle's loop and the distal tubule, and in the proximal tubule (Figs 1.216–1.218). Standard immunofluorescence may show IgM and C3 in mesangial areas. By electron microscopy, inclusions in lysosomes are widespread, and may be present in all renal cells. The inclusions vary in size and structure, and have been called myelin bodies, whorled or lamellated inclusions or zebra bodies (Figs 1.219–1.221). The lamellated inclusions show alternating dark and light layers with a periodicity of 35–50Å. These inclusions are most prominently present in glomerular visceral epithelial cells, but also are variably present in endothelium, particularly of the peritubular capillary, tubules, and

Fig. 1.219   Fabry's disease. Lysosomal inclusions with lamellated structure are abundantly present in the glomerular visceral epithelial cells. The glomerular basement membrane itself (upper left) is intact (TEM, ×12 000).

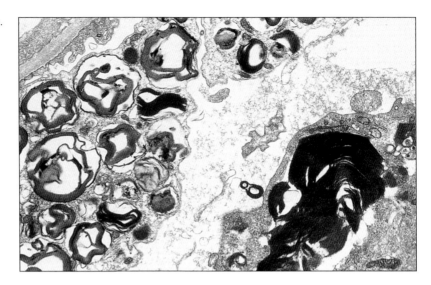

Fig. 1.220   Fabry's disease. Lysosomal inclusion with so-call 'myelin body appearance' in the glomerular visceral epithelial cell (TEM, ×34 000).

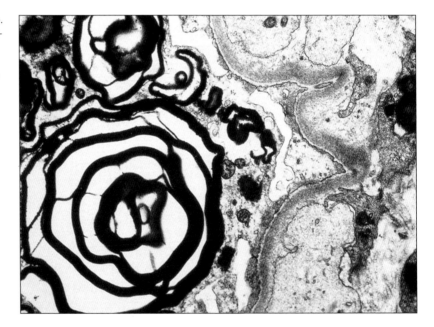

interstitial cells. Decreased peritubular capillary inclusions correlated with improvement after replacement enzyme therapy.

Etiology/pathogenesis

Fabry's disease is an X-linked recessive disease due to a deficiency of alpha-galactosidase. Disease occurs due to accumulation of intra-

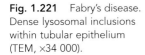

Fig. 1.221 Fabry's disease. Dense lysosomal inclusions within tubular epithelium (TEM, ×34 000).

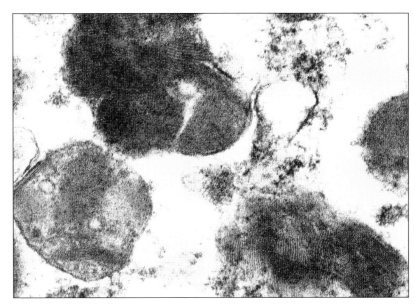

cellular glycosphingolipid globotriaosylceramide (Gb3). This enzyme is present in lysosomes throughout the body, and thus the disease manifestations are systemic. Its frequency is approximately 1:40 000 in the USA. Heterozygous females may also be affected, although typically with milder manifestations. Most recently, genetically engineered alpha-galactosidase A has been used to treat patients with Fabry's disease, resulting in decreased disease manifestations with decreased mesangial expansion and better preservation of GFR over the 1-year course of treatment. Renal disease has been postulated to be related to podocyte injury consequent to the marked accumulation of Gb3 in these cells.

Selected reading

Alroy J, Sabnis S, Kopp J B 2002 Renal pathology in Fabry disease. Journal of the American Society of Nephrology 13(Suppl 2):S134–S138.

Branton M H, Schiffmann R, Sabnis S G et al 2002 Natural history of Fabry renal disease: influence of alpha-galactosidase A activity and genetic mutations on clinical course. Medicine (Baltimore) 81(2):122–138.

Faraggiana T, Churg J 1987 Renal lipidoses: a review. Human Pathology 18:661–679.

Faraggiana T, Churg J, Grishman E et al 1981 Light and electron microscopic histochemistry of Fabry's disease. American Journal of Pathology 103:247–262.

Farge D, Nadler S, Wolfe L S et al 1985 Diagnostic value of kidney biopsy in heterozygous Fabry's disease. Archives of Pathological Laboratory Medicine 109:85–88.

Ojo A, Meier-Kriesche H U, Friedman G et al 2000 Excellent outcome of renal transplantation in patients with Fabry's disease. Transplantation 69:2337–2339.

Schiffmann R, Kopp J B, Austin H A 3rd et al 2001 Enzyme replacement therapy in Fabry disease: a randomized controlled trial. Journal of the American Medical Association 285:2743–2749.

Sessa A, Meroni M, Battini G et al 2001 Renal pathological changes in Fabry disease. Journal of Inherited Metabolic Disease 24(Suppl 2):66–70.

Thurberg B L, Rennke H, Colvin R B et al 2002 Globotriaosylceramide accumulation in the Fabry kidney is cleared from multiple cell types after enzyme replacement therapy. Kidney International 62(6):1933–1946.

Lipoprotein glomerulopathy

Lipoprotein glomerulopathy is a disorder with apparent autosomal recessive inheritance in some kindreds, with proteinuria and steroid resistant nephrotic syndrome. Most described patients have been Japanese, but the disease has also been described in patients of other ethnicities. Males outnumber females. Patients are usually adult at presentation, although some patients were children. Patients typically have increased beta-lipoprotein and pre-beta lipoprotein with elevated apoE. Glomerular lesions identical to those observed in these patients also occur in patients with type-III hyperlipoproteinemia. Approximately one-third of patients show slowly progressive renal disease, and the lesions may recur in renal transplants.

The characteristic light microscopic lesion is one of intracapillary lipoprotein thrombi distending and enlarging glomeruli (Fig. 1.222). The mesangium may show mesangiolysis. In areas that do not show mesangiolysis, there is increased mesangial cellularity and matrix. The capillary wall can be thickened or split in response to this injury. The lipoprotein thrombi stain only lightly with PAS, and typically are vacuolated and laminated. The material stains positively for Oil red O and Sudan stain (Fig. 1.223). There may be associated segmental sclerosis, but in contrast to LCAT deficiency, there usually is not predominant foam cell change in the glomerulus, unless sclerosis has occurred. The tubulointerstitial changes are proportionate and follow glomerulosclerosis. There are no specific vascular lesions. By immunofluorescence, there may be IgM, C1q and fibrinogen surrounding the lipoprotein thrombi, which contain beta-lipoprotein, apoB and apoE. By electron microscopy, there are

Fig. 1.222 Lipoprotein glomerulopathy. There are massive intraluminal pale lipid thrombi in the glomerular capillaries, distending the capillary lumens, with segmental GBM splitting (Jones' silver stain, ×200). (Case 1.222–1.225 kindly provided by Dr Barry Stokes).

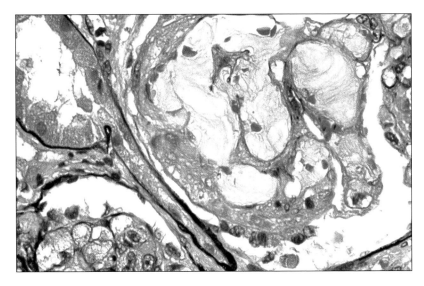

Fig. 1.223 Lipoprotein glomerulopathy. The intra-capillary thrombi stain brightly positive for lipid (oil Red O stain, ×200).

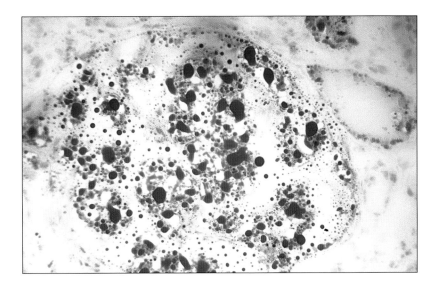

vacuolated or granular electron dense or lucent deposits and thrombi, often with a concentric, laminated pattern with small lipid vacuoles (Fig. 1.224). The splitting of the capillary wall is determined by electron microscopy to be due to segmental lipid material between the endothelial cell and the GBM, with segmental mesangial interposition (Fig. 1.225).

Fig. 1.224 Lipoprotein glomerulopathy. The intra-capillary thrombi have a concentric, laminated pattern with small lipid vacuoles (TEM, ×8000).

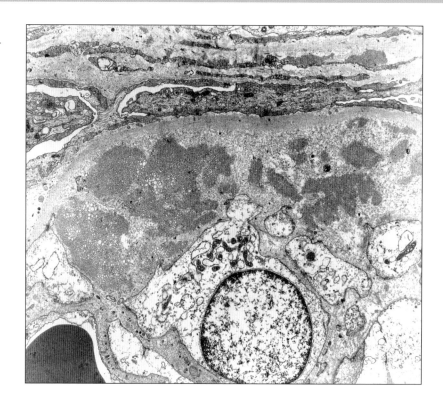

Fig. 1.225 Lipoprotein glomerulopathy. Occasional subendothelial/intramembranous deposits, with lipid vacuoles are present (TEM, ×18 000).

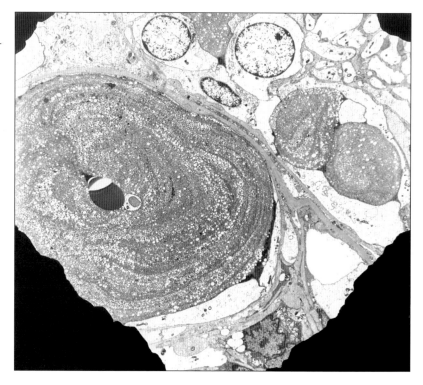

Selected reading

Faraggiana T, Churg J 1987 Renal lipidosis: A review. Human Pathology 18:661–679.

Saito T, Sato H, Kudo K et al 1989 Lipoprotein glomerulopathy: Glomerular lipoprotein thrombi in a patient with hyperlipoproteinemia. American Journal of Kidney Disease 132:148–153.

Watanabe Y, Ozaki I, Yoshida F et al 1989 A case of nephrotic syndrome with glomerular lipoprotein deposition with capillary ballooning and mesangiolysis. Nephron 521:265–270.

Lecithin-cholesterol acyltransferase deficiency

This systemic disorder is due to deficiency of lecithin-cholesterol acyltransferase (LCAT), due to a mutation of the gene, which is on the long arm of chromosome 16. The disease was originally described in Scandinavian patients, but occurs worldwide, and is inherited as an autosomal recessive trait with varying plasma levels of lecithin-cholesterol acyltransferase in different kindreds. Patients have proteinuria, anemia, hyperlipidemia, corneal opacities and accelerated atherosclerosis. Early kidney disease manifests as proteinuria, increasing in severity by the fourth and fifth decades, frequently progressing to nephrotic syndrome and end stage renal disease.

Light microscopy shows thickened capillary walls with irregular bubble appearance of the basement membranes (Figs 1.226–1.229). The mesangium is expanded, often with a bubble appearance, with a variable foam cell infiltrate in capillaries and mesangial areas

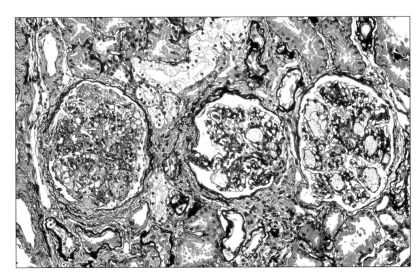

Fig. 1.226 LCAT deficiency. There may be non-specific sclerosis and tubulointerstitial fibrosis. The glomerular basement membrane is irregular and thickened. The mesangium is expanded, and there is variable foam cell infiltrate within capillary lumens and in mesangial areas, as seen on the left (Jones' silver stain, ×100).

(Figs 1.227–1.229). Foam cells may also be present in vessels and interstitium. In advanced cases, segmental sclerosis and hyalinosis are present. There are no immune complexes by immunofluorescence. Variable results have been reported with lipid stains. Electron microscopy reveals lacunae in basement membranes and mesangium containing dense structures that appear solid or lamellar, or contain

Fig. 1.227 LCAT deficiency. The focal prominent endocapillary foam cell infiltration is evident, with only minimal foam cells in the glomerulus on the left (PAS, ×200).

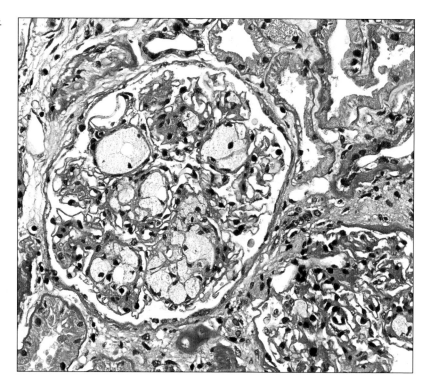

Fig. 1.228 LCAT deficiency. Segmental irregular peripheral capillary basement membranes are present, with prominent intracapillary and mesangial foam cells (H&E, ×400).

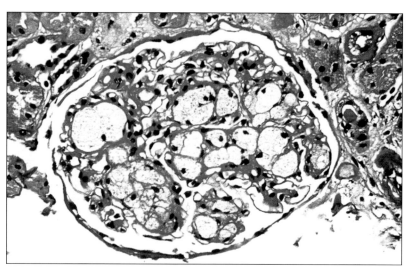

dense particles ('striated membranous structures'). Cells contain lipid inclusions (Fig. 1.230). The foot processes are effaced.

Etiology/pathogenesis

LCAT is a catalyst for esterification of free cholesterol bound to low-density lipoprotein. LCAT deficiency is due to mutation of the gene. The different mutations result in varying enzyme levels, ranging

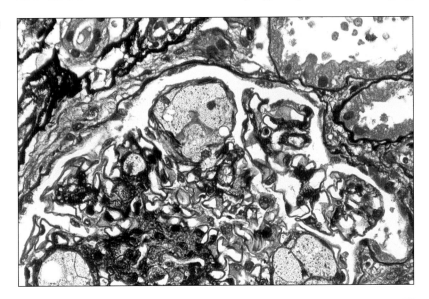

Fig. 1.229 LCAT deficiency. The glomerular basement membrane is thickened, with occasional splitting (bottom left). There are prominent intracapillary foam cells, with rare lipid vacuoles, and increased mesangial matrix (Jones' silver stain, ×400).

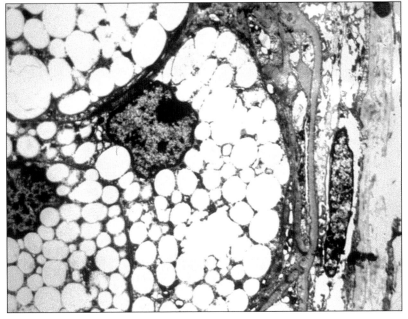

Fig. 1.230 LCAT deficiency. In the basement membrane, there may be lacuna, or solid or lamellar dense structures (not shown). Numerous lipid inclusions are seen within the intracapillary foam cells by EM (TEM, ×8000).

from absolute absence in some kindreds, to 10%–20% in some homozygotes. Heterozygotes may also have diminished LCAT activity. The gene frequency is about 2% in Scandinavia. Decreased LCAT activity results in abnormal lipid metabolism and accumulation of unesterified cholesterol, triglycerides and phosphatidylcholine throughout the body. Lipid accumulations have been documented in aorta, other arteries, liver, spleen and cornea. No effective therapy has been identified. Recently, knockout mice have been generated, creating a method for testing new gene therapy approaches. Renal transplantation does not restore normal lipid metabolism. Deposition of these lipid-related materials with foam cells in glomeruli recurs as early as 6 months after transplantation although renal function is usually maintained.

Selected reading

Faraggiana T, Churg J 1987 Renal lipidosis: A review. Human Pathology 18: 661–679.

Gjøne E 1981 Familial lecithin:cholesterol acyltransferase deficiency: a new metabolic disease with renal involvement. Advances in Nephrology 10:167–185.

Hovig T, Gjøne E 1974 Familial lecithin:cholesterol acyltransferase deficiency. Scandinavian Journal of Clinical Laboratory Investigation 33:135–146.

Imbasciati E, Paties C, Scarpioni L et al 1986 Renal lesions in familial lecithin-cholesterol acyltransferase deficiency: ultrastructural heterogeneity of glomerular changes. American Journal of Nephrology 6:66–70.

Lager D J, Rosenberg B F, Shapiro H et al 1991 Lecithin cholesterol acyltransferase deficiency: ultrastructural examination of sequential renal biopsies. Modern Pathology 4:331–335.

Lambert G, Sakai N, Vaisman B L et al 2001 Analysis of glomerulosclerosis and atherosclerosis in lecithin cholesterol acyltransferase-deficient mice. Journal of Biological Chemistry 276:15090–15098.

Diseases associated with nephritic syndrome or RPGN: immune mediated

Lupus nephritis

Both autopsy and biopsy studies of patients with the clinical diagnosis of systemic lupus erythematosus (SLE) have documented that renal involvement is a frequent and serious complication of the disease, making renal biopsy an important part of the clinical management of these patients. The nature of the lesion on renal biopsy gives direct information relating to the severity of the autoimmune response within the kidney and aids in the selection of appropriate therapies and the prediction of both short- and long-term outcome in individual patients. The various patterns of lupus nephritis (Fig. 1.231) must be considered in the context of the potential pathogenetic mechanisms that are involved in their evolution. Analysis in this way not only gives a basis to correlate with clinical outcome but also offers a rationale for therapeutic manipulation. For these reasons, many clinicians advocate renal biopsy as a routine part of the evaluation for all patients with SLE.

The classification scheme for lupus nephritis as developed by the World Health Organization (WHO) provides a basis clinical application. (Table 1.5) It combines all morphologic modalities of biopsy interpretation, including light, immunofluorescence and

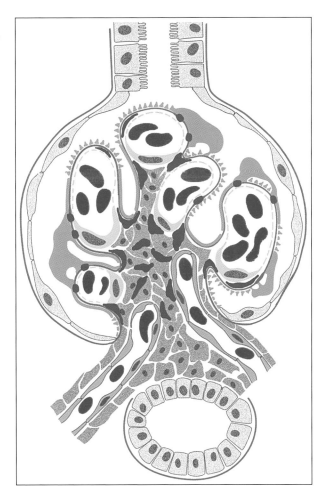

Fig. 1.231 (a) Lupus nephritis manifests in various forms. Mesangial lupus nephritis (WHO Type II) is characterized by predominantly mesangial proliferation and is due to mesangial deposits, with rare possible deposits in other compartments.

Fig. 1.231—cont'd
(b) Lupus nephritis may also present as a proliferative lesion when there are subendothelial deposits, with endocapillary proliferation and GBM splitting. In lupus nephritis of the proliferative type, there will frequently be small, scattered subepithelial deposits as well.

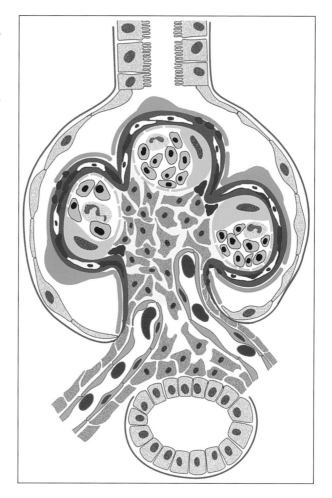

electron microscopic findings, and it thus represents a major improvement over previous classifications. The classification system, along with a semiquantitative assessment of severity and chronicity, is now in general use and has been accepted by clinical nephrologists and renal pathologists alike. A more detailed subclassification has been suggested by the pathology advisory group of the International Study of Kidney Diseases in Children (ISKDC), but this seems to be of greater value for investigative purposes than for general clinical use. A recent modification has been proposed by a joint committee of the International Society of Nephrology and the Renal Pathology Society which is more comprehensive (Table 1.6). It eliminates a class for biopsies with no significant findings and emphasizes the role of immunofluorescence and electron microscopy. These classifications do have the limitation of focusing on the glomerular

Fig. 1.231—cont'd
(c) In the membranous form of lupus nephritis, there are global subepithelial deposits, as in idiopathic membranous glomerulonephritis, with additional mesangial deposits.

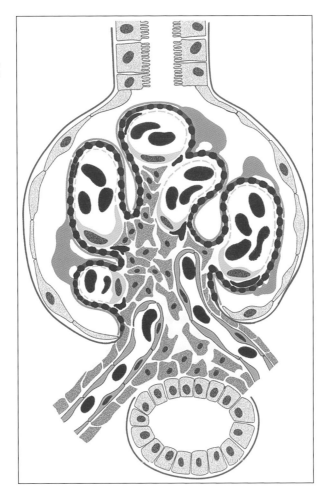

lesions while attributing much less significance to tubular, interstitial, and vascular lesions.

Histopathology

In this presentation the histopathologic findings of the most recent version of the RPS/ISN classification will be described as outlined in Table 1.6.

Class I

Class I contains lesions with minimal or no significant changes by light microscopy. Immunofluorescence, however, presents evidence of immune deposits that are confined to the mesangium, and

TABLE 1.5   1995 Modified Original Classification of Lupus Glomerulonephritis

I.   Normal Nil

II.   Pure mesangiopathy
A.   Normal by light microscopy but deposits present
B.   Moderate mesangial hypercellularity

III.   Segmental and focal proliferative glomerulonephritis
A.   Active necrotizing
B.   Active and sclerosing
C.   Sclerosing

IV.   Diffuse proliferative glomerulonephritis
A.   Without segmental necrotizing lesions
B.   With segmental necrotizing lesions
C.   With segmental active and sclerotic lesions
D.   Inactive, sclerotic

V.   Diffuse membranous glomerulonephritis
A.   Pure membranous
B.   Associated with lesions in group IIA or IIB

VI.   Advanced sclerosing glomerulonephritis

TABLE 1.6   2002 WHO/ISN/RPS Classification of Lupus Glomerulonephritis

Class I	Minimal mesangial lupus glomerulonephritis (LGN) Normal glomeruli by LM, but mesangial immune deposits by IF and/or EM
Class II	Mesangial proliferative LGN Purely mesangial hypercellularity of any degree and/or mesangial matrix expansion by LM with immune deposits, predominantly mesangial with none or few, isolated subepithelial and/or subendothelial deposits by IF and/or EM not visible by LM
Class III	Focal LGN (involving less than 50% of the total number of glomeruli) Active or inactive focal, segmental and/or global endo- and/or extracapillary GN, typically with focal, subendothelial immune deposits, with or without focal or diffuse mesangial alterations
	Class III (A) Purely active lesions: active focal proliferative LGN
	Class III (A/C) Active and chronic lesions: active and sclerotic focal proliferative LGN

TABLE 1.6—cont'd

	Class III (C) Chronic inactive with glomerular scars: inactive sclerotic focal LGN
	*Indicate proportion of glomeruli with active and with sclerotic lesions *Indicate the proportion of glomeruli with fibrinoid necrosis and/or cellular crescents
Class IV	Diffuse segmental (IV-S) or global (IV-G) LGN (involving 50% or more of the total number of glomeruli either segmentally or globally) Active or inactive diffuse, segmental or global endo- and/or extracapillary GN with diffuse subendothelial immune deposits, with or without mesangial alterations. This class is divided into diffuse segmental (IV-S) when >50% of the involved glomeruli have segmental lesions, and diffuse global (IV-G) when >50% of the involved glomeruli have global lesions. Class IV (A) Active lesions: diffuse segmental or global proliferative LGN Class IV (A/C) Active and chronic lesions: diffuse segmental or global proliferative and sclerotic LGN Class IV (C) Inactive with glomerular scars: diffuse segmental or global sclerotic LGN *Indicate the proportion of glomeruli with active and with sclerotic lesions *Indicate the proportion of glomeruli with fibrinoid necrosis and/or cellular crescents
Class V	Membranous LGN Numerous global or segmental subepithelial immune deposits or their morphologic sequelae by LM and/or IF and/or EM with or without mesangial alterations *May occur in combination with III or IV in which case both will be diagnosed
Class VI	Advanced sclerotic LGN 90% of glomeruli globally sclerosed without residual activity

Recommend that all renal biopsy include description and semiquantification of active and sclerosing glomerular lesions, grading of tubular atrophy, interstitial inflammation and fibrosis, severity of arteriosclerosis or other vascular lesions.

electron microscopy will reveal corresponding electron-dense deposits in this location (Figs 1.232, 1.233).

Class II

In Class II, light microscopy shows definite glomerular mesangial hypercellularity that is confined to the centrilobular areas away from the vascular pole (Fig. 1.234). There is no involvement of the peripheral glomerular capillary walls. Immunofluorescence reveals mesangial immunoglobulin deposition (Fig. 1.235), and electron microscopy discloses dense deposits that are confined to the mesangial regions (Fig. 1.236). In some cases deposits occasionally are seen in the paramesangial subendothelial areas. Tubular, interstitial, and vascular changes are usually insignificant.

Patients with class II lesions generally have minimal clinical evidence of renal involvement, with mild to moderate proteinuria and/or hematuria and little or no evidence of renal insufficiency.

Class III

Class III is characterized by light microscopic findings of a focal and segmental glomerulonephritis. Less than 50% of the glomeruli that are involved show only focal damage occupying less than 50%

Fig. 1.232 Class I or minimal lupus glomerulo-nephritis (LGN). There is only minimal mild segmental mesangial widening. Peripheral capillary loops are entirely normal (H&E, ×400).

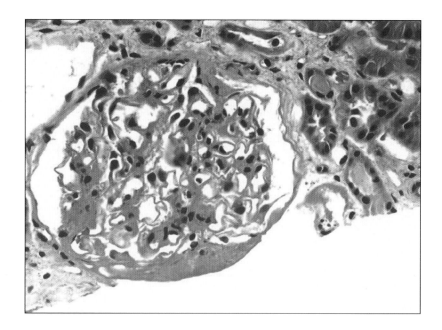

Fig. 1.233 Class I, minimal LGN. (a) Immunofluorescence of Class I shows immunoglobulin deposits in the mesangium. Most often this is IgG and may be accompanied by a similar pattern of deposition of C3 (anti-IgG immunofluorescence, ×400). (b) Electron microscopy in Class I reveals open peripheral capillary loops with well preserved foot processes and endothelial cells. The mesangium contains an increase in mesangial matrix and small mesangial electron dense deposits (TEM, ×4000).

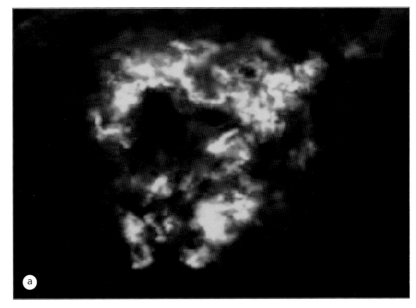

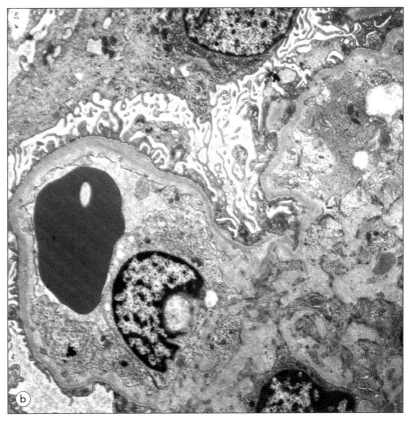

Fig. 1.234   Class II or mesangial proliferative LGN. There is more prominent mesangial widening than in Class I and there is a definite increase in mesangial cellularity. The peripheral capillary loops are normal. The adjacent tubules in inter-stitium are often uninvolved (H&E, ×400).

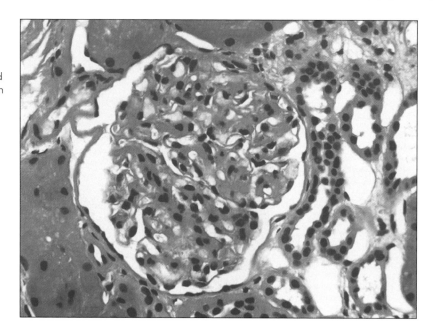

Fig. 1.235   Class II or mesangial proliferative LGN. Immunofluorescence of Class II reveals mesangial immunoglobulin deposition. The immunoglobulins deposited in lupus almost always include IgG but a full house of immunoglobulin deposition involving multiple immunoglobulins and complement is charac-teristic of lupus nephritis (anti-IgG immunofluo-rescence, ×400).

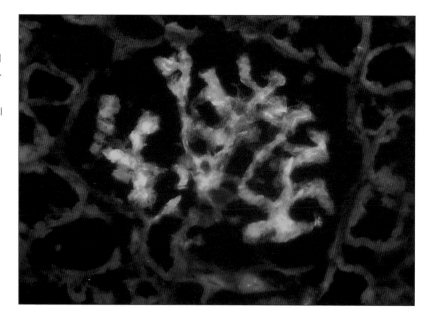

of the glomerular surface. The segmental changes can be prolifer-ative, necrotizing, sclerosing, or a combination of these alterations (Fig. 1.237). Segmental intracapillary and extracapillary cell proliferation with obliteration of the capillary lumina sometimes is found in addition to generalized mesangial widening. Segmental

Fig. 1.236   Class II or mesangial proliferative LGN. Electron microscopy of Class II shows definite mesangial changes with abundant mesangial electron dense deposits accompanying the increase in mesangial matrix. The electron dense deposits correspond to the deposition of immunoglobulins and complement seen by immunofluorescence (TEM, ×5000).

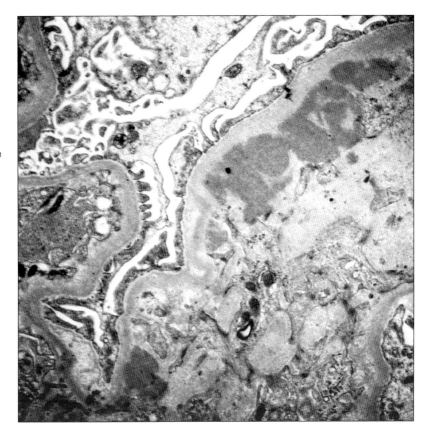

Fig. 1.237   Class III or focal and segmental lupus glomerulonephritis is characterized by focal involvement of glomeruli in which there are segmental lesions as demonstrated here with one entirely normal appearing glomerulus adjacent to glomerulus with a segmental area of adhesion and necrosis (H&E, ×200).

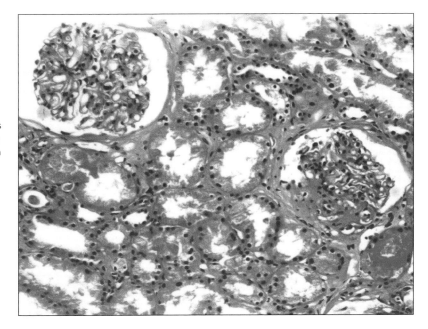

necrotic lesions may be associated with crescent formations that progress to segmental scars with focal capsular adhesions. These segmental lesions usually are superimposed on a minimal degree of mesangial hypercellularity (Fig. 1.238).

Immunofluorescence reveals peripheral granular as well as mesangial deposits of immunoglobulins (Fig. 1.239), and electron microscopy demonstrates subendothelial deposits in addition to

Fig. 1.238   LGN. (a) Segmental changes can be merely proliferative or as demonstrated here necrotizing with adhesion to Bowman's capsule loss of the normal architecture. (b) In some instances, this progresses to the presence of epithelial crescents associated with collapse of the normal glomerular architecture (a, H&E ×400; b, Masson trichrome, ×400).

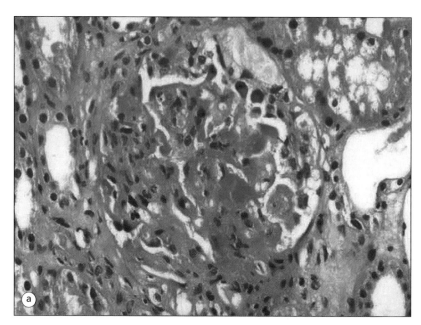

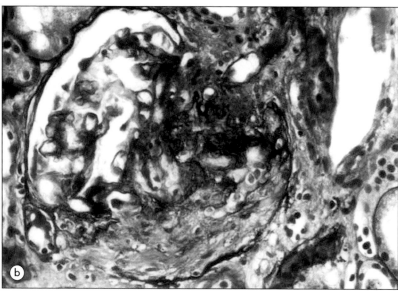

Fig. 1.239 LGN, Class III. The mesangial and peripheral capillary deposition of immunoglobulins appears more prominent than in Class II (anti-IgG immunofluorescence, ×400).

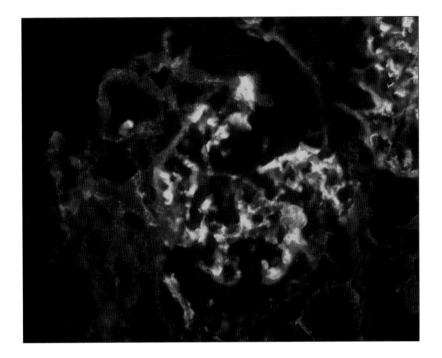

the presence of mesangial deposits (Fig. 1.240). The similarity of the immunofluorescence and electron microscopic findings of Class III lesions with those of Class IV suggests that these two classes actually may be variations of the same immunopathologic lesion, and that the focal nature of Class III represents a quantitative rather than a qualitative difference.

Class III has been broken down into three subclasses: (1) active necrotizing lesions, (2) necrotizing and sclerosing lesions, and (3) purely sclerosing lesions. The clinical significance of this subclassification is not clear, however. The natural history of patients with class III lesions is similar to that of patients with class IV lesions, again suggesting that these two classes are a continuum of the same lesion.

Class IV

Class IV is the most common form of active lupus nephritis, and it is characterized by a diffuse global or segmental proliferative glomerulonephritis. Most, or all, of the glomeruli are involved, and each glomerulus shows diffuse IV-G or segmental IV-S hypercellularity often in a lobular pattern (Fig. 1.241). As with Class III lesions, segmental areas of necrosis occasionally associated with focal areas of crescent formation can occur. Nuclear debris represented by hematoxyphil bodies also can be seen. Some segments of peripheral capillary loop can be dramatically thickened to form the so-called wire loop lesion. Occasionally extensive deposits of immune complexes are seen as hyaline thrombi in the capillary loops. Segmental areas of sclerosis are an indicator either of previous segmental necrosis or of chronicity.

The variety of lesions that can be encountered in this class range from diffuse mesangial hypercellularity without necrosis to a severe necrotizing and crescentic glomerulonephritis. Focal and global areas of sclerosis may be present. The new subclassification is useful in separating these different patterns into: IV(A), proliferative lesions with evidence of activity such as focal necrosis; IV(A/C), proliferative lesions with necrosis and sclerosis; and IV(C), proliferative lesions with sclerosis (Fig. 1.242). About one-quarter of cases exhibit lobular accentuation with mesangial extension around the

Fig. 1.240 Class III, LGN. Electron microscopy in Class III is similar to the findings in Class IV. (a) Subendothelial deposits are present in addition to mesangial deposits as seen in Classes I and II (TEM, ×4000).

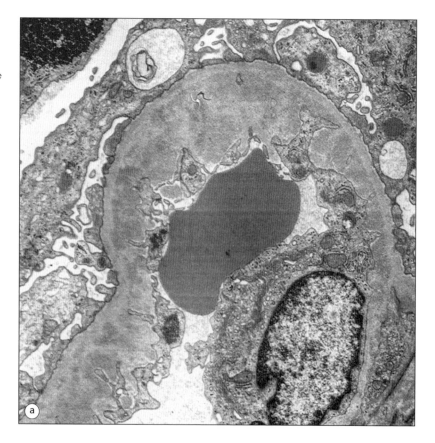

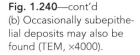

Fig. 1.240—cont'd
(b) Occasionally subepithelial deposits may also be found (TEM, ×4000).

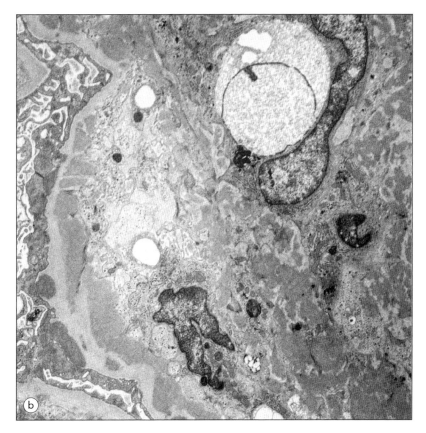

peripheral loops, forming a pattern similar to that of other forms of mesangiocapillary glomerulonephritis.

Immunofluorescence microscopy reveals a coarsely granular pattern of immunoglobulin deposition both in the mesangium and in the peripheral capillary walls (Fig. 1.243). Multiple immunoglobulins frequently are encountered and generally are accompanied by evidence of the activation of inflammatory mediators, such as a deposition of complement components, fibrinogen and properdin. This pattern has been termed a full house pattern of immunoglobulin deposition.

Electron microscopic examination is similar to that seen with Class III lesions (Fig. 1.244). Abundant subendothelial deposits are accompanied by large mesangial deposits. These deposits generally are larger and more abundant than in other classes of lupus nephritis. Epimembranous deposits often are present. Mesangial hypercellularity with circumferential mesangial interposition is associated

with the light microscopic pattern of a mesangiocapillary glomerulonephritis. Occasionally, the electron-dense deposits show an
organized (Fig. 1.244e) or crystalline pattern, which has been termed
a fingerprint pattern. This organized appearance most frequently is
seen in the presence of abundant endothelial deposits, but it can be

Fig. 1.241   Class IV, LGN.
(a) Class IV or diffuse lupus
glomerulonephritis by light
microscopy involves most
or all of the glomeruli.
In general, there is a marked
increase in mesangial cellularity with lobular accentuation and mesangialization
of the peripheral capillary
loops (H&E, ×400). (b) Silver
methenamine (Jones) stains
demonstrate the mesangialization and demonstrate the
presence of subendothelial
deposits lining along the
capillary loops (×400).

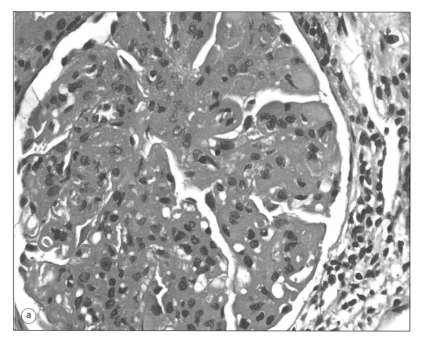

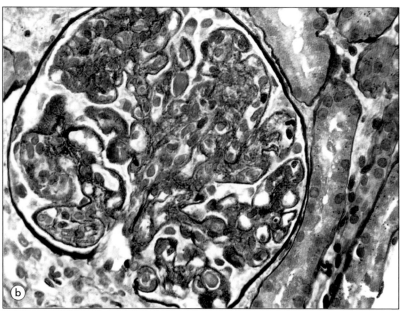

Fig. 1.241—cont'd
(c) The capillaries can contain hyaline thrombi and may be thickened to the point to be considered 'wire loop' lesions (H&E, ×400). (d) Segmental areas of necrosis are often associated with the presence of epithelial crescents (Masson trichrome, ×400).

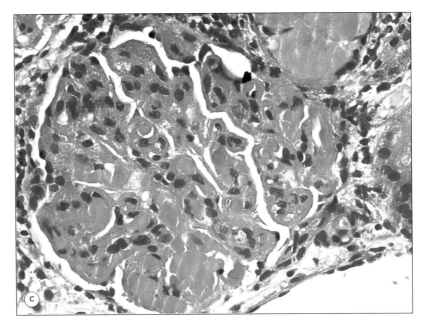

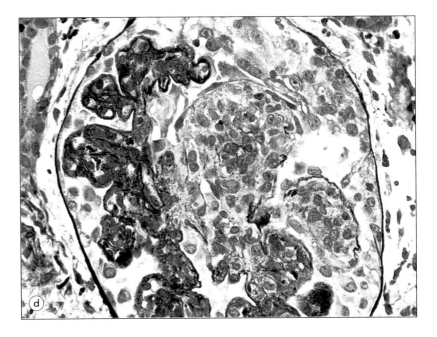

present in all classes of lupus nephritis. The crystalline structure is thought by some to represent the presence of cryoglobulins, because similar structures are seen in patients with idiopathic mixed cryo-globulinemia. They also might represent a pattern of crystalline DNA. Endothelial cell swelling and proliferation are prominent,

Fig. 1.242 Class IV, LGN.
(a,b) These active lesions
will eventually become
sclerotic and are sub-
classified as IVc namely
proliferative lesions with
sclerosis (Masson trichrome,
a, ×200; b, ×400).

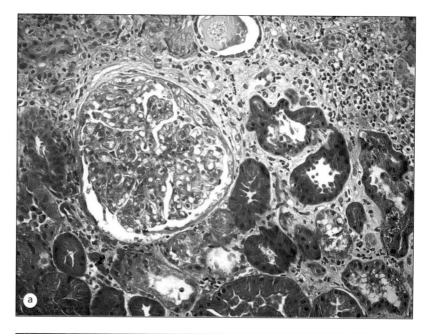

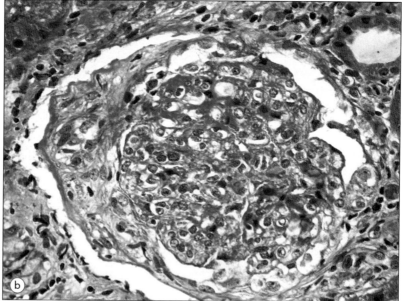

and occasional mitotic figures of glomerular cellular components
suggest active proliferation and regeneration secondary to activation
of inflammatory cytokines in growth factors. Intraendothelial tubular reticular inclusions (TRIs) resembling myxoviruses (Fig. 1.245)
have been identified in a majority of patients with lupus nephro-

Fig. 1.243 Class IV, LGN. Immunofluorescence reveals coarsely granular deposition of immunoglobulin in both the mesangium and in the peripheral capillary walls (anti-IgG immunofluorescence, ×200).

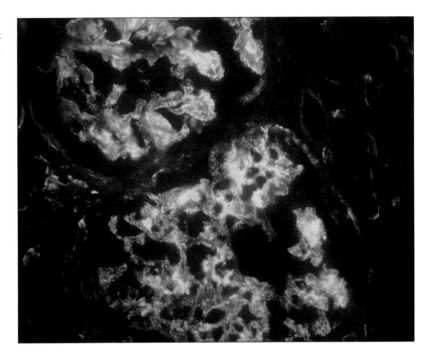

Fig. 1.244 Class IV, LGN. (a) Electron microscopy reveals the presence of abundant subendothelial deposits lining all capillary loops. These are occasionally accompanied by subepithelial deposits in varying degrees (TEM, ×1500).

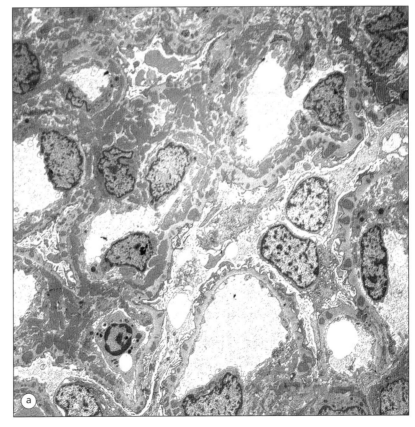

Fig. 1.244—cont'd
(b) Mesangialization of the peripheral capillary loops and leukocytic infiltration are also demonstrated (TEM, ×5000).

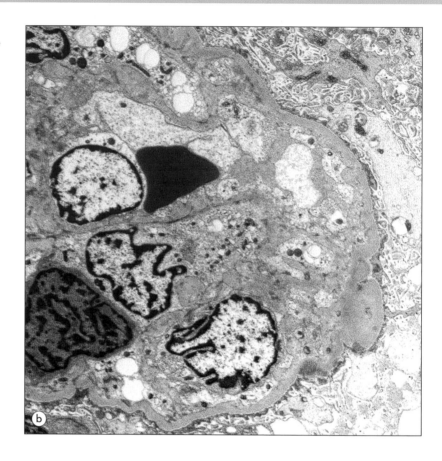

pathy. The significance of these structures is unclear, but some evidence suggests that they are induced by the cytokine α-interferon.

Class III and IV lesions represent the most severe form of glomerular involvement in patients with lupus, because the subendothelial immune complexes have access to the humoral and cellular mediators of inflammation that are present in the circulation. Patients with Class III or IV pathologic lesions usually have evidence of significant clinical renal disease, including proteinuria (frequently in the nephrotic range), renal insufficiency and an active urinary sediment. In some individual cases these lesions constitute the initial presentation of lupus erythematosus, and in rare instances, these lesions are silent. The nature of the immunopathogenesis underlying the renal lesion in patients with Class III or IV lesions suggests an unfavorable prognosis, with a high percentage of such patients eventually progressing to renal failure despite aggressive treatment. A major consequence of severe glomerular

Fig. 1.244—cont'd
(c) Foci of necrosis can be seen with disruption of the basement membrane and extrusion of the endothelia cell through the gap (TEM, ×10,000).

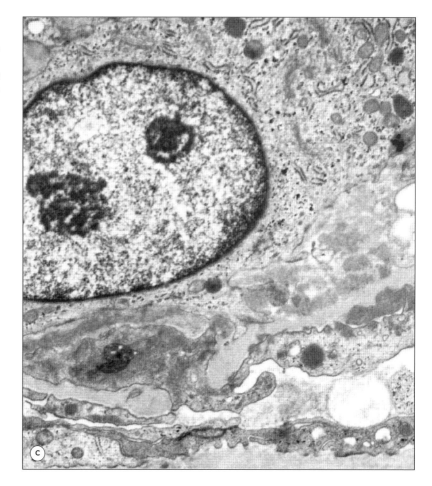

inflammation with necrosis is the development of both glomerular scarring and sclerosis, which results in decreasing glomerular filtration surface and contributes to progressive renal scarring and loss of function.

Class V

The Class V lesion is a diffuse, membranous glomerulonephropathy. Light microscopy reveals a generalized diffuse thickening of the peripheral capillary walls, which on silver methenamine-Masson stains exhibits a so-called spike and dome pattern (Fig. 1.246). The spikes are outward projections of membrane-like material between domes that correspond to the subepithelial and intramembranous deposits that are seen on immunofluorescence and electron micro-

Fig. 1.244—cont'd
(d) The capillary lumen can contain large deposits which correspond to the hyaline thrombus seen on light microscopy. (e) The electron dense deposits seen on electron microscopy often have an organized appearance sometimes taking a fingerprint pattern (TEM, ×6000, ×10,000).

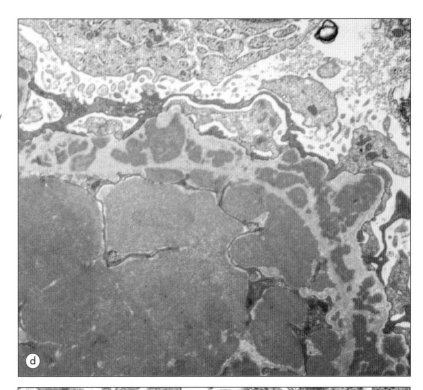

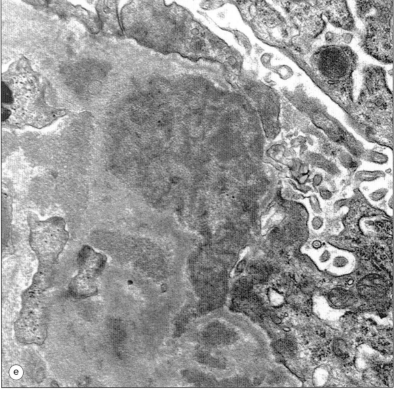

Fig. 1.245 Lupus GN. In the majority of patients with lupus, the endothelial cells contain tubular reticular inclusions. The significance of these structures is still unclear but some evidence suggests that they are induced by the cytokine alpha-interferon (TEM, ×15,000).

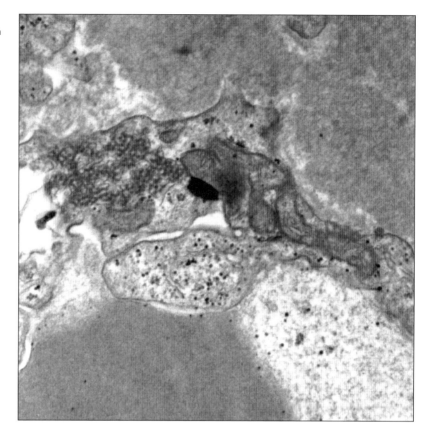

scopy. A variable degree of mesangial widening may be present, involving both an increase of mesangial cells and mesangial matrix.

Immunofluorescence demonstrates a classic confluent peripheral granular deposition of immunoglobulins and, occasionally, mesangial granular deposits (Fig. 1.247). Electron microscopy reveals a typical epimembranous nephropathy, with subepithelial and intramembranous deposits of varying electron density (Fig. 1.248). The pattern is essentially identical to that seen in idiopathic membranous glomerulonephropathy, except that mesangial deposits occasionally are present.

Some centers use a subclassification to separate biopsies with prominent subepithelial deposits into Va, pure membranous nephritis, Vb, associated with lesions of Class II, Vc, associated with lesions of Class III, Vd, associated with lesions of Class IV. While this classification is of interest from a morphological view, it is not helpful from a clinical standpoint as patients with Vc and Vd should be treated as aggressively as patients with pure Class III or Class IV.

Fig. 1.246 (a) Class V lesion or lupus membranous glomerulopathy. There is diffuse thickening of the peripheral capillary walls associated with an increase in mesangial matrix. Lobular accentuation is sometimes seen but is not associated with an increase in cellularity (H&E, ×400). (b) Silver methenamine (Jones) stains reveal a spike and dome pattern to be present along the peripheral capillary loops where the wall of the capillaries cut tangentially; there is a moth-eaten appearance of the capillary wall (Jones, ×400).

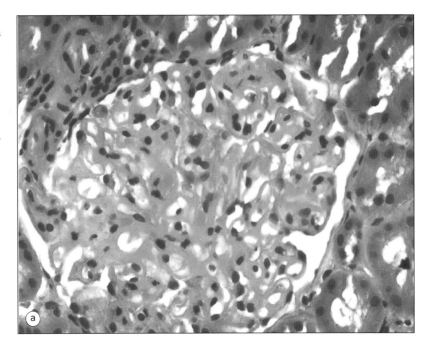

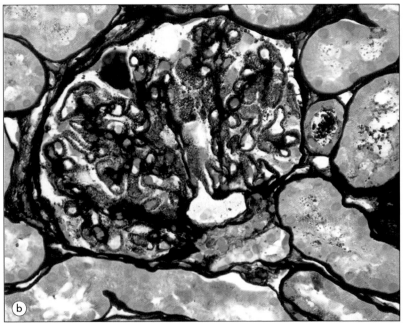

Class VI

This Class is essentially end stage renal disease. Light microscopy reveals advanced glomerulosclerosis and interstitial fibrosis. Often it cannot be distinguished from chronic sclerosing lesions from

Fig. 1.247 Class V LGN. Immunofluorescence reveals a peripheral granular deposition of immunoglobulin (anti-IgG immunofluorescence, ×400).

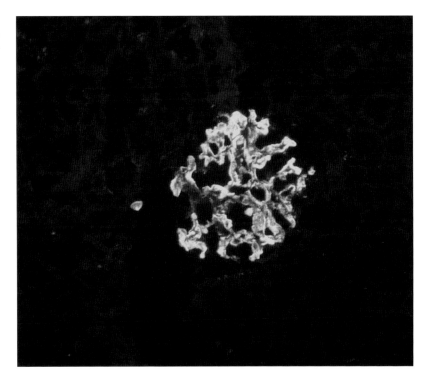

Fig. 1.248 Class V LGN. (a) Electron microscopy reveals that there are numerous subepithelial deposits scattered throughout the peripheral capillary loops. There are no subendothelial deposits present. Mesangial deposits can be seen (TEM, ×4000).

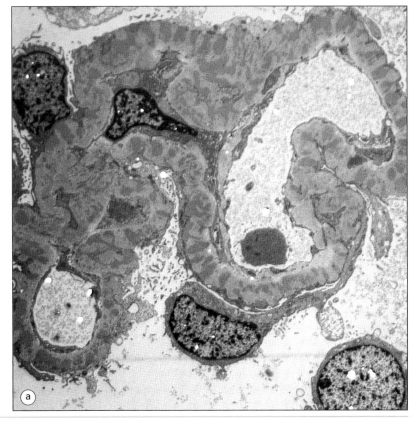

Fig. 1.248—cont'd
(b) In more advanced forms, some of the deposits may be totally intramembranous and show evidence of resorption (TEM, ×8000).

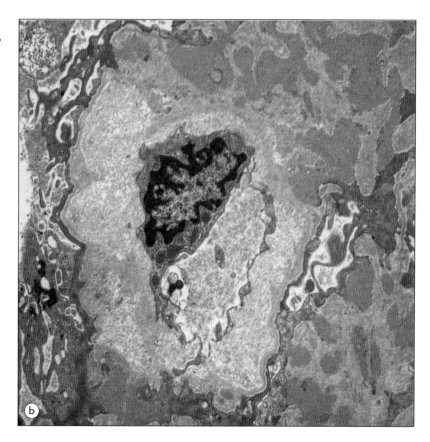

other etiologies. The presence of immune deposits by immuno-fluorescence and electron microscopy is the only way of ascertaining the diagnosis of Lupus nephritis.

Mixed patterns and transformation

Given the variability in the clinical and immunologic expression of disease that occurs in lupus erythematosus, these classes and sub-classes likely are not absolutely distinct clinical pathologic entities but rather represent different points in a continuum of disease. This is particularly evident in that transformation of renal lesions from one class to another can occur both spontaneously and as a result of treatment. The exact incidence of spontaneous transformation is difficult to determine, however, as relatively few serial biopsy studies have been performed in untreated patients. A number of studies do suggest that transformation occurs commonly and is particularly noted after various treatment protocols. Transformation from Class III to Class IV disease has been reported so frequently that most nephropathologists consider these classes to be morphologic variants of a single class of lesion with common immunofluorescence and electron microscopic patterns. Transformation of diffuse proliferative glomerulonephritis to a predominantly membranous glomerulonephropathy or a mesangial pattern has been observed in patients undergoing remission during the course of treatment.

Immunofluorescence microscopic features

One factor that has not been given enough consideration in the histopathologic evaluation of the glomerular lesion of patients with lupus nephritis is the role of immunoglobulin isotype and subclass. Most studies of the immunofluorescence microscopic findings in lupus nephritis have emphasized the deposition rather than the classes of immunoglobulins found.

In our own series of patients with lupus nephritis, IgG was most frequently present, followed by IgM and IgA. Less often, IgE is detected and usually is confined to the peripheral capillary wall. In WHO Class III and IV, peripheral granular and mesangial deposits appear concurrently. With equal frequency, IgM and IgG are detected in Class II and V disease. IgE is identified most frequently in Class IV lupus nephritis and appears to be associated with necrosis in Class IVB and C. These findings are similar to those of other studies.

IgG and IgM are the classes of immunoglobulin that most commonly are deposited, and although IgA is found frequently, it is not as common, nor is its distribution as extensive, as that of the other two immunoglobulins. In one study, IgG2 was found more frequently than other subclasses. Because subclasses IgG2 and IgG4 do not readily activate complement, a mild lesion would be expected to occur with these subclasses rather than with IgG1 or IgG3. This analysis, however, showed a poor correlation between IgG subclass and the severity of the morphologic lesion. Deposition of IgE usually has not been identified specifically. When reported, however, it has been found infrequently and been thought to reflect part of the general autoimmune response associated with this clinical syndrome of systemic lupus erythematosus. Some recent reports have suggested that IgE deposits in lupus nephritis are associated with a poor prognosis.

The so-called full house pattern of multiple immunoglobulin deposition is characteristic of SLE and does not indicate any difference in severity of the lesion from a pattern of one immunoglobulin alone. Complement components, including the membrane attack complex, fibrinogen, and properdin, usually are associated with the presence of immunoglobulins, particularly in the more severe classes of disease. Less frequently, C4 is found in Class II and IV disease, which correlates with a lower activity index. The pattern of deposition usually is coarsely granular and corresponds to the dense deposits that are seen on electron microscopy. Occasionally, a purely linear pattern similar to that seen with antiglomerular basement membrane antibody is found, but no pathologic or clinical implications for this type of deposition have been identified.

Additional pathologic features

Although the WHO classification is based primarily on the glomerular changes, it should be recognized that tubular interstitial and vascular lesions are an important part of the renal involvement and can contribute to the clinical picture. These additional pathologic features include vascular thrombosis and proliferative and sclerotic vascular lesions, including inflammatory vasculitis and tubular interstitial lesions. These complicating lesions occasionally are the predominant ones leading to clinical evidence of renal involvement. In addition, these lesions may become active or progress independently of the primary glomerular lesion. Thus, they should be evaluated independently as additional comorbid factors that may relate to specific additional therapeutic maneuvers or that have different prognostic significance.

Vascular lesions

Vascular lesions were not considered in the establishment of the WHO classification or in the currently used activity and chronicity indices. Vascular lesions are common and may include intravascular thrombosis, arterial and arteriolosclerosis, and necrotizing vasculitis. Of particular importance is the occurrence of glomerular capillary thrombosis signifying intravascular coagulation (Fig. 1.249). A pattern

Fig. 1.249 Lupus nephritis. One of the most prominent vascular lesions seen in association with lupus nephritis is the presence of intracapillary thrombi. This is associated with the presence of anti-phospholipid antibodies or lupus anti-coagulant (Jones, ×400).

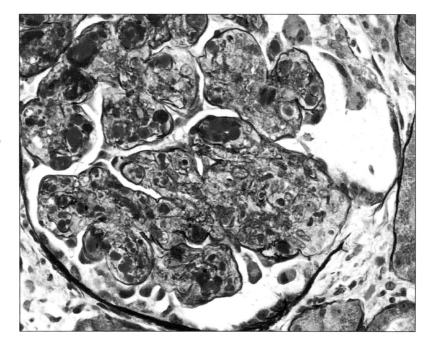

similar to that seen in adult hemolytic uremic syndrome, with multiple capillary and arteriolar thrombi containing fibrinogen, has been associated with the clinical course of rapidly progressive renal failure and been termed lupus vasculitis. Plasminogen activators are depressed in some of these patients, in whom inhibitors of plasminogen activators are elevated. Studies have shown low levels of tissue-type plasminogen activator and elevated levels of plasminogen inhibitor in patients with lupus nephropathy that is associated with glomerular capillary deposition of fibrin or thrombus formation. Because these alterations in plasma levels of tissue plasminogen activator and 2-antiplasmin would be expected to retard fibrinolysis, they were corrected by administration of the fibrinolytic agent ankyroid to patients with lupus glomerulonephritis. Together with solution of the fibrin deposits by biopsy, it is proposed that the disorder in fibrinolysis predisposes some patients with SLE to renal microvascular thrombi. Others have confirmed the association of glomerular thrombi with the presence of antiphospholipid antibodies. Patients with this lupus anticoagulant in their serum are subject to glomerular thrombosis, which might be independent of the presence of glomerular inflammation. In such patients, the glomerular thrombosis sometimes is the primary pathogenic event and likely causes the progression of renal disease without participation of the accompanying immune responses.

Necrotizing vasculitis with vascular necrosis and leukocyte infiltration is a rare finding, but it appears to be a marker of poor prognosis in patients with lupus nephritis (Fig. 1.250a). The lesions can resemble the necrotizing arteriolitis that is seen with malignant hypertension and hemolytic uremic syndrome or a true vasculitis characterized by fibrinoid necrosis of small arteries and arterioles surrounded by an inflammatory infiltrate of the vessel wall. Electron microscopy sometimes reveals immune complex deposition in the vessel wall (Fig. 1.250b). These lesions, which are reported in as many as 10% of patients with lupus nephritis, generally are considered to be an additional morbid factor. Nephrosclerotic lesions with intimal fibroplasia and hyaline arteriolar sclerosis are encountered, particularly in hypertensive patients. These lesions also are a major comorbid factor, contributing not only to the progression of renal failure but possibly also having an adverse effect on patient survival. Renal venous thrombosis is another vascular complication of lupus nephritis, but it is seen almost exclusively in patients with membranous lupus nephropathy complicated by nephrotic syndrome.

Tubulointerstitial disease

Interstitial inflammation, fibrosis, and tubular epithelial changes frequently are encountered in lupus nephritis (Fig. 1.251). Severe active tubulointerstitial nephritis most commonly is seen in patients with Class III or IV glomerular lesions. Although in most instances the interstitial inflammation is composed of lymphocytes and plasma cells, granulocytes and eosinophils also frequently are found and probably reflect the more active lesion. Immunofluorescence microscopy occasionally reveals granular peritubular deposits or, rarely, a linear deposition, suggesting an antitubular basement membrane antibody. In most instances, the presence of interstitial disease without immune deposits suggests that several different mechanisms may be involved in the pathogenesis of this component of lupus nephritis. Of interest is the observation that tubular interstitial disease may progress independently of

Fig. 1.250 Lupus nephritis. (a) Rarely, a vasculitis is seen in patients with lupus. The vasculitis resembles that of microscopic polyarteritis and shows transmural necrosis associated with an inflammatory infiltrate (Masson trichrome, ×200). (b) Immunofluorescence of these vessels often reveals deposition of immuno-globulins (anti-IgG immunofluorescence, ×400).

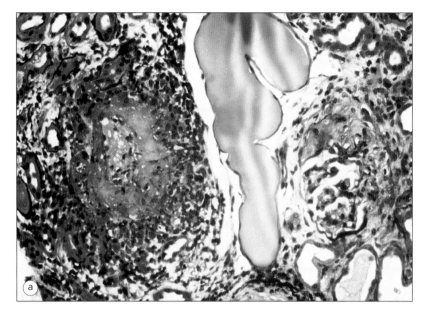

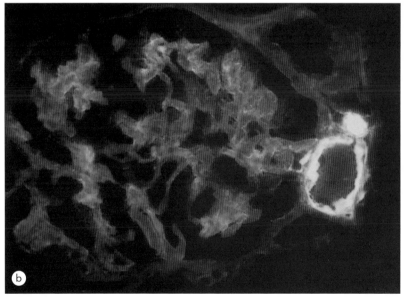

glomerular disease in some patients. It has been suggested that the infiltrate of T cells and monocytes may be an important deter-minant of the pathogenesis and progression of chronic injury in lupus nephritis by mediating interstitial injury.

Fig. 1.251 Lupus nephritis. A tubular interstitial nephritis in which there is evidence of tubulitis with lymphocytes invading the tubular epithelium sometimes accompanies the glomerular lesion. The eosinophils are often prominent in the infiltrate. The tubular interstitial disease in some instances progresses independently of the glomerular disease and can in and of itself lead to end stage renal disease (H&E, ×400).

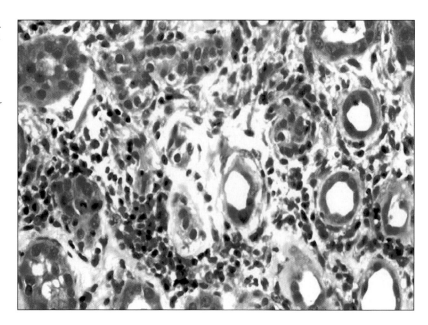

Assessment of severity and chronicity

Several studies have emphasized the importance of using semiquantitative biopsy analyses to assess the activity and severity of lupus nephritis. Disease activity has been related to the presence of necrosis, crescent formation, endocapillary and mesangial cellular proliferation, glomerular leukocytic infiltration, hyaline thrombi, and glomerular and interstitial inflammation (Table 1.2). Chronicity has been graded according to the degree of glomerulosclerosis and fibrosis as well as the amount of interstitial scarring and tubular atrophy. Although some authors have questioned the value of these indexes and their reproducibility, such an approach has been useful in studies of large groups of patients, and recent studies have suggested that quantification may be of value in assessing the prognosis for individual patients. Because application of these indexes is both observer and institution dependent, variations can occur between institutions. Within an institution, however, where greater standardization for the application of criteria can be accomplished, these indices are of value in following patients, particularly those who undergo serial or repeat biopsies.

The clinical value of renal biopsy in lupus nephritis appears to be well established. Some still question its usefulness, whereas others recommend it for every patient, even in the absence of clinical and laboratory data indicating renal involvement. On the other hand, most investigators agree that it is impossible to predict the types of severity and activity of renal lesions from any combination of clinical and laboratory findings alone. Further advances are needed in the treatment of severe lupus erythematosus both to reduce the current mortality rate of 10% to 20% after 10 years and to decrease the development of renal insufficiency during dialysis, which occurs in nearly 25% of patients. Close collaboration between the clinical nephrologist and the renal pathologist is most important in making appropriate therapeutic decisions in the application of new strategies. To the extent that findings from renal biopsy provide a rationale for the use of potentially toxic drugs, the procedure appears to be more than worthwhile. This team approach will help to reduce the current mortality rate and to decrease the development of renal insufficiency requiring dialysis.

Etiology/pathogenesis

The above lesions of Lupus correspond to the experimental lesions produced by immune complex deposition. The pathogenesis varies with the class of the lesion. The generation of relatively small numbers of stable immune complexes of intermediate size with antibodies having high affinity and high avidity accumulate in the mesangium as a result of the mesangial clearing system for removal of macromolecules. The relatively small number of complexes, which is characteristic of Class II, prevents the mesangial system from becoming overloaded and allows the complexes to be sequestered in the mesangium, where they are subject to degradation and removal rather than remaining at sites where they could initiate an inflammatory response Fibronectin is an important component of the mesangial matrix, and given its capacity to interact with aggregates of immunoglobulins and immune complexes in the circulation, its presence in the mesangium may play a role in this type of localization.

The localization of immune complexes to the subendothelial region as seen in Class III and IV have access to plasma inflammatory mediators initiating the severe glomerular nephritis that is seen in these forms of lupus nephropathy. Large numbers of intermediate-size complexes or large complexes that are formed by high-affinity antibodies likely overcome the mesangial ability to clear these macromolecules. As a result, these complexes accumulate in a paramesangial subendothelial location, and then ultimately in the peripheral capillary loops. The nature of the antigen and antibody also may contribute to the predominance of subendothelial localization in this class. Characteristics of certain antibodies, such as cationic charge, could permit binding of complexes that contain such antibodies to negative charges within the glomerular capillary wall, thus accounting for the nephrotropism. If the complexes are large and highly cationic, they will bind and fix to the closest anionic charges that are encountered at the subendothelial location. Following the initial binding of what might only be a small population of nephrotropic antibodies, activation of inflammatory cytokines can increase the permeability of the capillary wall, thus allowing other complexes to deposit.

The pathogenetic mechanism leading to membranous pattern of Lupus likely results from *in situ* formation of immune complexes. This suggests an immune response that is characterized by the presence of small, unstable, circulating immune complexes formed by low-avidity and low-affinity antibodies in the presence of antigen excess. Under such conditions, complexes may disassociate with the antigen or antibody lodging in the glomerular capillaries. Subsequently, complexes are formed *in situ* attaching to the target protein, which has been planted in the outer aspect of the glomerular basement membrane. Of particular importance is that histones are highly cationic and, potentially, have a high affinity for the anionic sites of the glomerular basement membrane. Once bound to the glomerular basement membrane, they can act as a target antigen and a focus for *in situ* complex formation. Because such epimembranous deposits also are sequestered from access to circulating inflammatory mediators, an inflammatory component with cellular infiltration is not present.

Selected reading

Appel G B, Radhakkrishnan Jai, D'Agati, V 2003 Secondary glomerular disease in the kidney, 7th edn. Saunders, London.

D'Agati, Vivette D 1998 Renal disease in systemic lupus erythematosus. In: Jennette J C, Olson J L, Schwartz M M, Silva F G (eds) Heptinstall's pathology of the kidney, 5th edn, Lippincott Raven, London.

Kashgarian M 2002 Lupus nephritis: Pathology, pathogenesis, clinical correlations and prognosis. In: Wallace D J, Hahn BH (eds) Dubois's lupus erythematosus, 6th edn. Lippincott Williams & Wilkins, London.

Diseases associated with the nephritic syndrome or RPGN

Henoch-Schoenlein purpura

Henoch-Schoenlein purpura is a form of IgA nephropathy with prominent extrarenal involvement. The clinical picture is that of an acute nephritis and is associated with the presence of purpuric lesions of the skin, arthritis and gastrointestinal hemorrhage. It is a multiorgan systemic vasculitis, which is immune complex-mediated by IgA rich immune complexes. It is largely a disease of children but reports of Henoch-Schoenlein purpura have encompassed the entire age range. Clinical manifestations of Henoch-Schoenlein purpura mimic those of systemic vasculitis of various types.

The histomorphology of Henoch-Schoenlein purpura is similar to that of other immune complex-mediated diseases. The lesions associated with Henoch-Schoenlein purpura are varied and range from a pure mesangial proliferative glomerulonephritis to a focal segmental necrotizing glomerulonephritis to a diffuse crescentic glomerulonephritis and a pattern similar to that of membrano-proliferative glomerulonephritis (Figs 1.252–1.258). The variety of lesions seen in Henoch-Schoenlein purpura is similar to that seen in lupus glomerulonephritis. Immunofluorescence microscopy is characterized by the deposition of IgA in glomeruli and depending on the severity of the lesion the pattern of the lesion may range from a mesangial distribution to a peripheral capillary distribution (Figs 1.259, 1.260). A feature which distinguishes Henoch-Schoenlein purpura from other forms of IgA nephropathy is the frequent presence of IgG and occasionally IgM. Complement components and fibrinogen coexist with the immunoglobulins. Electron microscopy is also varied. Abundant mesangial electron dense deposits are the most characteristic finding but subepithelial deposits and mesangial interposition are also present in severe cases (Figs 1.261–1.264).

Etiology/pathogenesis

Henoch-Schoenlein purpura is an immune complex disease characterized by the presence of immune complexes of IgA antibody and exogenous antigens. Exogenous antigens from food, drugs, and infections have all been implicated. Mucosal infec-

Fig. 1.252 Henoch-Schoenlein purpura. The glomerulus shows evidence of lobular accentuation, mesangial hypercellularity and focal thickening of the peripheral capillary walls (H&E, ×400).

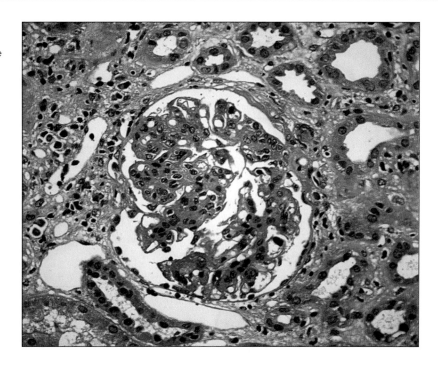

Fig. 1.253 Henoch-Schoenlein purpura. Glomerulus demonstrates moderate diffuse mesangial proliferation with an early epithelial crescent (PAS, ×400).

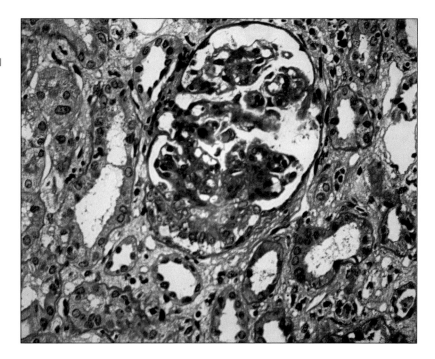

Fig. 1.254 Henoch-Schoenlein purpura. There is an adhesion to Bowman's capsule, early crescent formation and an increase in mesangial matrix. The pattern is segmental (Jones, ×400)

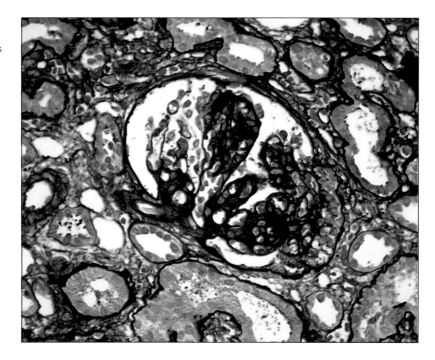

Fig. 1.255 Henoch-Schoenlein purpura. There is segmental necrosis with accumulation of fibrinoid material. The remainder of the glomerulus shows mesangial hypercellularity and an increase in matrix (Trichrome, ×400).

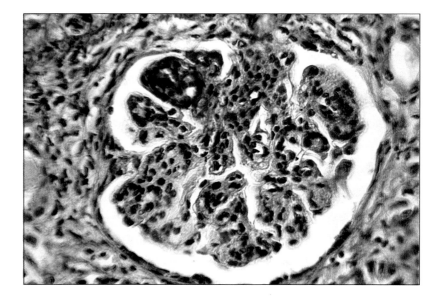

Fig. 1.256 Henoch-Schoenlein purpura. A later stage demonstrates more extensive mesangial sclerosis in addition to the continued presence of fragmented red blood cells and leukocytes within the capillary lumina (Trichrome, ×400).

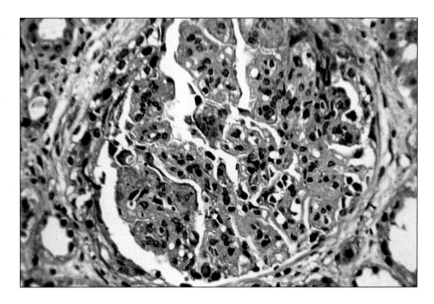

Fig. 1.257 Henoch-Schoenlein purpura. Segmental sclerosis is prominent with loss of the normal architecture. The remainder of the glomerulus appears to have a somewhat less degree of hypercellularity (Trichrome, ×400).

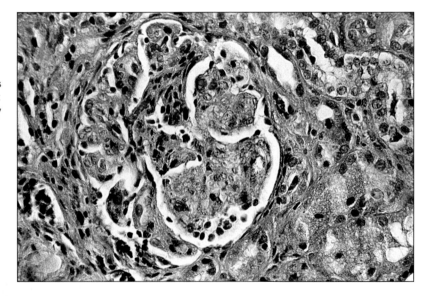

Fig. 1.258 Henoch-Schoenlein purpura. A more severe example where global glomerular necrosis is present with abundant fibrin within Bowman's space (Jones, ×400).

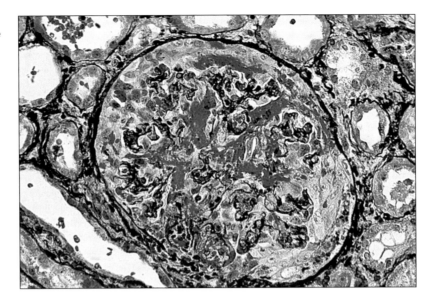

Fig. 1.259 Henoch-Schoenlein purpura. Immunofluorescence demonstrates diffuse deposition of IgA. (anti-IgA immunofluorescence, ×400).

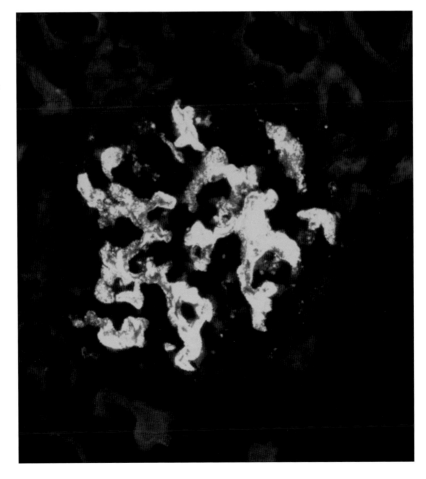

Fig. 1.260 Henoch-Schoenlein purpura. IgG is also present in a similar diffuse pattern (anti-IgG immunofluorescence).

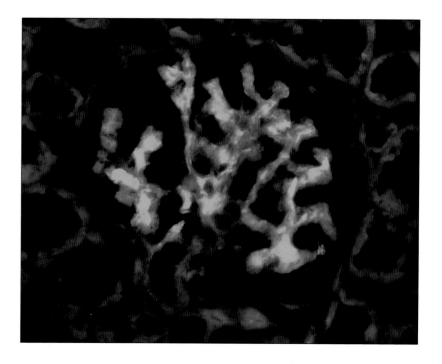

Fig. 1.261 Henoch-Schoenlein purpura. Electron microscopy reveals an increase in mesangial cellularity with the presence of mesangial deposits. The capillary lumina are occluded by the presence of numerous leukocytes (TEM, ×3000).

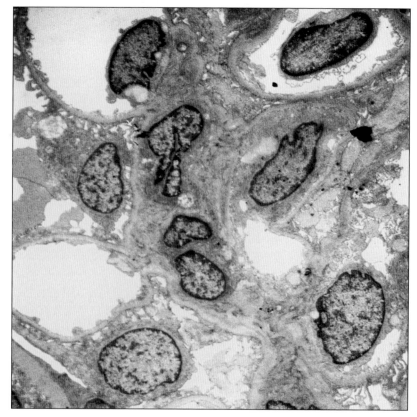

Fig. 1.262 Henoch-Schoenlein purpura. The endothelial cells are swollen and there are subendothelial electron dense deposits corresponding to IgA, IgG deposits seen on immunofluorescence (TEM, ×5000)

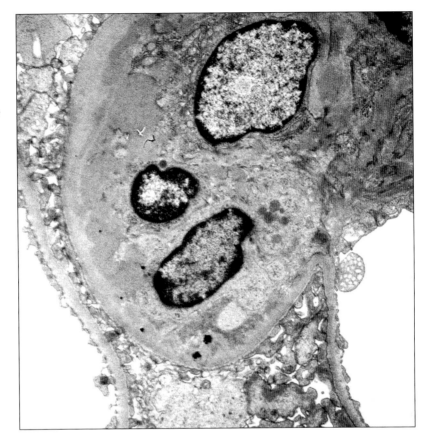

tions of the upper respiratory tract and gastrointestinal tract have been of special interest as these are the sites of IgA-mediated immunity.

Selected reading

Pillebout E, Thervet E, Hill G et al 2002 Henoch-Schoenlein purpura in adults: Outcome and prognostic factors. Journal of the American Society of Nephrology 13:1271–1278.

Fig. 1.263 Henoch-Schoenlein purpura. Subepithelial deposits resembling humps are also occasionally seen. The capillary lumen demonstrates a leukocyte, which has stripped the endothelium away from the basement membrane (TEM, ×5000).

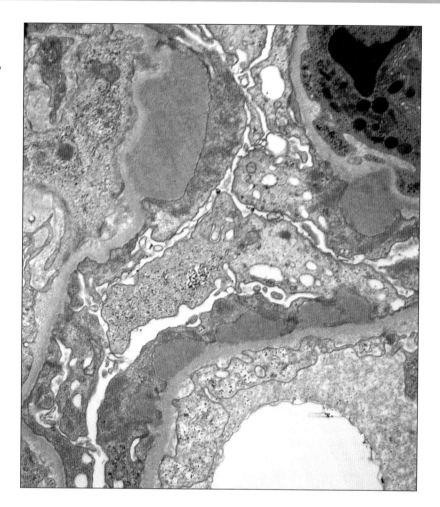

Fig. 1.264 Henoch-Schoenlein purpura. Mesangial deposits are universally present. In this image, a leukocyte can be seen in the mesangial area as well as the presence of subendothelial deposits in the adjacent capillary loop with endothelial cell swelling. There is also focal effacement of the epithelial foot processes (TEM, ×5000).

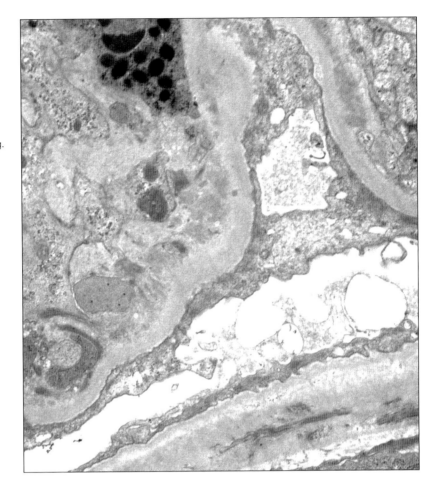

Diseases associated with the nephrotic/nephritic syndrome

Mixed connective tissue disease

Mixed connective tissue disease (MCTD) is an overlap syndrome carrying features of systemic lupus erythematosus (SLE), progressive systemic sclerosis (PSS) and polymyositis. Serologically, it is distinguished from SLE and PSS by high titer antinuclear antibodies and antibodies to a saline extractable nuclear antigen that is ribonuclease sensitive. Clinical features include a variety of systemic manifestations, similar to SLE and PSS. Renal manifestations are relatively uncommon. The clinical manifestations of renal involvement are variable in degrees of proteinuria including a full-blown nephrotic syndrome. A few patients have marked hypertension and microangiopathic hemolytic anemia.

The most common pattern of renal pathology in MCTD is a membranous nephropathy (Figs 1.265–1.269). As in lupus, there are usually mesangial deposits and some degree of mesangial proliferation. Immunofluorescence studies typically reveal granular capillary

Fig. 1.265 Membranous nephropathy in mixed connective tissue disease (MCTD). The pattern is similar to that seen in lupus with lobular accentuation and diffuse thickening of the basement membranes (H&E, ×400).

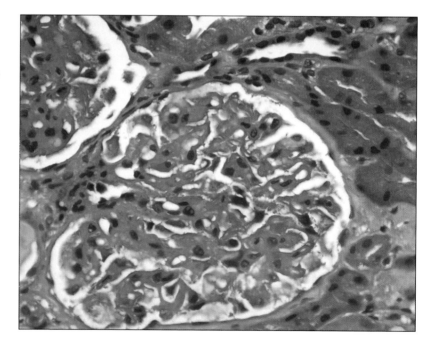

Fig. 1.266 Membranous nephropathy in MCTD. Silver methenamine Masson stain demonstrates thickening of the capillary walls and a typical spike and dome appearance (Jones, ×400).

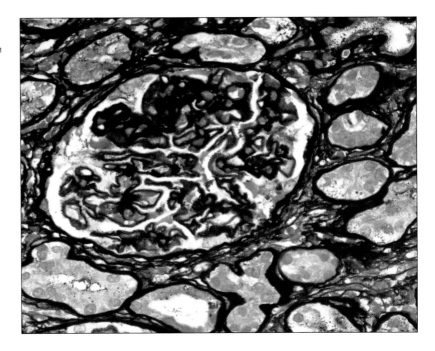

Fig. 1.267 Membranous nephropathy in MCTD. Trichrome stain demonstrates diffuse thickening and the presence of eosinophilic deposits in the basement membranes (Trichrome, ×400).

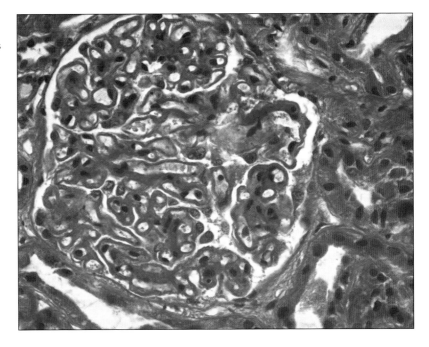

Fig. 1.268 Membranous nephropathy in MCTD. Electron micrograph demonstrates diffuse thickening of the basement membrane with patent capillary loops. Numerous subepithelial and intramembranous deposits are present (TEM, ×3000).

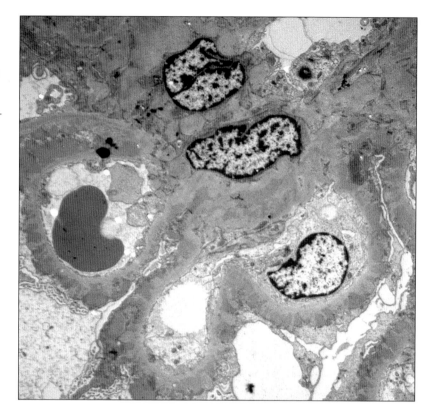

staining for IgG and C3 and occasionally IgA and IgM (Fig. 1.270). Less commonly, the renal lesion is a diffuse mesangial proliferative glomerulonephritis (Figs 1.271, 1.272). Rarely, a few cases demonstrate subendothelial deposits and have a more diffuse membranoproliferative pattern (Figs 1.273–1.275). The renal findings essentially parallel those in lupus with a more prominent involvement of membranous lesions. Vascular lesions are similar to those of systemic sclerosis (Fig. 1.276).

Etiology/pathogenesis

Mixed connective tissue disease is an autoimmune disease with prominent development of antibodies to ribonuclear proteins. The etiology and pathogenesis of the renal lesions are essentially similar to that of lupus nephritis (see section on SLE).

Fig. 1.269 Membranous nephropathy in MCTD. High-powered electron micrograph demon-strates the presence of numerous electron dense deposits (TEM, ×10,000).

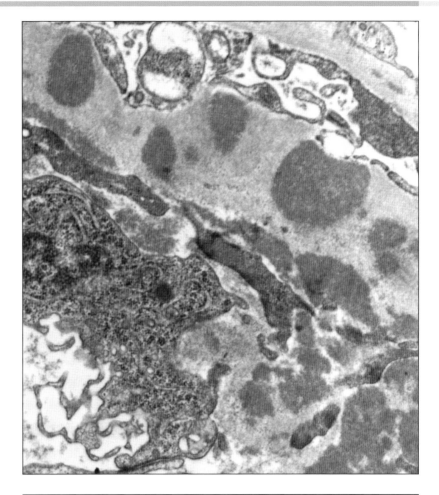

Fig. 1.270 Membranous nephropathy in MCTD. Immunofluorescence studies typically reveal a peripheral granular staining for IgM and IgA (anti-IgM immunofluorescence, ×400).

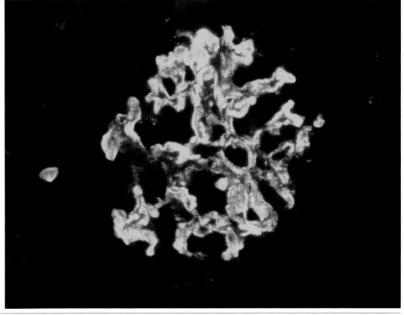

Fig. 1.271 Mesangial proliferative glomerulonephritis in mixed connective tissue disease. There is diffuse mesangial hyperplasia, peripheral capillary loops are well preserved, leukocytic infiltration is not prominent (HPS, ×200).

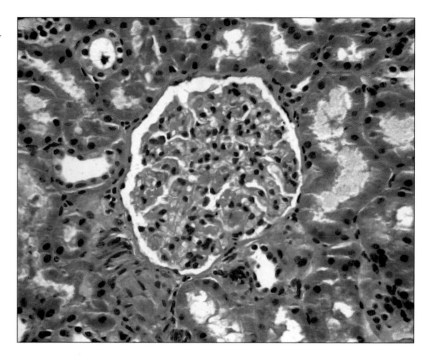

Fig. 1.272 Mesangial proliferative GN in MCTD. There is increase in mesangial cellularity and matrix. (PAS, ×200).

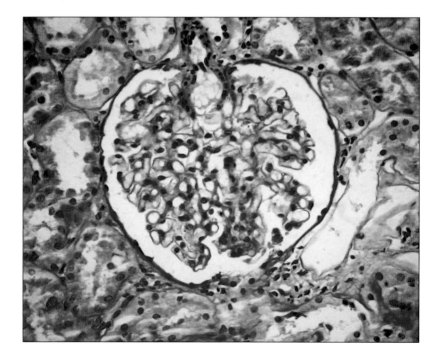

Fig. 1.273 Membranoproliferative glomerulonephritis in mixed connective tissue disease. The pattern here is similar to that seen in lupus erythematosus with lobular accentuation increase in mesangial cellularity and matrix and mesangialization of the peripheral capillary loops (PAS, ×400).

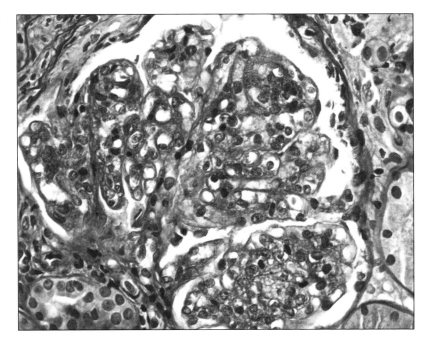

Fig. 1.274 MPGN in MCTD. Immunofluorescence demonstrates the presence of immunoglobulins in a mesangial and peripheral capillary pattern (anti-IgG immunofluorescence, ×200).

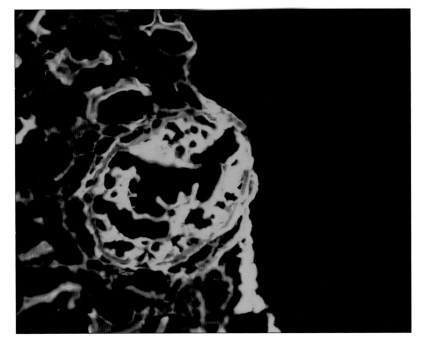

Fig. 1.275 MPGN in MCTD. Electron microscopy demonstrates mesangial deposits and paramesangial subendothelial deposits (TEM, ×5000).

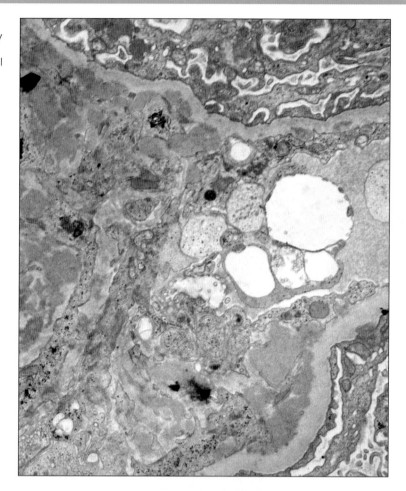

Fig. 1.276 MCTD. The vascular changes are similar to those of systemic sclerosis with concentric hyperplasia of the media (H&E, ×400).

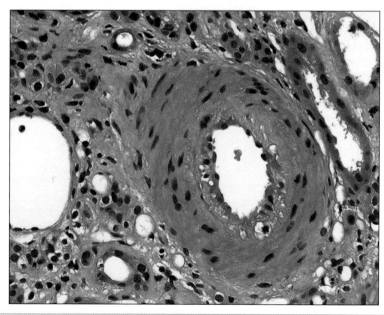

Selected reading

Cohen A H, Weiss M A 1986 Renal pathology forum. American Journal of Nephrology 6:51–56.

Kobayashi S, Nagase M, Kimura M et al 1985 Renal involvement in MCTD. American Journal of Nephrology 5:282–291.

Diseases associated with the nephritic syndrome

Mixed cryoglobulinemia

Three types of cryoglobulinemic disease have been described, two of which are related to monoclonal antibodies including monoclonal IgM and are described elsewhere. Mixed cryoglobulinemia or Type III is the result of the presence of polyclonal antibodies involving both components of the cryoglobulin.

By light microscopy, the pattern is identical to that seen in Type I membranoproliferative glomerulonephritis (Figs 1.277, 1.278). The glomeruli are enlarged, have lobular accentuation and have varying degrees of leukocytic infiltration. Double contours of the peripheral capillaries can be seen and capillary lumina contain eosinophilic deposits that correspond to the circulating cryoglobulins (Fig. 1.279). They are often referred to as hyaline thrombi or cryo plugs. There are

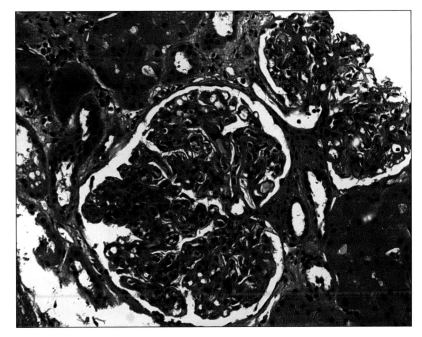

Fig. 1.277 Mixed Cryoglobulinemia. Glomerulus from the biopsy of a patient with cryoglobulinemia. There is lobular accentuation of the glomerular architecture with an increase in mesangial cellularity and matrix. The capillaries are pushed to the periphery and mesangialization of the capillaries can be identified (H&E, ×400).

Fig. 1.278 Mixed cryoglobulinemia. Trichrome stain shows the lobular accentuation, evidence of mesangialization with capillaries filled with leukocytes. Hyaline thrombi area also seen within some capillary lumina (Trichrome stain, ×400).

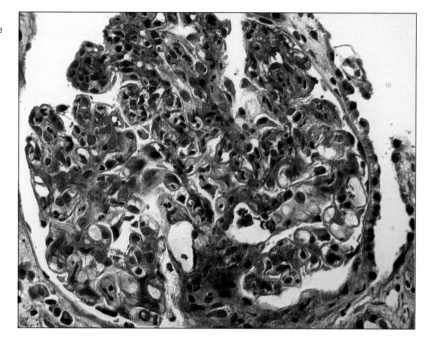

Fig. 1.279 Mixed cryoglobulinemia. Silver stains show evidence of reduplication of the capillary basement membrane consistent with mesangialization of the peripheral capillary loops (Jones, ×400).

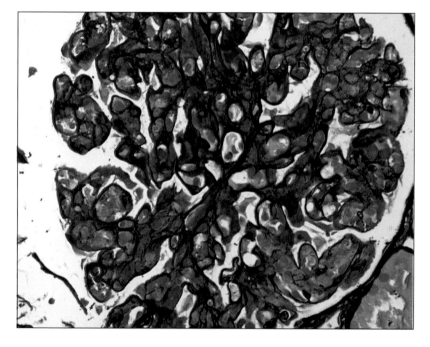

no distinguishing morphologic features to separate Type III mixed cryoglobulinemia from the other forms. Immunofluorescence microscopy demonstrates the presence of IgM and IgG as well as complement components. In cryoglobulin-related GN, IgM may be more prominent than other Igs. When a monoclonal component is present, there may be predominance of either kappa or lambda (Figs 1.280–1.282). Electron microscopy reveals a pattern similar to that seen with Type I membranoproliferative glomerulonephritis

Fig. 1.280 Mixed cryoglobulinemia. Immuno-fluorescence demonstrates the presence of IgM in a peripheral capillary and mesangial pattern. The peripheral capillary pattern is markedly granular (anti-IgM immunofluorescence, ×400).

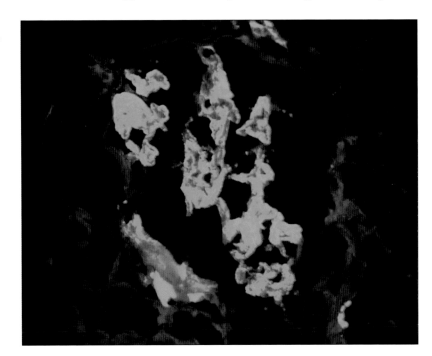

Fig. 1.281 Mixed cryoglobulinemia. Immuno-fluorescence microscopy also demonstrates the presence of IgG. Comple-ment is present in a similar pattern (anti-IgG immuno-fluorescence, ×400).

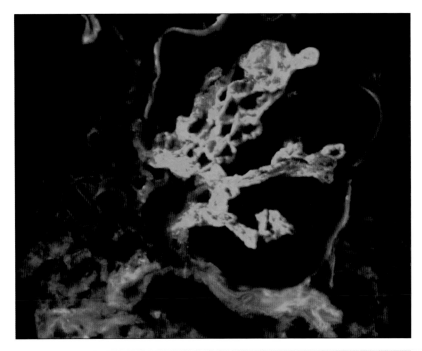

Fig. 1.282 Mixed cryoglobulinemia. When a monoclonal component is present, either kappa or lambda chain staining is seen in a similar peripheral pattern (anti-kappa immunofluorescence, ×400).

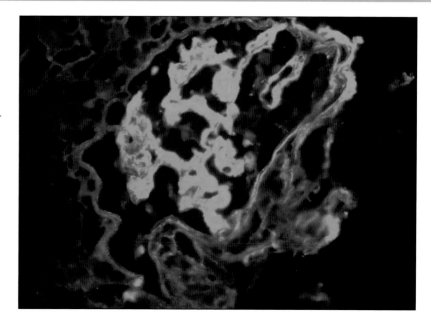

Fig. 1.283 Mixed cryoglobulinemia. Electron microscopy reveals evidence of mesangialization of the peripheral capillary loops with the presence of abundant subendothelial deposits. The capillary lumina are filled with leukocytes (TEM, ×3000).

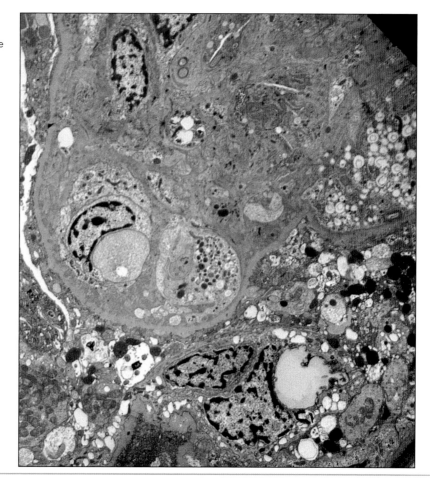

(Figs 1.283–1.285). One distinguishing feature seen in cryoglobulinemia is the presence of organized deposits. Deposits have a crystalline structure and sometimes a tubular configuration (Figs 1.286, 1.287). Once again, there are no distinguishing features to separate out Type III cryoglobulinemia on a morphologic basis and the diagnosis of the specific type of cryoglobulin is made on analysis of the serum cryoglobulins.

Etiology/pathogenesis

The pathogenesis of the renal lesions is similar to that of the other types of cryoglobulin-associated disease but is distinguished by the presence of antibodies which are polyclonal and specific for an antigen. Mixed cryoglobulins have been described in a variety of connective tissue diseases, infections, and malignancies. A link with hepatitis C infection has emerged in the last several years.

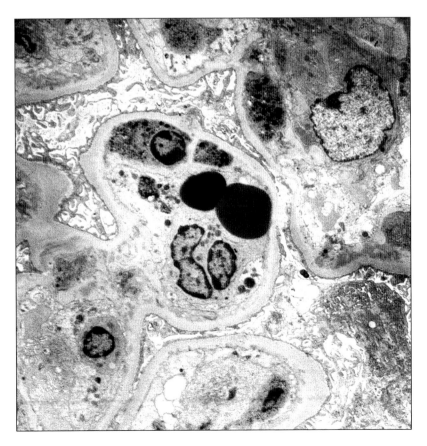

Fig. 1.284 Mixed cryoglobulinemia. Leukocytic infiltration with occlusion of the capillary lumen is prominent (TEM, ×3000).

Fig. 1.285 Mixed cryoglobulinemia. There is marked endothelial cell swelling and the sub-endothelial deposits have an irregular organized appearance (TEM, ×8000).

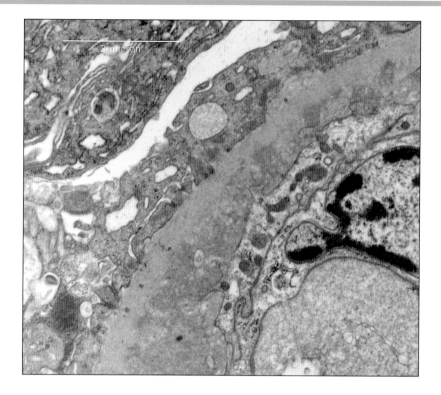

Fig. 1.286 Mixed cryoglobulinemia. The hyaline thrombi seen on light microscopy consist of large deposits with an organized tubular appearance by EM. (TEM, ×12,000).

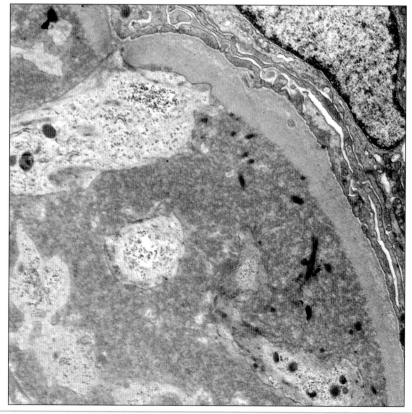

Fig. 1.287 Mixed cryoglobulinemia. The sub-endothelial deposits have the organized appearance characteristic of cryoglobulinemia (TEM, ×6000).

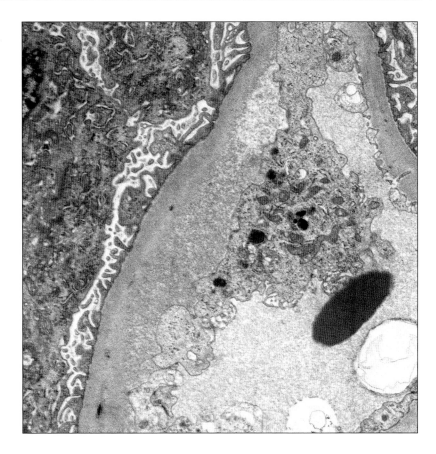

Selected reading

Brouet J C, Clauvel J P, Danon F et al 1974 Biological and clinical significance of cryoglobulins. A report of 86 cases. American Journal of Medicine 57:775–788.

D'Amico G, Colasanti G, Ferrario F, Sinico RA 1989 Renal involvement in mixed cryoglobulinemia. Kidney International 35:1004–1014.

Anti-GBM-antibody mediated glomerulonephritis

Patients with anti-GBM-antibody mediated glomerulonephritis typically present with rapidly progressive glomerulonephritis. Patients may have isolated renal disease and inconspicuous or absent pulmonary symptoms. The antibody may cross-react in some patients with alveolar basement membranes and cause pulmonary hemorrhage (Goodpasture's syndrome). Men are affected more commonly than women. The disease occurs at any age, but is more common in adults aged 20–40 years. A flu-like illness may precede the onset of Goodpasture syndrome.

By light microscopy, the glomeruli show breaks of the GBM due to fibrinoid necrosis (Figs 1.288–1.290). In very early disease, crescents may not be apparent. This early stage is typically seen in patients who present with severe, life-threatening lung disease, who undergo renal biopsy for more specific and sensitive diagnosis of Goodpasture syndrome than possible by lung biopsy. Cellular crescents develop consequent to the GBM breaks (Fig. 1.291). The glomerular basement membrane shows ischemic corrugation with ruptures, with no apparent deposits or proliferation (Fig. 1.292). With ongoing disease, Bowman's capsule ruptures, and there is periglomerular fibrosis and organization of the cellular crescent to a fibrocellular and ultimately fibrous crescent (Fig. 1.293). The interstitium shows lymphoplasmacytic infiltrate particularly around crescentic glomeruli with Bowman's capsule rupture and interstitial

Fig. 1.288 There is segmental necrosis with a break of the glomerular basement membrane, and fibrinoid necrosis and PMNs in this area, with a cellular crescent developing in response to this GBM break. The remainder of the glomerulus is unremarkable without proliferation and without deposits. Differentiation from other causes of crescentic glomerulonephritis without evident proliferation by light microscopy is made by immunofluorescence, which demonstrates linear staining for IgG in anti-GBM antibody-mediated disease.

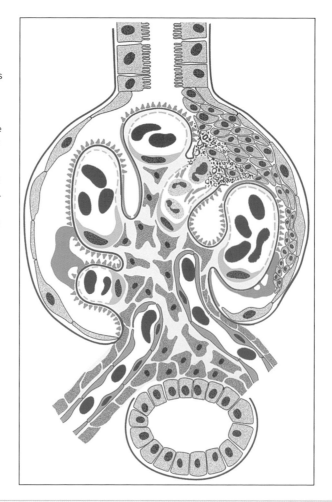

Fig. 1.289 Anti-GBM antibody-mediated glomerulonephritis. There is evident segmental necrosis in both glomeruli, with uninvolved segments of the glomeruli showing no proliferation or evidence of immune complexes. There is early cellular crescent formation (Jones' silver stain, ×100).

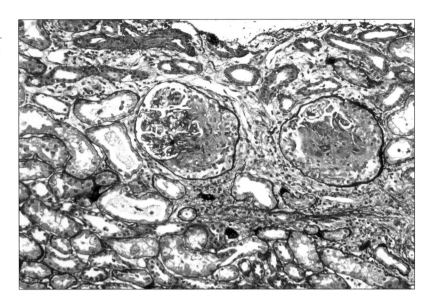

Fig. 1.290 Anti-GBM antibody-mediated glomerulonephritis. Early segmental fibrinoid necrosis is present, with glomerular basement membrane rupture. There is not yet a cellular crescentic reaction. The remaining portion of the glomerulus shows no proliferation or evidence of immune complexes (Jones' silver stain, ×400).

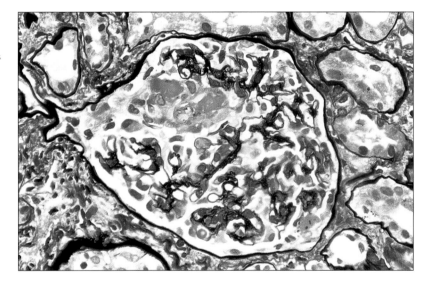

fibrosis and tubular atrophy developing. Although fibrinoid necrosis may extend from the glomerular tuft to the arteriole at the hilum, the interlobular and larger arteries do not show vasculitic lesions.

Immunofluorescence microscopy is diagnostic, revealing strong, linear glomerular basement membrane staining for IgG (Fig. 1.294). C3 is positive in nearly all cases, but is usually weaker than IgG and may be discontinuous or even granular (Fig. 1.295). Very rare cases

Fig. 1.291 Anti-GBM antibody-mediated glomerulonephritis. There is fibrinoid necrosis with karyorrhexis and ruptured fragments of GBM, with a small remaining intact portion of the glomerulus at the top. There is surrounding cellular crescent formation, and periglomerular inflammatory infiltrate (Jones' silver stain, ×400).

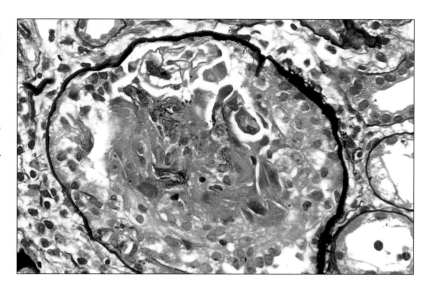

Fig. 1.292 Anti-GBM antibody-mediated glomerulonephritis. The right half of the glomerulus is completely preserved, while the left half shows glomerular basement membrane ruptures, with corrugation and cellular crescent (Jones' silver stain, ×400).

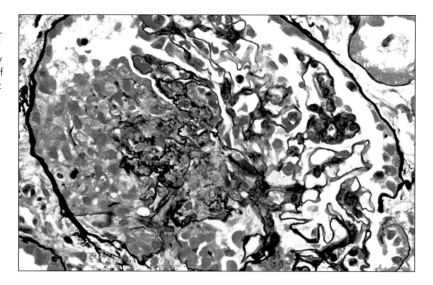

of other immunoglobulin anti-GBM antibodies have been described, with case reports of linear IgA or IgM in apparent anti-GBM-antibody mediated glomerulonephritis. Occasionally, anti-GBM antibodies may cross-react with tubular basement membranes, resulting in linear tubular basement membrane staining (Fig. 1.296). This may contribute to an interstitial nephritis.

By electron microscopy, no deposits are detected (Fig. 1.297). This may reflect the uniform distribution of the antigen, the non-collagenous (NC1) domain of alpha 3(IV) collagen, and/or that

Fig. 1.293 Anti-GBM antibody-mediated glomerulonephritis. In this more advanced lesion, there is corrugation and rupture of glomerular basement membrane with early fibrocellular organization of the crescent and rupture of Bowman's capsule with corresponding fibrinoid necrosis and surrounding periglomerular inflammation (Jones' silver stain, ×400).

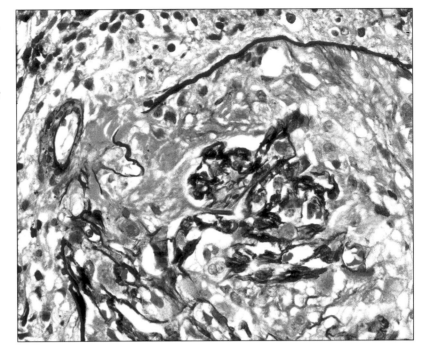

Fig. 1.294 Anti-GBM antibody-mediated glomerulonephritis. Linear glomerular basement membrane staining with IgG is diagnostic of this disease in this setting (anti-IgG immunofluorescence, ×400).

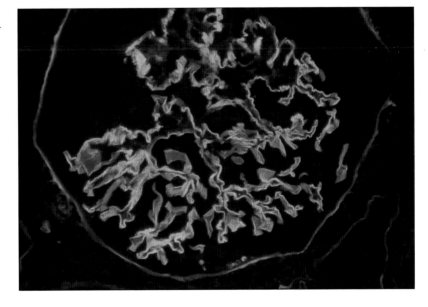

these uniformly distributed deposits have the same density as the GBM. IgG antibody has been identified along the lamina interna of the GBM by immuno-electron microscopy. Breaks in the glomerular basement membrane may be detected by EM (Fig. 1.298), along with fibrin tactoids reflecting the segmental fibrinoid necrosis.

Fig. 1.295 Anti-GBM antibody-mediated glomerulonephritis. Linear staining for C3 typically accompanies the IgG staining in cases of anti-GBM antibody-mediated glomerulonephritis, a useful feature to distinguish from the linear accentuation and staining with IgG that may occur in diabetic nephropathy (anti-C3 immunofluorescence, ×400).

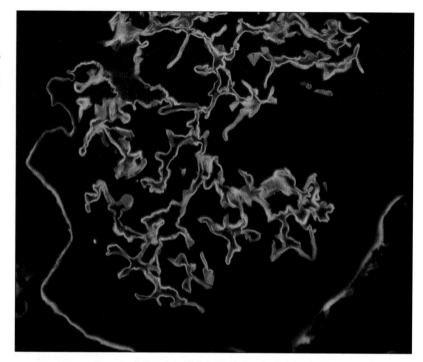

Fig. 1.296 Anti-GBM antibody-mediated glomerulonephritis. The antibody directed against the GBM may sometimes cross-react with the tubular basement membrane, as in this case, and may then be causal in an associated interstitial nephritis and tubular injury (anti-IgG immunofluorescence, ×400).

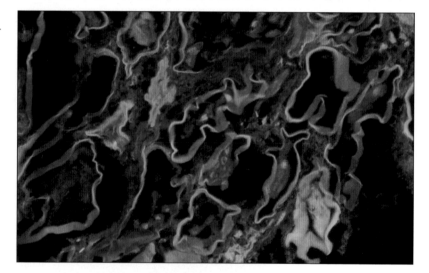

Etiology/pathogenesis

Anti-GBM-antibody mediated glomerulonephritis is due to the development of autoantibody against the noncollagenous C-terminal (NC1) domain of alpha 3(IV) collagen. The antibody to glomerular basement membrane cross-reacts with lung basement membrane, giving rise in some patients to combined pulmonary and renal

Fig. 1.297 Anti-GBM antibody-mediated glomerulonephritis. Electron microscopy shows no discrete immune complexes since the antigen, the noncollagenous domain of α3 collagen, is a diffusely distributed integral part of the type IV collagen of the glomerular basement membrane. Only mild foot process effacement and segmental corrugation are present in this glomerulus (TEM, ×6000).

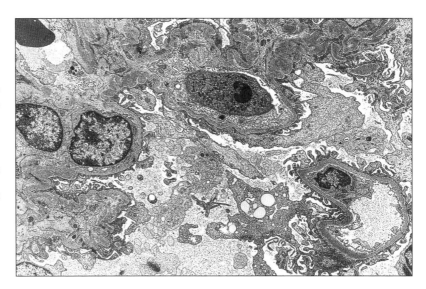

Fig. 1.298 Anti-GBM antibody-mediated glomerulonephritis. Electron microscopy may sometimes demonstrate the glomerular basement membrane breaks also seen by light microscopy, as demonstrated here. There are associated fibrin tactoids (TEM, ×8000).

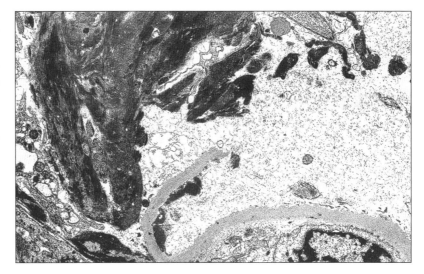

lesions. The development of disease sometimes is preceded by a flu-like illness or hydrocarbon or solvent exposure, suggesting the possibility that alveolar antigens may have become exposed and caused an autoimmune response. A similar histologic pattern may occur in some patients with Alport syndrome and renal transplantation, who develop autoantibodies against normal type IV collagen in the transplanted kidney (see Alport syndrome). Anti-GBM-antibody mediated glomerulonephritis can rarely recur in the transplant, usually when antibody titers remain high (Fig. 1.299).

Fig. 1.299 Anti-GBM antibody-mediated glomerulonephritis. When antibody titers persist at time of transplantation, this disease may occasionally recur in the transplant, as in this case, where linear anti-GBM antibody staining was associated with mild glomerular injury. Note the associated linear tubular basement membrane staining (anti-IgG immunofluorescence, ×200).

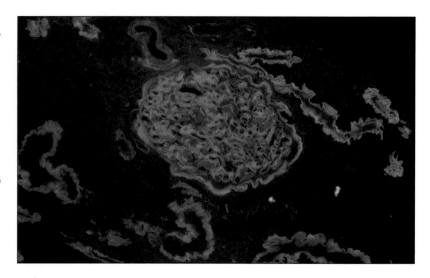

Interestingly, the appellation Goodpasture's syndrome by Drs Stanton and Tange did not meet with Dr Goodpasture's approval, in that he deduced that the young man whom he described with pulmonary-renal syndrome during the 1919 influenza epidemic did not have anti-GBM-antibody-mediated disease.

Selected reading

Couser W G 1988 Rapidly progressive glomerulonephritis: classification, pathogenetic mechanisms, and therapy. American Journal of Kidney Disease 11(6):449–464.

Goodpasture W 1919 The significance of certain pulmonary lesions in relation to the etiology of influenza. American Journal of Medical Science 158:863–870.

Levy J B, Lachmann R H, Pusey C D 1996 Recurrent Goodpasture's disease. American Journal of Kidney Disease 27(4):573–578.

Saus J, Wieslander J, Langeveld J P et al 1988 Identification of the Goodpasture antigen as the alpha 3(IV) chain of collagen IV. Journal of Biology and Chemistry 263(26):13374–13380.

Savage C O, Pusey C D, Bowman C et al 1986 Antiglomerular basement membrane antibody mediated disease in the British Isles 1980–4. British Medical Journal 292(6516):301–304.

Stanton M C, Tange J D 1958 Goodpasture's syndrome (pulmonary haemorrhage associated with glomerulonephritis). Aust Ann Med 7:132–144.

Wilson C B, Dixon F J 1973 Anti-glomerular basement membrane antibody-induced glomerulonephritis. Kidney International 3(2):74–89.

Diseases associated with the nephritic syndrome or RPGN: pauci-immune- or non-immune-mediated

Introduction

Rapidly progressive glomerulonephritis is a variant of the acute nephritic syndrome in which patients initially present with acute glomerulonephritis associated with a rapid onset of severe acute renal failure. The onset of the disease is characterized by oliguria, advancing azotemia, proteinuria of varying amounts, hematuria with cellular casts and hypertension which is sometimes in the malignant range. The nephrotic syndrome is occasionally present. In a few patients, renal function eventually stabilizes at an impaired level after several weeks, but in most patients, progression to end-stage renal insufficiency occurs. The clinical pathologic entity can be divided into three subgroups. These include patients with post-infectious immune complex glomerulonephritis of a severe nature and patients with an antibody to glomerular basement membranes. These are discussed elsewhere in this atlas. The third group has been termed pauci-immune in that antibody deposition is not present and no definite relationship to a particular antigen has been identified, although 80% of patients in this group have the presence of an anti-neutrophil cytoplasmic antibody (ANCA) directed against either myeloperoxidase or serine protease in their serum. Pauci-immune glomerulonephritis with positive serum ANCA encompasses four subgroups. These include patients with renal involvement alone, patients with renal and systemic involvement by microscopic polyangiitis, patients with Wegener's granulomatosis (Fig. 1.300) and patients with Churg-Strauss syndrome. The histopathology is similar in all forms of pauci-immune glomerulonephritis.

Wegener's granulomatosis/microscopic polyangiitis

Light microscopy demonstrates the presence of a necrotizing glomerulonephritis accompanied with an active interstitial nephritis (Figs 1.301–1.303). Vascular necrosis may also be present with a transmural vasculitis (Figs 1.304, 1.305). Glomerular necrosis may be focal and segmental or diffuse and global (Figs 1.306, 1.307). Glomerular necrosis is uniformly accompanied by crescents.

Fig. 1.300 Pauci-immune crescentic glomerulonephritis. There is segmental necrosis with a break of the glomerular basement membrane, and fibrinoid necrosis and PMNs in this area, with a cellular crescent developing in response to this GBM break. The remainder of the glomerulus is unremarkable without proliferation and without deposits.

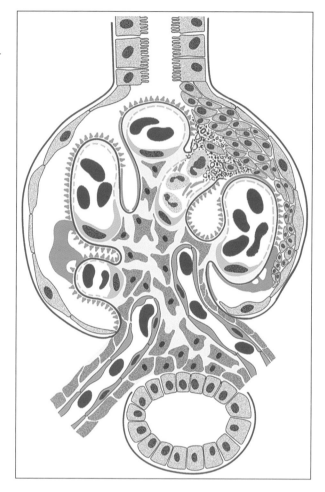

The crescents may be cellular or fibrous depending on the stage of evolution of the glomerular lesion (Fig. 1.308). The crescents consist of accumulations of cells derived from the parietal epithelium and infiltrating monocytes in Bowman's space and they appear to be initiated by the deposition of fibrin across gaps or disruptive lesions of the glomerular capillary with extrusion of fibrin into Bowman's space. As the crescents mature, fibroblasts with collagen begin to replace the cells and become fibroepithelial and finally fibrous crescents are formed. Segmental areas of necrosis of the glomerular capillaries are usually present as well as areas of glomerular capillary collapse and focal increases in mesangial matrix. The necrosis and inflammation may extend through Bowman's capsule and form a granulomatous glomerulonephritis (Fig. 1.309). The light microscopic picture is similar in all three types of pathogenic mechanisms

Fig. 1.301 Wegener's granulomatosis. There is a diffuse interstitial infiltrate with marked tubular epithelial changes. A vessel shows evidence of vascular necrosis within the wall. The glomeruli show evidence of focal necrosis with adhesion and crescent formation (H&E, ×100).

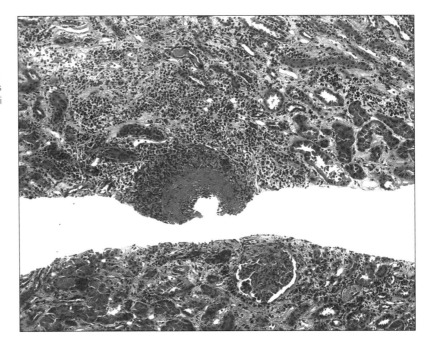

Fig. 1.302 Wegener's granulomatosis. Two glomeruli demonstrating evidence of glomerular necrosis with dense inflammatory reaction extending into the interstitium with a granulomatous appearance (H&E, ×200).

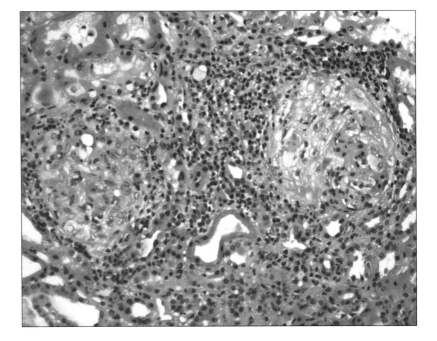

that are better characterized on the basis of immunofluorescence and electron microscopy. However, immune complex-related crescentic disease typically shows mesangial or endocapillary proliferation, depending on the underlying condition, whereas the pauci-

Fig. 1.303 Wegener's granulomatosis/microscopic polyangiitis. The interstitial inflammatory infiltrate consists of mononuclear cells and has an abundant eosinophilic component with evidence of tubulitis (H&E, ×200).

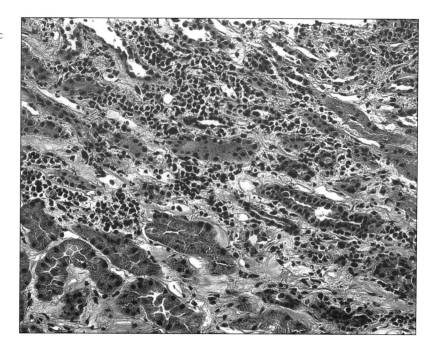

Fig. 1.304 Wegener's granulomatosis/microscopic polyangiitis. Vessel showing focal transmural necrosis extending into the interstitium with a granulomatous interstitial infiltrate (Trichrome, ×200).

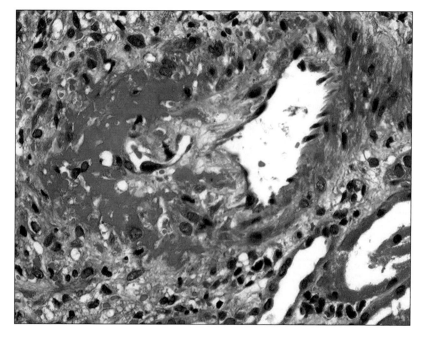

immune disease does not show significant proliferation of uninvolved glomeruli or segments thereof. Of note, granulomas do not typically occur in the kidney in Wegener's granulomatosis, but rather are present in bronchioles. Thus, microscopic polyangiitis

Fig. 1.305 Wegener's granulomatosis/microscopic polyangiitis. Vessel with transmural necrosis involving the vessels circumferentially with a significant inflammatory infiltrate with mixed polymorphonuclear leukocytes and mononuclear cells (H&E, ×200).

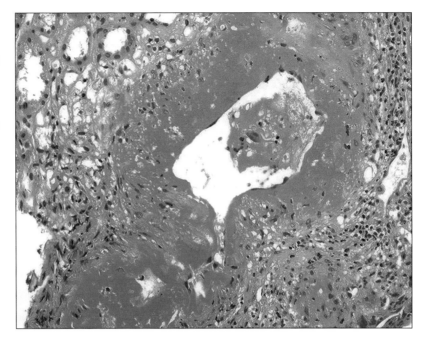

Fig. 1.306 Wegener's granulomatosis/microscopic polyangiitis. Glomerulus demonstrating focal and segmental necrosis with adhesion to Bowman's capsule and proliferation of parietal epithelium (HPS, ×400).

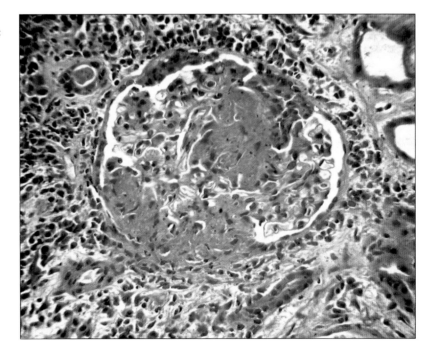

Fig. 1.307 Wegener's granulomatosis/microscopic polyangiitis. A globally necrotic glomerulus with total obliteration of the architecture and infiltration with numerous leukocytes (H&E, ×400)

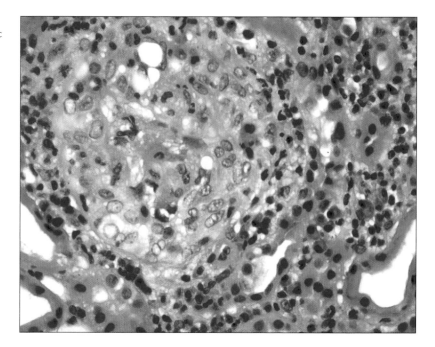

Fig. 1.308 Wegener's granulomatosis/microscopic polyangiitis. Trichrome stain demonstrates the residual portions of the glomerulus and the entire Bowman's space is filled with proliferating epithelial cells and infiltrating monocytes (Trichrome, ×400).

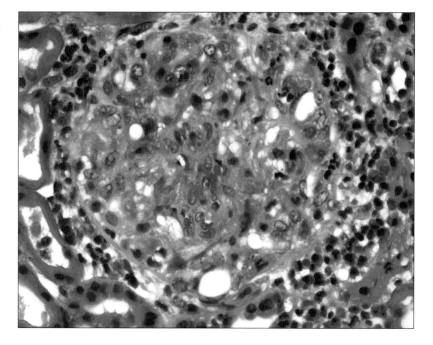

and Wegener's granulomatosis appear identical in the kidney and must be distin-guished based on clinical criteria.

By immunofluorescence the findings are variable. No specific immunoglobulin deposition is identified by immunofluorescence microscopy. Complement components and fibrinogen may be present focally and are usually seen in association with the crescents (Figs 1.310–1.312). This relative lack of immunoglobulin deposition has given rise to the term pauci-immune.

Fig. 1.309 Wegener's granulomatosis/microscopic polyangiitis. A glomerulus with global necrosis surrounded by a granulomatous inflammatory infiltrate. (H&E, ×400).

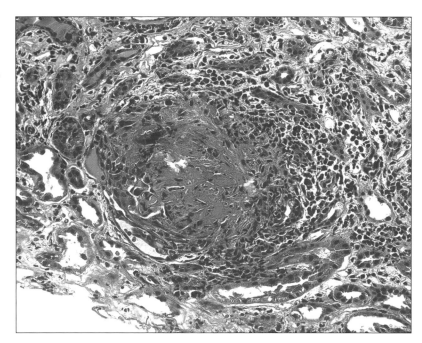

Fig. 1.310 Wegener's granulomatosis/microscopic polyangiitis. Immunofluorescence reveals that the crescent is associated with abundant fibrin deposition (anti-fibrin immunofluorescence, ×400).

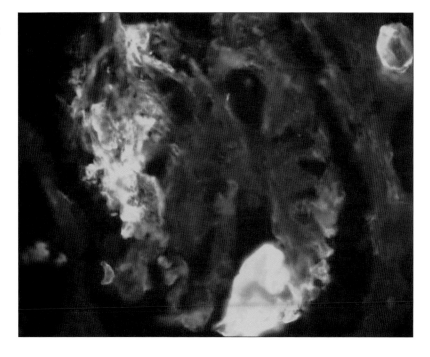

Fig. 1.311 Wegener's granulomatosis/microscopic polyangiitis. Fibrin deposition is also present in a segmental fashion in the capillaries (anti-fibrin immunofluorescence, ×400).

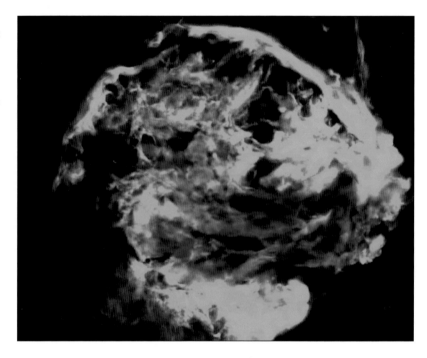

Fig. 1.312 Wegener's granulomatosis/microscopic polyangiitis. Complement is also occasionally seen in association with necrosis and fibrin deposition (anti-C3 immunofluorescence, ×400).

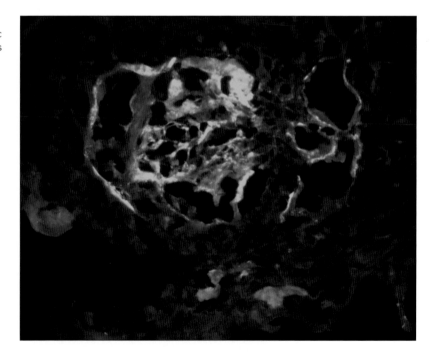

Electron microscopy findings are also variable. Patients with pauci-immune disease do not demonstrate electron dense deposits. In most instances, fibrin deposition is prominent and is often associated with breaks within the capillary wall and the basement membrane (Figs 1.313–1.315). Electron microscopy is also helpful in separating primary forms of crescentic glomerulonephritis from the miscellaneous immune complex-associated diseases described elsewhere, which also can display crescents by light microscopy.

Etiology/pathogenesis

The role of anti-neutrophil cytoplasmic antibody (ANCA) in the pathogenesis of glomerulonephritis is still incompletely understood. *In vivo* and *in vitro* studies indicate that the pathogenesis of ANCA-associated glomerulonephritis involves activation of neutrophils and monocytes via the binding of ANCA to target antigens on

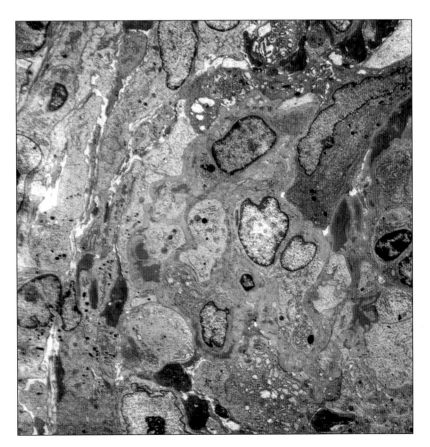

Fig. 1.313   Wegener's granulomatosis/microscopic polyangiitis. Electron microscopy reveals the crescent to consist of a variety of cell types including mononuclear cells and epithelial cells (TEM, ×4000).

Fig. 1.314 Wegener's granulomatosis/microscopic polyangiitis. Abundant fibrin tactoids are also interspersed with the cells of the crescent (TEM, ×3000).

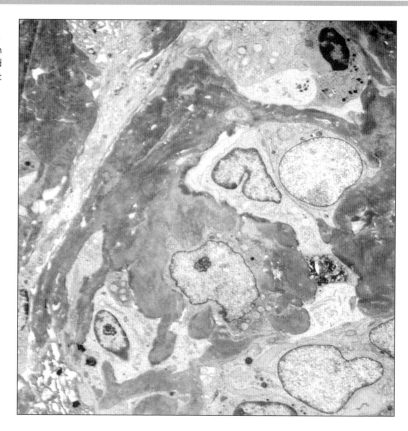

Fig. 1.315 Wegener's granulomatosis/microscopic polyangiitis. There is endothelial cell swelling associated with accumulation of fibrin within the capillary lumen and numerous leukocytes are also present (TEM, ×3000).

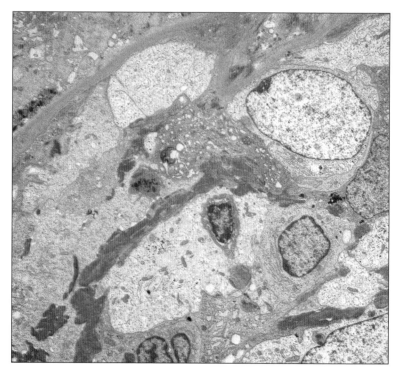

or near the surface of neutrophils and monocytes. Experimental studies in mice have produced lesions similar to those in humans by injection of anti myeloperoxidase IgG alone in immune deficient animals. The most convincing evidence is the clinical association of these antibodies with crescentic glomerulonephritis and small vessel vasculitis.

Selected reading

Falk R J, Jennette J C 1997 ANCA small vessel vasculitis. Journal of the American Society of Nephrology 8:314–322.

Jennette J C, Falk R J 1998 Pathogenesis of the vascular and glomerular damage in ANCA positive vasculitis. Nephrology, Dialysis and Transplantation 13(Suppl. 1):16–20.

Xiao H, Heeringa P, Hu P et al 2002 Antineutrophil cytoplasmic autoantibodies specific for myeloperoxidase cause glomerulonephritis and vasculitis in mice. Journal of Clinical Investigation 110:955–963.

Polyarteritis nodosa (PAN)

This is a rare disease, which primarily affects medium size arteries with 'blow-out', pseudoaneurysmal, vasculitic lesions, which give rise to the nodose appearance of these vessels. Organs affected include the heart, liver, kidney and mesenteric arteries. Radiographic studies show typical beaded appearance. In the kidney, large vessels show a transmural vasculitis (Fig. 1.316). Glomeruli are not affected. There are no immune complexes by IF or EM. There are associated hemorrhagic infarcts related to the large vessel lesions.

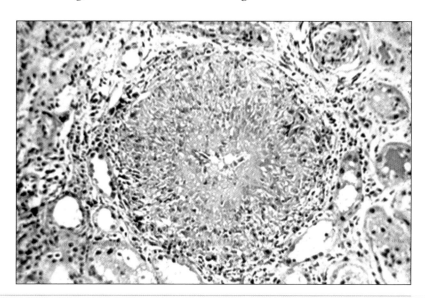

Fig. 1.316 PAN. Periarteritis involving an intrarenal artery. There is a transmural inflammatory infiltrate, which extends into the interstitium (Trichrome, ×200).

Etiology/pathogenesis

Polyarteritis nodosa has been associated with hepatitis B infection. The precise etiology is not known.

Selected reading

Jennette J C, Falk R J 1994 The pathology of vasculitis involving the kidney. American Journal of Kidney Disease 24:130–141.

Churg-Strauss syndrome

Clinically, patients have asthma and eosinophilia, and often have pulmonary-renal syndrome or only rapidly progressive glomerulo-nephritis. Renal lesions are similar, but tend to be milder, than those seen in Wegener's granulomatosis or microscopic polyangiitis. Glomeruli may also show varying mesangial proliferation, and there may not even be a crescentic component. There are no immune complexes by either IF or EM. Despite the eosinophilia, there may not be prominent eosinophils in the renal inflammatory infiltrate, and indeed, this finding is not a required criterion to make the diagnosis of Churg-Strauss syndrome. Specific diagnosis rests on clinicopathologic criteria.

Etiology/pathogenesis

The etiology is unknown. The prominent eosinophilia and clinical setting suggests a hypersensitivity component.

Selected reading

Jennette J C, Falk R J 1994 The pathology of vasculitis involving the kidney. American Journal of Kidney Disease 24:130–141.

Diseases of the basement membrane

Alport syndrome

Classical Alport syndrome is inherited in an X-linked dominant pattern and is the most common form of Alport syndrome (85% of cases). It is due to mutation of alpha 5 type IV collagen. The overall incidence of Alport syndrome in the USA is between 1:5000 to 1:10 000. Hematuria is the initial renal presentation of disease in childhood, although some proteinuria may also be present. Other manifestations of Alport syndrome in affected men include hearing loss and ocular defects. Hearing loss typically does not manifest until adulthood. Ocular defects occur in up to one-third of patients. Anterior lenticonus is the most common eye defect. Nephrotic syndrome may develop in as many as 30%–40% of patients with severe disease due to more extensive abnormality of the mutated type IV collagen. Chronic renal failure develops in 30%–40% of patients. Female carriers of X-linked classic Alport syndrome have hematuria and only rarely develop progressive renal disease. Males and females both can develop chronic renal insufficiency when Alport syndrome is caused by rare autosomal mutations of type IV collagen genes (alpha 3 or 4 type IV collagen chains, see below).

Light microscopy is unremarkable in the early stage in males with X-linked disease, and in carrier females (Fig. 1.317). At later stages, secondary, nonspecific glomerulosclerosis, interstitial fibrosis and prominent interstitial foam cells are typical in males with X-linked disease, or in either gender with autosomal disease (Fig. 1.318). These foam cells are not specific for this disease, and are found in numerous proteinuric states.

Standard immunofluorescence may show only non-specific trapping of IgM. Immunofluorescence for type IV collagen molecules in either skin or kidney biopsy is useful for diagnosis. Type IV

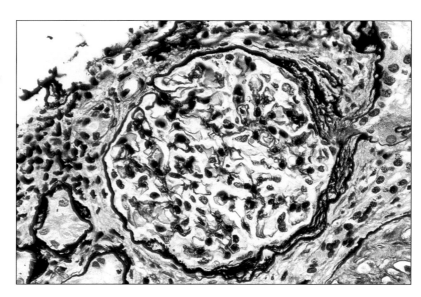

Fig. 1.317 Alport syndrome. The glomerular basement membrane irregularities in Alport syndrome are not detectable by light microscopy. Early in the course, the glomeruli may be unremarkable. In this case, there is early periglomerular fibrosis (Jones' silver stain, ×200).

Fig. 1.318 Alport syndrome. There is periglomerular fibrosis and tubular interstitial fibrosis and atrophy. Secondary sclerotic lesions in a segmental distribution can develop in classic, X-linked Alport syndrome when the patient is in his 20s, as in this patient (PAS, ×100).

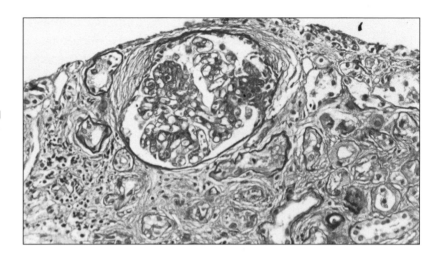

collagen organizes in heterotrimers composed of various combinations of alpha 1–6 collagen chains. The epidermal basement membrane normally contains alpha 1, alpha 2, alpha 5 and alpha 6(IV) collagen, but not alpha 3 or alpha 4(IV) collagen. Skin biopsy staining to demonstrate the absence of alpha 5(IV) collagen has been suggested as a tool to distinguish patients with X-linked Alport syndrome from those with other causes of hematuria. In the kidney, the GBM consists of alpha 3, 4, 5 (IV) heterotrimers, while Bowman's capsule and the distal tubule contain alpha 1, 1, 2 and 5, 5, 6 heterotrimers. In kidney biopsies, about 70%–80% of males with X-linked Alport lack staining of GBM, distal tubular basement membrane and Bowman's capsule for alpha 5(IV) chains. Alpha 3 and alpha 4(IV) collagen staining is also lacking in the GBM in patients with classic Alport syndrome, because the molecular defect in alpha 5(IV) collagen results in defective incorporation of the alpha 3 and alpha 4 chains. In autosomal recessive Alport, the kidney GBMs also show no expression of alpha 3, 4 or 5(IV) collagen, because a defect in any one of the molecules of the heterotrimer prevents its formation. However, in contrast to X-linked cases, autosomal recessive cases show strong expression of alpha 5 in Bowman's capsule, distal tubular basement membrane and skin, reflecting the normal incorporation of the non-mutated alpha 5(IV) collagen in the alpha 5, 5, 6(IV) heterotrimers of these basement membranes. Female heterozygotes for X-linked Alport syndrome frequently show mosaic staining of GBM and distal TBM for alpha 3, alpha 4 and alpha 5(IV) chains, and skin mosaic staining for alpha 5(IV) (Fig. 1.319). Patients with autosomal dominant Alport have not been studied immunohistochemically.

Thus, the co-absence of alpha 3 and alpha 5(IV) collagen is a major diagnostic clue to the diagnosis of Alport syndrome, because it has so far not been described in other glomerular diseases, including the thin basement membrane lesion underlying 'benign familial hematuria'. However, the sensitivity and specificity of skin or renal biopsy IF studies in the diagnosis of Alport syndrome have not been proven, and occasional cases with Alport syndrome clinically and by renal biopsy showed normal alpha 5(IV) collagen pattern of skin IF staining. About 20% of male classic Alport patients and affected homozygous autosomal recessive Alport patients show faint or even normal staining of the GBM for alpha 3 and alpha 5(IV) collagen. This is thought to reflect a mutation that still leaves intact the epitope recognized by the commercially available antibodies. Thus, an apparent normal staining pattern in either skin or kidney does not definitively rule out Alport syndrome. The possible continuum of Alport syndrome with some cases of apparent benign familial hematuria with thin basement membranes, caused by mutations in COL4A3 or COL4A4 further complicates interpretation of staining patterns (see 'Thin Basement Membrane').

By electron microscopy, the diagnostic lesion consists of irregular thinned and thickened areas of the glomerular basement membranes

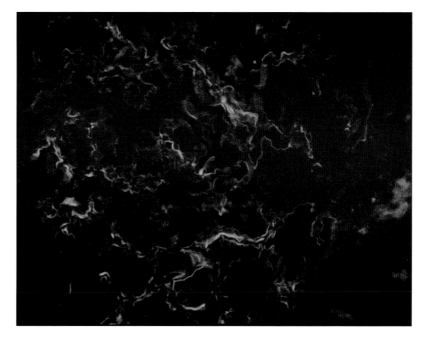

Fig. 1.319 Alport syndrome. Mosaic staining for alpha5 (IV) collagen is present along the GBM, strongly supporting a heterozygous carrier state of X-linked Alport syndrome. By EM, this female patient showed only diffuse thinning of the GBM (anti-alpha 5(IV) collagen immunofluorescence, ×400).

with splitting and irregular multilaminated appearance of the lamina densa, with thin fibrils amidst irregular lucent thickened areas of the lamina densa, with short stubs of fibrils at right angles to the GBM, resulting in a 'basket weaving' pattern (Figs 1.320–1.323). In between these lamina, granular, mottled material is present. At early stages of disease, i.e. in children or carrier females, the basement membrane may show only thinning rather than thickening (Fig. 1.320). To further complicate matters, some kindreds with typical Alport's syndrome clinically have only manifested basement membrane thinning as a morphologic change, even at advanced stages. Ultra-structural features do not strictly correlate with type of mutation, in that some patients with major gene rearrangements had no significant lesions, and varying ultrastructural abnormalities were present even within the same kindred.

Etiology/pathogenesis

The alpha 5(IV) collagen chain (COL4A5) gene is mutated in classic, X-linked Alport syndrome. Rare mutations of alpha 3 or alpha 4 type IV collagen genes (COL4A3 or COL4A4) cause autosomal

Fig. 1.320 Alport syndrome. The definitive diagnosis of Alport syndrome is made by electron microscopy. Early in the course, there is only thinning of the GBM, with segments of irregular thickening due to a loose, mottled, so-called 'basketweaving' appearance of the GBM. There is only minimal effacement of the overlying foot processes (TEM, ×3000).

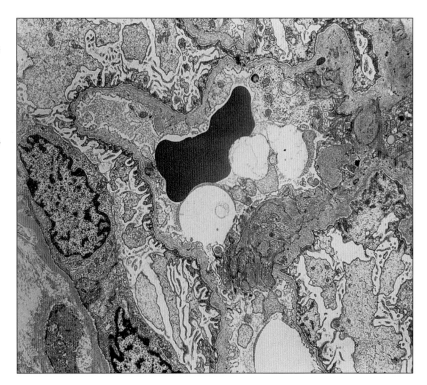

Fig. 1.321 Alport syndrome. There is irregular thickening of the glomerular basement membrane with a loose, basketwoven appearance. The overlying foot processes are blunted and partially effaced (TEM, ×17 125).

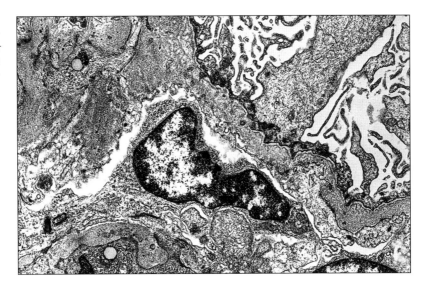

Fig. 1.322 Alport syndrome. Alternating areas of extreme thinning of the glomerular basement membrane (~120 nm) with thick, irregular areas with basketweaving are shown (TEM, ×7000).

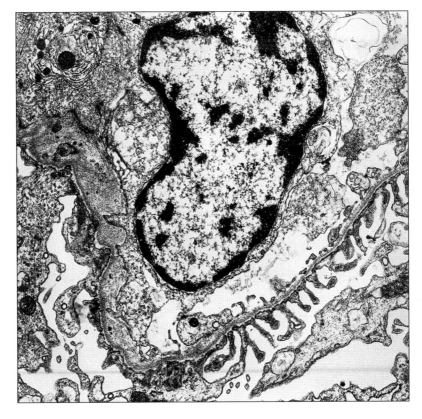

Fig. 1.323 Alport syndrome. The irregular mottled appearance of the basketweaving lesion is illustrated. There are no immune deposits and over-lying foot processes are only partially effaced. The lamellated appearance is highly characteristic of Alport syndrome, but may be seen in very small to very minor degree in small areas in other scarring conditions (TEM, ×9750).

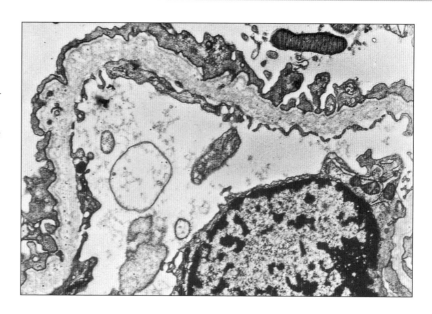

recessive Alport syndrome, or very rarely autosomal dominant Alport syndrome.

The organs involved reflect sites where these collagen chains are normally highly expressed. Alpha 3, alpha 4, and alpha 5(IV) collagen chains are normally highly expressed in the kidney, eye, and ear and organize as the alpha 3,4,5(IV) heterotrimer of the GBM. The abnormal alpha 5(IV) collagen prevents incorporation of alpha 3(IV) and alpha 4(IV) into these heterotrimers. *In situ* hybridization and immunostaining reveals normal mRNA transcription of COL4A3 and COL4A4 and normal alpha 3(IV) staining in podocytes in Alport patients, implicating events downstream to transcription, RNA processing and protein synthesis in the absent staining in X-linked Alport patients.

Transplantation in patients with Alport syndrome has shed additional light on the molecular basis for this disease. Each Alport kindred reported thus far has presented its own unique mutation. The rate of progression to end stage and deafness are mutation dependent. Large deletions, nonsense mutations or mutations that changed the reading frame were associated with 90% risk of end stage renal disease before age 30 in affected males with X-linked Alport, with only 50% risk for patients with missense and 70% risk for those with splice site mutations. Risk for hearing loss before age 30 was 60% in patients with missense mutations, versus 90% risk for all other mutations. Some patients with Alport receiving kidney transplants, probably around 5%–10%, develop antibodies to the normal glomerular basement membrane in the transplant (Fig. 1.324). These antibodies may cross-react with the tubular basement membrane (Fig. 1.325). Occurrence of this post-transplant anti-GBM disease appears more frequent in patients with

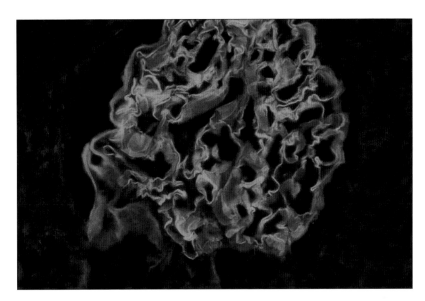

Fig. 1.324 Alport syndrome. In some patients with Alport syndrome receiving a transplant, there is an antibody response to the normal type IV collagen of the transplanted kidney resulting in anti-GBM antibody-mediated glomerulonephritis with linear staining for IgG by immunofluorescence, as in this case (anti-IgG immuno-fluorescence, ×400).

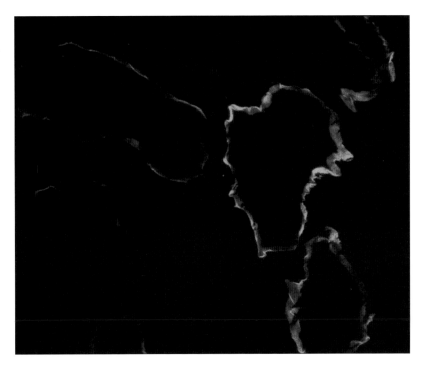

Fig. 1.325 Alport syndrome. The anti-GBM antibody developing against the transplant in some patients with Alport may also cross-react with tubular basement membranes, and thus give rise to a tubulitis. This tubulitis must be distinguished from acute rejection, by correlating with glomerular findings and clinical course (anti-IgG immunofluorescence, ×400).

more extensive deletion of the COL4A5 gene. The antibody binding results in a necrotizing, crescentic lesion, usually resulting in loss of the graft (Figs 1.326, 1.327).

Fig. 1.326 Alport syndrome. Early in the course of anti-GBM antibody-mediated glomerulonephritis occurring in the Alport patient post-transplant, there may only be subtle, very early segmental fibrinoid necrosis and glomerular basement membrane breaks as shown here. Immunofluorescence is key in evaluating this lesion and making the correct diagnosis (see Figs 1.324 and 1.325) (Jones' silver stain, ×400).

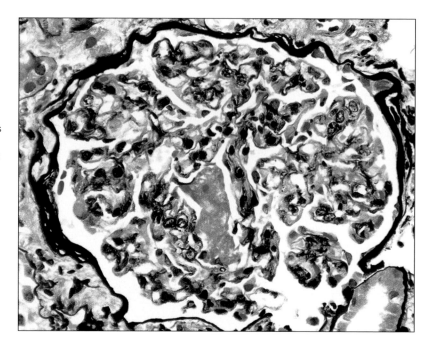

Fig. 1.327 Alport syndrome. The early necrotizing lesion shown in Figure 1.326 does, with time, give rise to a frank crescentic glomerulonephritis, associated with linear immunofluorescence, as in this case (Jones' silver stain, ×200).

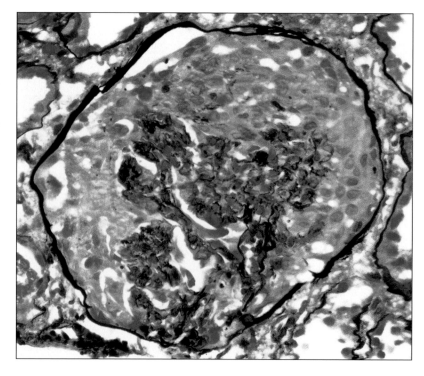

Selected reading

Bodziak K A, Hammond W S, Molitoris B A 1994 Inherited diseases of the glomerular basement membrane. American Journal of Kidney Disease 23:605–618.

Churg J, Sherman R L 1973 Pathologic characteristics of hereditary nephritis. Archives of Pathology 95:374–379.

Ding J, Kashtan C E, Fan W W et al 1994 A monoclonal antibody marker for Alport syndrome identifies the Alport antigen as the α5 chain of type IV collagen. Kidney International 45:1504–1506.

Jais J P, Knebelmann B, Giatras I et al 2000 X-linked Alport syndrome: natural history in 195 families and genotype-phenotype correlations in males. Journal of the American Society of Nephrology 11:649–657.

Kashtan C E 2000 Alport syndromes: phenotypic heterogeneity of progressive hereditary nephritis. Pediatric Nephrology 14:502–512.

Kashtan C E, Gubler M C, Sisson-Ross S et al 1998 Chronology of renal scarring in males with Alport syndrome. Pediatric Nephrology 12:269–274.

Lemmink H H, Nillesen W N, Mochizuki T et al 1996 Benign familial hematuria due to mutation of the type IV collagen α4 gene. Journal of Clinical Investigation 98:1114–1118.

Liapis H, Gokden N, Hmiel P et al 2002 Histopathology, ultrastructure, and clinical phenotypes in thin glomerular basement membrane disease variants. Human Pathology 33(8):836–845.

Mazzucco G, Barsotti P, Muda A O et al 1998 Ultrastructural and immunohistochemical findings in Alport's syndrome: a study of 208 patients from 97 Italian families with particular emphasis on COL4A5 gene mutation correlations. Journal of the American Society of Nephrology 9:1023–1031.

Nakanishi K, Yoshikawa N, Iijima K et al 1996 Expression of type IV collagen α3 and α4 chain mRNA in X-linked Alport syndrome. Journal of the American Society of Nephrology 7:938–945.

Pirson Y 1999 Making the diagnosis of Alport's syndrome. Kidney International 56:760–775.

Thin basement membranes

This basement membrane abnormality underlies the condition of 'benign familial hematuria.' This term has been used to distinguish these families from Alport's syndrome since affected individuals have been thought to have a benign prognosis. However, morphology alone does not allow one to make specific prognostic inferences. Kindreds may show autosomal dominant or apparent autosomal recessive inheritance. The clinical manifestation is that of hematuria, either macroscopic and microscopic, intermittent or continuous. This lesion is common, and is present in 20%–25% of patients biopsied for persistent isolated hematuria in some series. Thin basement membranes (without lamellation) may also be an early or only manifestation in some kindreds with Alport syndrome (see Alport syndrome discussion). Thus, the presence of thin basement membranes cannot *per se* be taken to categorically indicate a benign prognosis. Of note, thin glomerular basement membranes may also be seen in sporadic cases of hematuria. The lesion may also coexist with other glomerular disease, commonly diabetic nephropathy changes (alternating very thin and thick GBM), or IgA nephropathy. Occasionally patients with thin basement membranes have nephrotic range proteinuria, with 5 of 8 reported cases showing superimposed FSGS lesions.

Light microscopy shows no specific lesion, and standard immunofluorescence studies are negative (Figs 1.328, 1.329). The diagnosis of thin basement membranes is thus based on morphometric measurements from electron microscopic examination, revealing marked thinning of the lamina densa of the glomerular basement membranes (Figs 1.330, 1.331). Diagnosis of thinning must be made by comparison to age-matched controls, because the glomerular basement membrane thickness normally increases with age. Normal thickness in adults in one series was 373 ± 42 nm in men versus 326 ± 45 nm in women. Glomerular basement thickness <250 nm has been used as a cutoff in many series. In children, the diagnosis of thin basement membranes must be made with special care, establishing normal age-matched controls within each laboratory. In our laboratory, we found a range of GBM thickness in normal

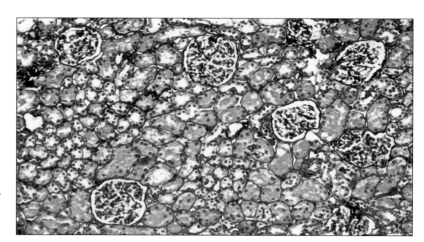

Fig. 1.328 Thin basement membrane lesion. There are no light microscopic abnormalities in thin basement membrane lesion. This lesion is common, and may therefore be found superimposed on other diseases, such as IgA nephropathy or diabetic nephropathy. When occurring with diabetic nephropathy, there are alternate segments of thick and very thin GBM with very sudden transition (Jones' silver stain, ×100).

Fig. 1.329 Thin basement membrane lesion. The thin glomerular basement membrane cannot be detected by light microscopic examination (Jones' silver stain, ×200).

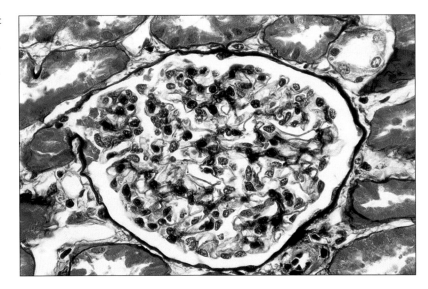

Fig. 1.330 Thin basement membrane lesion. When thin basement membranes are associated with benign familial hematuria, a carrier state of Alport or early in the course of Alport, the lesion is diffuse and global. Very segmental areas of thinning may occur non-specifically (TEM, ×9750).

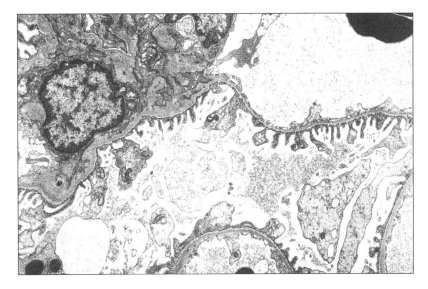

children, from approximately 110 nm at age 1 year, to 222 ± 14 nm in 7 year olds.

Etiology/pathogenesis

There is no understanding of the molecular defect underlying many, but perhaps not all, cases of 'benign familial hematuria'. Mutation of the α4 type IV collagen gene segregated with hematuria in a

Fig. 1.331 Thin basement membrane lesion. Diagnosis of thin basement membrane is made specifically by measurements of the electron microscopic images and must be compared with the normal for age, as GBM thickness normally increases from childhood to adulthood. However, the relative thickness of the base of the intact foot process versus the GBM gives an approximate guide to the GBM thickness. In the adult, the normal GBM is 2–3 times the thickness of the base of the podocyte (TEM, ×20 250).

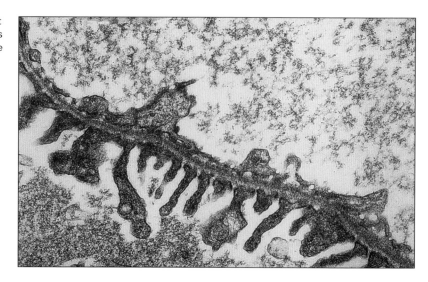

kindred with apparent benign familial hematuria. The index patient had electron microscopic changes typical of Alport syndrome by renal biopsy at age 5 years, i.e. areas of lamellation alternating with areas of thinning. This boy's parents both had microscopic hematuria and family histories of benign hematuria without progression in any members. In contrast, the boy developed proteinuria at age 16 years. These findings suggest that this patient may have inherited a disorder manifest by hematuria from both parents, resulting in a more severe phenotype. Further, the findings in this kindred suggest the possibility that autosomal recessive Alport syndrome and 'benign familial hematuria/thin basement membrane disease' may be the severe and mild forms of different molecular defects in the same gene. Recent genotypic studies indeed indicate that these diseases are part of a spectrum, with mutations of COL4A3 or COL4A4 genes discovered in patients who clinically had benign familial hematuria.

Further, 'benign familial hematuria' may not be entirely benign. Some patients with thin basement membranes on renal biopsies showed increased global sclerosis, and later increased hypertension and late onset of renal insufficiency. However, these patients were not defined molecularly and were presumed to not have Alport based on absence of hearing or eye abnormalities. Renal disease also developed over the follow-up in some relatives. It is possible that a second process, such as hypertensive nephrosclerosis, was also present in these families, or that this represents a part of a continuum of basement membrane abnormalities. These observations further reiterate that the finding of thin basement membranes alone does not allow one to predict a 'benign' process.

Selected reading

Badenas C, Praga M, Tazon B et al 2002 Mutations in the COL4A4 and COL4A3 genes cause familial benign hematuria. Journal of the American Society of Nephrology 13:1248–1254.

Buzza M, Wang Y Y, Dagher H et al 2001 COL4A4 mutation in thin basement membrane disease previously described in Alport syndrome. Kidney International 60:480–483.

Cosio F G, Falkenhain M E, Sedmak D D 1994 Association of thin glomerular basement membrane with other glomerulopathies. Kidney International 46:471–474.

Hisano S, Kwano M, Hatae K et al 1991 Asymptomatic isolated microhaematuria: natural history of 136 children. Pediatric Nephrology 5:578–581.

Lemmink H H, Nillesen W N, Mochizuki T et al 1996 Benign familial hematuria due to mutation of the type IV collagen α4 gene. Journal of Clinical Investigation 98:1114–1118.

Longo I, Porcedda P, Mari F et al 2002 COL4A3/COL4A4 mutations: from familial hematuria to autosomal-dominant or recessive Alport syndrome. Kidney International 61:1947–1956.

Matsumae T, Fukusaki M, Sakata N et al 1994 Thin glomerular basement membrane in diabetic patients with urinary abnormalities. Clinical Nephrology 42:221–226.

Nieuwhof C M G, de Heer F, de Leeuw P et al 1997 Thin GBM nephropathy: Premature glomerular obsolescence is associated with hypertension and late onset renal failure. Kidney International 51:1596–1601.

Tiebosch A T M G, Frederik P M, van Breda Vriesman P J C et al 1989 Thin-basement-membrane nephropathy in adults with persistent hematuria. New England Journal of Medicine 320:14–18.

Yoshiokawa N, Matsuyama S, Iijima K et al 1988 Benign familial hematuria. Archives in Pathological Laboratory Medicine 112:794–797.

Nail-patella syndrome

Nail-patella syndrome is inherited in autosomal dominant fashion, and occurs in approximately 22/1 000 000. Patients show hypoplastic or absent patellae, dystrophic fingernails and toenails, and abnormalities of bones in the elbow and iliac horns. Renal disease occurs in less than one half of affected patients, and is quite variable, even within a given kindred. End-stage renal disease develops in ~10% of patients; only half of these patients manifest proteinuria, microhematuria, edema and hypertension. The disease has not been reported to recur in the transplant.

The light microscopic appearance is normal at early stages, with glomerulosclerosis developing as disease advances, with associated tubulointerstitial fibrosis. Immunofluorescence studies do not show immune complexes. The renal biopsy diagnosis is made at the ultrastructural level. Basement membranes show thickened GBM with irregular lucent areas with intervening clear zones and rarefied areas, resulting in a moth-eaten appearance. Some areas contain coarse fibrils that appear like cross-banded collagen (Fig. 1.332). Collagen fibrils are usually in the mid portion of the GBM but may occasionally be present in the subepithelial or subendothelial area, and rarely in the mesangium. Staining with phosphotungstic acid enhances these collagen bundles.

Etiology/pathogenesis

The gene mutated in nail-patella syndrome, LMX1B on chromosome 9, has now been identified. The gene encodes a LIM-homeodomain transcription factor. Mice null-mutated for the LMX1B gene develop a phenotype remarkably similar to human nail-patella syndrome, and have markedly decreased α3 and α4 collagen type IV expression in their GBM. These knockout mice also have abnormal podocytes lacking typical slit diaphragms. CD2AP and podocin, two key com-

Fig. 1.332 Nail-patella syndrome. Light microscopy is nonspecific, and the diagnosis is made by EM, which shows mottled, moth-eaten areas of the GBM, and banded collagen within the glomerular basement membrane (TEM, ×8000).

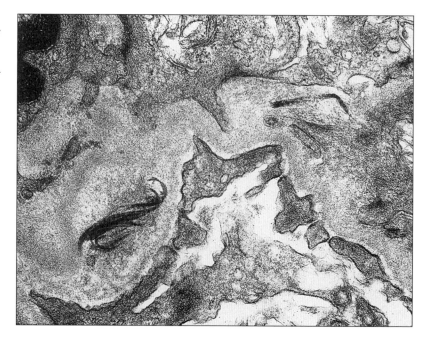

ponents of the slit diaphragm, were markedly reduced, although other podocyte genes such as nephrin, synaptopodin, ZO1, alpha-3 integrin and specific laminins were preserved. Thus, the LMX1b gene product plays an integral part in foot process development and integrity, pointing to important interactions of the podocyte and the underlying GBM. A total of 25 differing mutations of the LMX1B gene have been identified in 37 families screened, but with no correlation between aspects of the phenotype and specific mutations.

Selected reading

Chen H, Lun Y, Ovchinnikov D et al 1998 Limb and kidney defects in LmX1b mutant mice suggest an involvement of LMX1B in human nail patella syndrome. Nature Genetics 19:51–55.

McIntosh I, Dreyer S D, Clough M V et al 1998 Mutation analysis of LMX1B gene in nail-patella syndrome patients. American Journal of Human Genetics 1998 63:1651–1658.

Miner J H, Morello R, Andrews K L et al 2002 Transcriptional induction of slit diaphragm genes by LmX1b is required in podocyte differentiation. Journal of Clinical Investigation 109:1065–1072.

Morello R, Zhou G, Dreyer S D et al 2001 Regulation of glomerular basement membrane collagen expression by LMX1B contributes to renal disease in nail patella syndrome. Nature Genetics 27:205–208.

Morita T, Laughlin L O, Kawano K et al 1973 Nail-patella syndrome. Light and electron microscopic studies of the kidney. Archives of Internal Medicine 131:271.

Taguchi T, Takebayashi S, Nishimura M et al 1988 Nephropathy of nail-patella syndrome. Ultrastructural Pathology 12:175–183.

Glomerular involvement with bacterial infections

Subacute bacterial endocarditis

Subacute bacterial endocarditis (SBE) may result in glomerulonephritis regardless of the causative organisms (e.g. *Streptococcus viridans*, *Enterococci*, *Streptococcus aureus*). Patients have hematuria and proteinuria and may occasionally have acute nephritic or nephrotic syndrome. There is often associated hypocomplementemia, fever, rash, weakness and enlarged spleen.

By light microscopy, there is a focal segmental proliferative glomerulonephritis, often with crescents (Figs 1.333–1.337). In some patients, there may be more diffuse and global endocapillary proliferation. Crescents often occur along with the proliferative

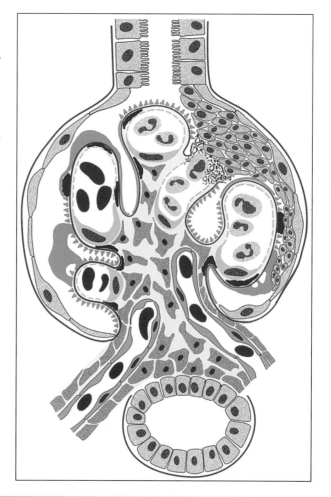

Fig. 1.333 Subacute bacterial endocarditis-associated GN. There is focal segmental proliferative glomerulonephritis, often with crescents, with predominant mesangial deposits and occasional subendothelial deposits associated with endocapillary proliferation, with only rare subepithelial deposits.

Fig. 1.334 Subacute bacterial endocarditis-associated glomerulonephritis. Kidney lesions may result from embolization of portions of the valve vegetations, resulting in multiple infarcts due to occlusion of interlobular arteries and arterioles.

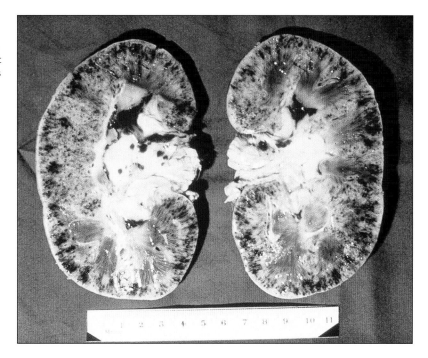

Fig. 1.335 Subacute bacterial endocarditis-associated glomerulonephritis. The glomeruli in subacute bacterial endocarditis show hypercellularity, often with a membranoproliferative pattern, but in a focal and segmental distribution. There is often coexistence of segmental sclerosis. This glomerulus shows widespread glomerular basement membrane splitting and only rare PMNs (Jones' silver stain, ×400).

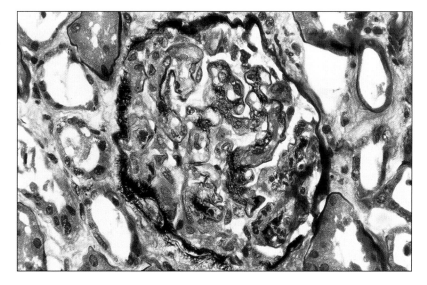

lesions (Fig. 1.338). Infiltrating cells are typically monocytes/macrophages, rather than PMNs as seen in acute postinfectious glomerulonephritis or shunt nephritis. Segmental thrombosis and necrosis may also be present, and with chronicity organize as segmental scars and adhesions. There is proportional tubulointerstitial

Fig. 1.336 Subacute bacterial endocarditis-associated glomerulonephritis. A global proliferative pattern is present in this glomerulus, with scattered PMNs (same case as Fig. 1.335, Jones' silver stain, ×400).

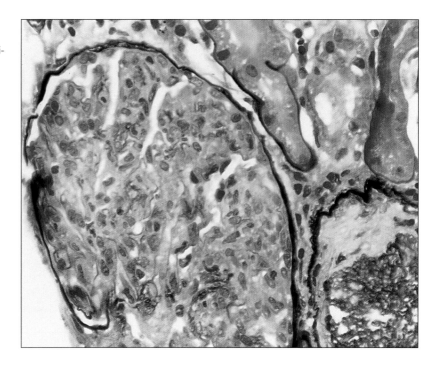

Fig. 1.337 Subacute bacterial endocarditis-associated glomerulonephritis. Crescents are often associated with proliferative lesion of subacute bacterial endocarditis. This glomerulus shows segmental proliferation and sclerosis with an associated fibrocellular crescent (Jones' silver stain, ×400).

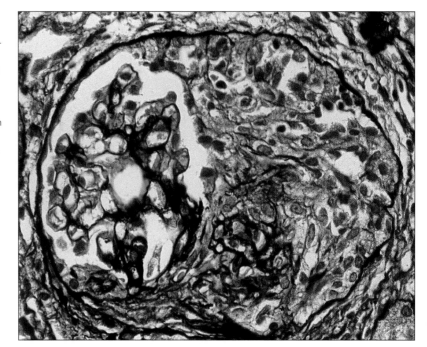

Fig. 1.338 Subacute bacterial endocarditis-associated glomerulonephritis. When the underlying valve lesion is not successfully treated, lesions may progress. In this case (same case as Fig. 1.335), the patient became septicemic and died weeks after renal biopsy. At autopsy, there was a diffuse proliferative glomerulonephritis with numerous PMNs (Jones' silver stain, ×400).

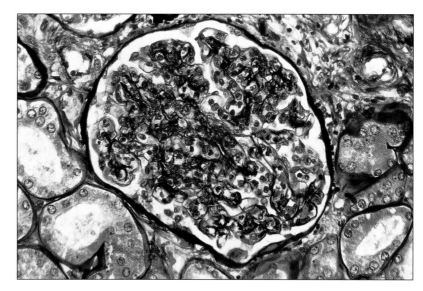

Fig. 1.339 Subacute bacterial endocarditis-associated glomerulonephritis. Immunofluorescence shows chunky deposits in the mesangial area, frequently extending to capillary loops, corresponding to subendothelial deposits in the diffuse, membranoproliferative forms of subacute bacterial endocarditis-associated glomerulonephritis. Deposits typically stain with IgG, IgM, C3 and C1q. This glomerulus (same case as Fig. 1.335) shows typical segmental accentuation of staining with mesangial and peripheral capillary loop deposits (anti-IgG immunofluorescence, ×200).

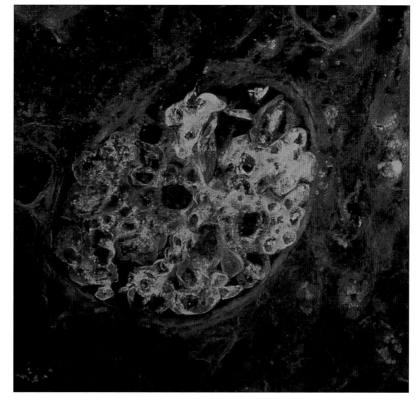

fibrosis. Vessels do not show any specific lesions. By immunofluorescence, there are diffuse mesangial granular deposits of IgG and C3, with rare other components (Figs 1.339, 1.340). Endocapillary proliferation is associated with peripheral loop deposits.

Fig. 1.340 Subacute bacterial endocarditis-associated glomerulonephritis. Chunky peripheral loop and mesangial deposits are evident in this case of subacute bacterial endocarditis-related glomerulonephritis. The smooth outer contours of some of the peripheral loop deposits correspond to their subendothelial location (anti-C3 immunofluorescence, ×400).

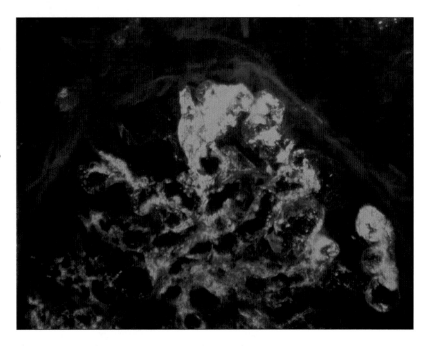

Fig. 1.341 Subacute bacterial endocarditis-associated glomerulonephritis. Bacterial endocarditis-associated post-infectious glomerulonephritis. There is diffuse endocapillary proliferation and scattered mesangial and small subendothelial deposits. The lumens are filled with proliferating monocytes and occasional PMNs along with resident endothelial and mesangial cells (TEM, ×3000).

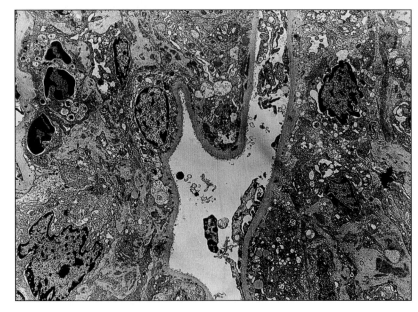

Electron microscopy shows the presence of mesangial deposits, with subendothelial deposits in those patients with endocapillary proliferation (Figs 1.341, 1.342). Subepithelial deposits are rare.

Fig. 1.342 Subacute bacterial endocarditis-associated glomerulonephritis. Bacterial endocarditis-associated post-infectious glomerulonephritis. Scattered small to medium mesangial deposits are seen underneath the paramesangial glomerular basement membrane (TEM, ×14 000).

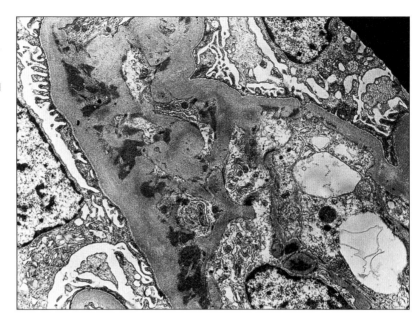

Etiology/pathogenesis

Although renal cortical infarcts may occur due to emboli from the valve lesions, these do not play a role in the pathogenesis of the glomerulonephritis (Fig. 1.334). Patients with glomerulonephritis associated with SBE typically have circulating immune complexes that deposit in the kidney. Early lesions may resolve if the infection is eradicated with appropriate antibiotic treatment.

Selected reading

Gutman R A, Striker G E, Gilliland B C et al 1972 The immune complex glomerulonephritis of bacterial endocarditis. Medicine (Baltimore) 51(1):1–25.

Morel-Maroger L, Sraer J D, Herreman G et al 1972 Kidney in subacute endocarditis. Pathological and immunofluorescence findings. Archives of Pathology 94(3):205–213.

Neugarten J, Gallo G R, Baldwin D S 1984 Glomerulonephritis in bacterial endocarditis. American Journal of Kidney Disease 5:371–379.

Shunt nephritis

Patients with nephritis due to infected shunts usually have coagulation-negative staphylococcus (*S. epidermidis*) infection. Deep visceral abscesses may give rise to a similar glomerulonephritis.

Rarely, other bacteria may be involved. Patients typically exhibit anorexia, anemia, malaise and fever, resulting from transient bacteremia. There may also be skin manifestations with purpura, arthralgias, hepatosplenomegaly, and lymphadenopathy. Renal signs include marked proteinuria, with over half exhibiting nephrotic syndrome, with hematuria and edema.

By light microscopy, there is a diffuse proliferative glomerulonephritis that may show membranoproliferative features, with mesangial and endocapillary proliferation and GBM splitting (Figs 1.343, 1.344). There are frequent intraglomerular PMNs (Figs 1.345, 1.346). Pure mesangial proliferation is less common (Fig. 1.347). In some patients, there is only focal segmental endocapillary proliferation. Crescents are not uncommon (Fig. 1.348). By immunofluorescence there is coarse, chunky, prominent C3 and also C1q and C4 deposits, in

Fig. 1.343 Shunt nephritis. There is a diffuse proliferative glomerulonephritis, with mesangial and endocapillary proliferation and occasional GBM splitting, due to mesangial, subendothelial, and rare subepithelial immune complex deposits.

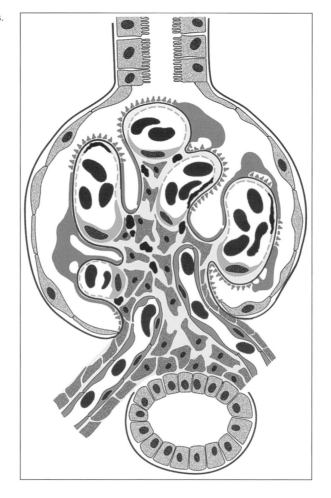

Fig. 1.344 Shunt nephritis. There typically are membranoproliferative features with predominant mesangial cells and macrophages, occasionally with scattered PMNs (PAS, ×200).

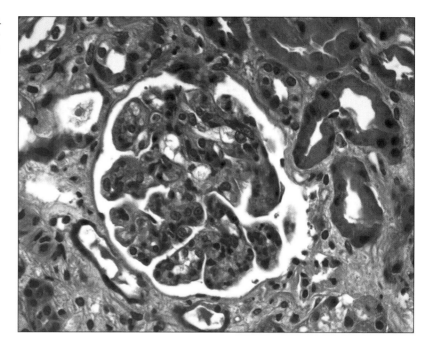

Fig. 1.345 Shunt nephritis. A predominant lobular pattern with numerous mononuclear cells and PMNs is present in this case of shunt nephritis (H&E, ×200).

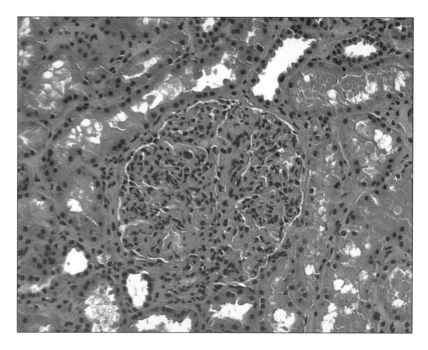

Fig. 1.346 Shunt nephritis. The marked lobular appearance is due to endocapillary proliferation with infiltrating mononuclear cells, including macrophages, and frequent PMNs, in addition to proliferating mesangial cells. There is interposition and reduplication of the peripheral capillary wall, better seen on silver stain (H&E, ×400).

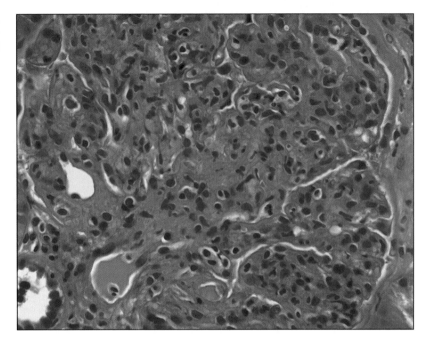

Fig. 1.347 Shunt nephritis. In some cases of shunt nephritis, there is only mesangial proliferation, with corresponding predominance of mesangial deposits by immunofluorescence and electron microscopy (Jones' silver stain, ×200).

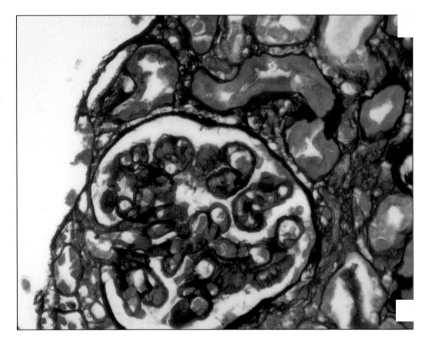

Fig. 1.348 Shunt nephritis. Crescents are occasionally present, particularly associated with proliferation. The underlying glomerulus shows endocapillary proliferation with frequent PMNs, and segmental reduplication of the capillary wall (Jones' silver stain, ×400).

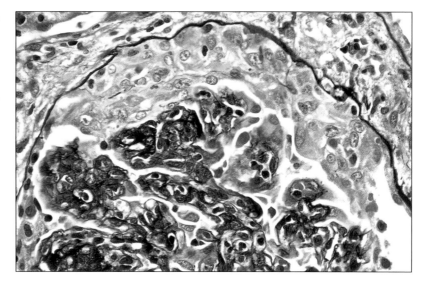

Fig. 1.349 Shunt nephritis. By immunofluorescence, there are chunky granular deposits of IgG, with very predominant C3 in mesangial areas and extending in an irregular, segmental distribution to peripheral loops (anti-IgG immunofluorescence, ×400).

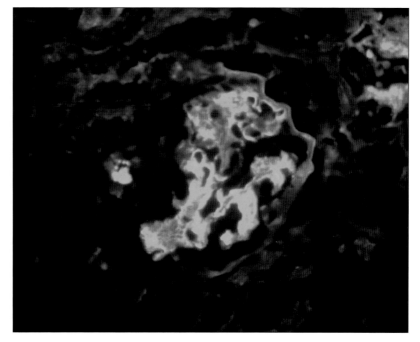

addition to IgG and IgM (Figs 1.349, 1.350). Deposits are present only in the mesangium in about half of patients, with some showing peripheral loop deposits corresponding to the common proliferative pattern found by light microscopy. When IgM is predominant, the possibility of a cryoglobulinemic response to the infection should be considered. By EM, the deposits most frequently are localized in

Fig. 1.350   Shunt nephritis. C3 is often very prominent in shunt nephritis, with chunky mesangial and peripheral loop deposits (same case as Figs 1.345 and 1.349). There is strong, chunky to granular mesangial staining with segmental irregular chunky peripheral loop staining (anti-C3 immunofluorescence, ×400).

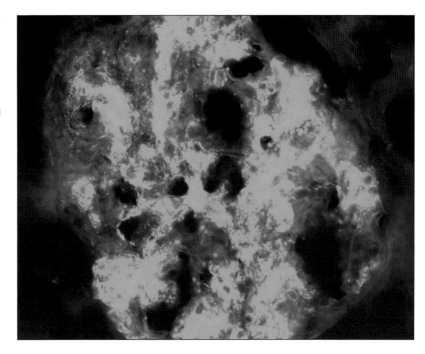

the mesangial and subendothelial areas, with rare intramembranous and subepithelial deposits (Figs 1.351–1.353). Reduplication of the glomerular basement membrane due to interposition and subendothelial deposits is present.

Etiology/pathogenesis

This glomerulonephritis may develop when ventriculoperitoneal, portocaval or other shunts become infected, most commonly with *Streptococcus epidermidis* although other bacteria may also cause shunt nephritis. The nephritis is related to immune complex deposition, with marked activation of the classic complement pathway. Thus, the majority of patients have reduced complement levels. Colonization of the shunt is typically present. There may be low-grade bacteremia, but cultures may also be sterile, with identification of the pathogen only possible when the shunt is removed. Specific diagnosis and removal of the infected shunt allow recovery in patients, usually within months. Antibiotic therapy alone has not been as effective, although in some case this has also led to resolution of disease.

Fig. 1.351 Shunt nephritis. Marked endocapillary proliferation fills up the capillary lumen, with rare, scattered small mesangial, subendothelial and small intramembranous deposits (TEM, ×3000).

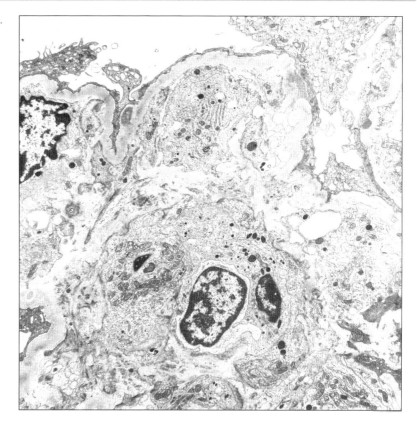

Fig. 1.352 Shunt nephritis. There may rarely be sub-epithelial or intramem-branous deposits. Typical hump-shaped deposits, as in acute post-infectious glomerulonephritis, are not a feature of shunt nephritis (TEM, ×7000).

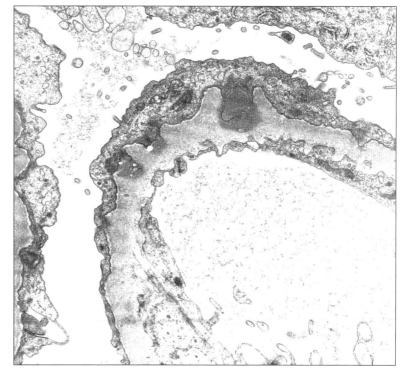

Fig. 1.353 Shunt nephritis. Small, sliver-like subendothelial deposits are present, along with marked endocapillary proliferation. There is extensive efface-ment of overlying foot processes (TEM, ×8000).

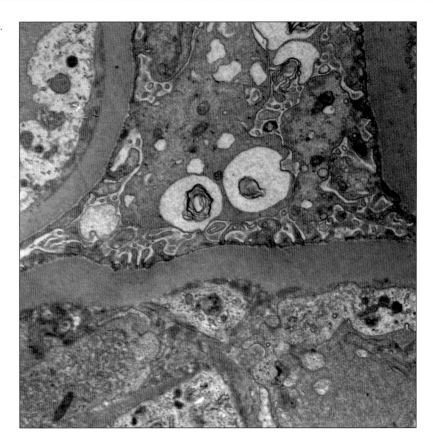

Selected reading

Arze R S, Rashid H, Morley R et al 1983 Shunt nephritis: Report of two cases and review of literature. Clinical Nephrology 19:48–53.

Beaufils M, Morel-Maroger L, Sraer J-D et al 1976 Acute renal failure of glomerular origin during visceral abscesses. New England Journal of Medicine 295:185–189.

7Dobrin R S, Day N K, Quie P G et al 1975 The role of complement, immunoglobulin and bacterial antigen in coagulase-negative staphylococcal shunt nephritis. American Journal of Medicine 59(5):660–673.

Fukuda Y, Ohtomo Y, Kaneko K et al 1993 Pathologic and laboratory dynamics following the removal of the shunt in shunt nephritis. American Journal of Nephrology 13(1):78–82.

Rames L, Wise B, Goodman J R et al 1970 Renal disease with *Staphylococcus albus* bacteremia. A complication in ventriculoatrial shunts. Journal of the American Medical Association 212(10):1671–1677.

Wakabayashi Y, Kobayashi Y, Shigematsu H 1985 Shunt nephritis: histological dynamics following removal of the shunt. Case report and review of the literature. Nephron 40(1):111–117.

Vascular Diseases

References to **Brenner & Rector's** *The Kidney* **7th edition** are given in parentheses below.

Diabetic nephropathy

Patients with diabetic nephropathy (DN) typically present with gradual progression of disease from microalbuminuria to proteinuria, usually around 15 years after onset of diabetes. Renal lesions are quite similar in type I and type II diabetes mellitus (DM), although the delay in clinical diagnosis of type II diabetes mellitus may give the appearance of shorter interval to DN in these patients. Type I diabetics with DN have a high incidence of retinopathy, while only slightly more than half of type II diabetics have retinopathy. Type II diabetes and obesity are increasing epidemically worldwide, in adults as well as in children. Type II DM is particularly prevalent in some Native American Indian tribes, such as the Pima. DN only develops in about 30% of diabetic patients. Patients with the typical course of DN usually do not undergo renal biopsy. Thus, the biopsied diabetic patient is clinically atypical. Lesions other than DN, either alone, or superimposed on DN, are common in this population. DN also occurs in the transplant; either as recurrent disease, or as a *de novo* lesion. DN develops more rapidly in this population than in native kidneys, with DN lesions present on average 6 years after transplant.

The earliest changes in diabetic patients' kidneys are renal enlargement, due to both hyperfiltration and hypertrophy. By light microscopy, glomerular hypertrophy, hyperplasia and thickened glomerular basement membranes are present as early as 2–8 years after onset of diabetes in some patients. Mesangial volume expansion can be detected even earlier by morphometry from EM examinations (Fig. 2.1). Progressive increase in mesangial matrix and cellularity ensue and may culminate in diffuse increase in mesangial matrix or nodular glomerulosclerosis with associated hyaline in arterioles and occasionally in Bowman's capsule ('capsular drop') (Figs 2.2–2.5). The nodules, so-called Kimmelstiel–Wilson nodules, have a lamel-

Fig. 2.1 Diabetic nephropathy. There is mesangial increase or nodular sclerosis, accompanied by hyalinosis of both afferent and efferent arterioles and thickening of the glomerular basement membrane lamina densa without deposits.

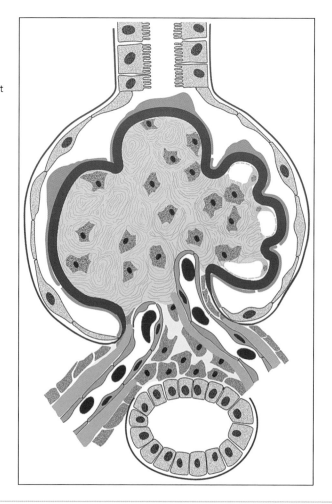

Fig. 2.2 Diabetic nephropathy. The lesions in diabetic nephropathy are characterized by arteriolar hyalinization, mesangial matrix expansion and glomerular basement membrane thickening. There is also associated tubular interstitial fibrosis (PAS, ×100).

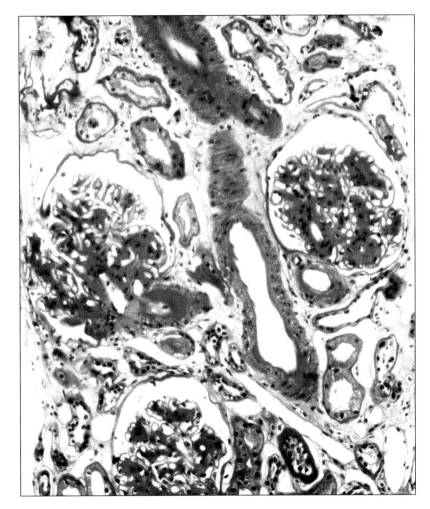

Fig. 2.3 Diabetic nephropathy. The arteriolar hyalinization in diabetes typically involves both afferent and efferent arterioles. The glomerulus shows diffuse mesangial matrix increase without formation of Kimmelstiel–Wilson nodules in this case. There is thickening of Bowman's capsule, and a small 'capsular drop', that is, hyalin within Bowman's capsule at the '6 o'clock' position (PAS, ×200).

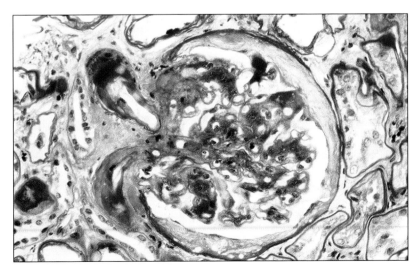

Fig. 2.4 Diabetic nephropathy. Diffuse mesangial matrix increase and basement membrane thickening are evident in this case of early diabetic nephropathy. A 'capsular drop' is seen at the bottom of Bowman's capsule. There is moderate increase in mesangial matrix and cellularity, with surrounding tubulointerstitial fibrosis. There are no deposits, splitting or irregularities of the basement membrane (Jones' silver stain, ×200).

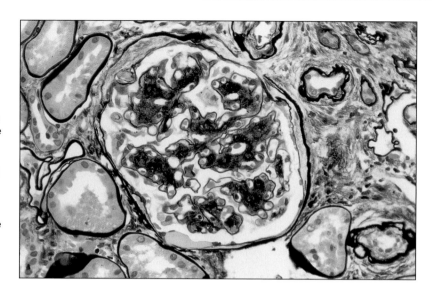

Fig. 2.5 Diabetic nephropathy. Diabetic nephropathy may manifest either as diffuse mesangial increase (as seen in Figs 2.3 and 2.4), or with nodular glomerulosclerosis as in this case. There are multiple nodules of mesangial matrix, surrounded by a small rim of intact capillaries. The glomerular basement membrane is prominent. The expanded nodules show a lamellated appearance, thought due to repeated injury with mesangiolysis and exuberant repair responses laying down increased matrix (PAS, ×200).

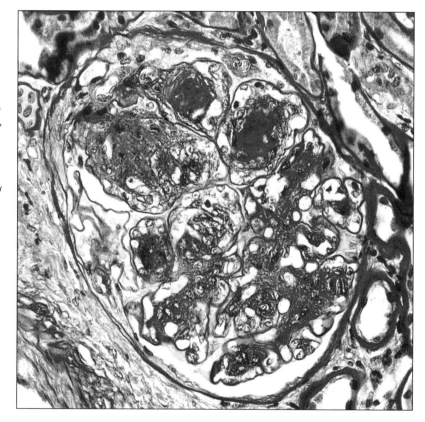

Fig. 2.6 Diabetic nephropathy. The lamellated appearance of the Kimmelstiel–Wilson nodule characteristic of the nodular sclerosis form of diabetic nephropathy is shown, along with arteriolar hyalinization and surrounding tubulointerstitial fibrosis (Jones' silver stain, ×200).

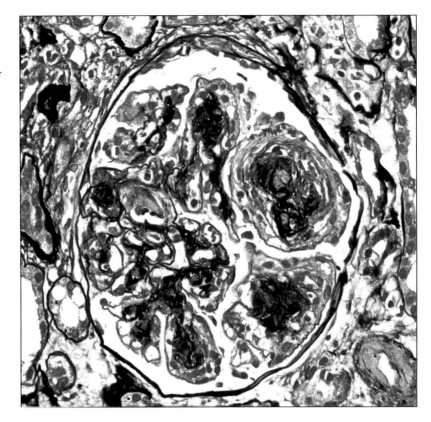

lated appearance on silver stains (Figs 2.6, 2.7). There often are dilated capillary aneurysms surrounding the expanded Kimmelstiel–Wilson nodules, resulting from mesangiolysis and loss of tethering of the capillary walls of the glomerular basement membrane to the mesangium (Figs 2.8–2.12). This repeated mesangiolysis with subsequent augmented mesangial matrix synthesis in a repair response gives rise to the laminated appearance. Occasionally, red blood cell fragments may be present in these nodules, thought to represent more severe localized microvascular injury.

The glomerular basement membrane is diffusely thickened without spikes or splitting on silver stains. Hyalinosis is common in diabetic nephropathy, resulting from insudation of plasma proteins. The term 'hyaline cap' (also called 'fibrin cap') is used to describe hyalinosis in peripheral segments of the glomerular tuft. The term 'capsular drop' is used to describe the appearance of hyaline material within Bowman's capsule. The latter lesion is quite rare, and highly specific, although not pathognomonic, for diabetic nephropathy.

Fig. 2.7 Diabetic nephropathy. The large Kimmelstiel–Wilson nodules contain small red blood cell fragments and frayed, irregular mesangial matrix, evidence of early mesangiolysis (Jones' silver stain, ×200).

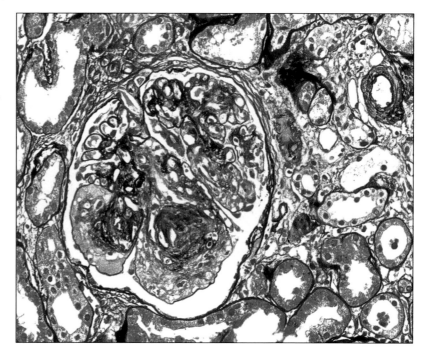

Fig. 2.8 Diabetic nephropathy. A large area of mesangial injury with red blood cell fragments and frayed, lucent-appearing mesangial matrix, indicative of mesangiolysis, are shown (Jones' silver stain, ×400).

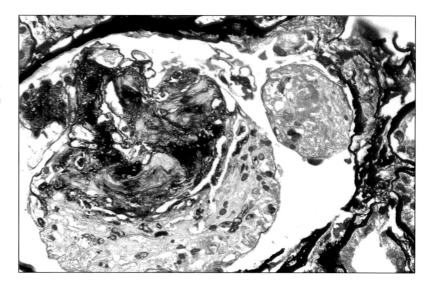

Fig. 2.9 Diabetic nephropathy. There is an area of mesangiolysis with foam cells with loss of matrix and breaks of attachments of the capillary loop. This loss of tethering of the mesangium is thought to give rise to microaneurysms. The glomerular basement membrane is also thickened, without evident deposits (Jones' silver stain, ×400).

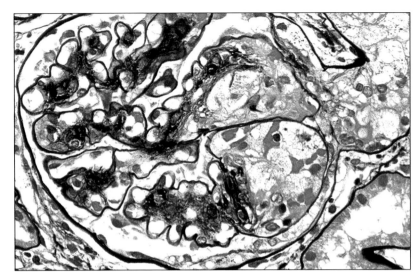

Fig. 2.10 Diabetic nephropathy. There is an area of mesangiolysis with fraying of the mesangium and loss of attachment of the mesangial area to the peripheral capillary loop. Red blood cell fragments are also present (Jones' silver stain, ×1000).

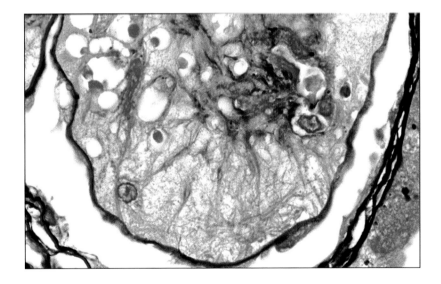

Fig. 2.11 Diabetic nephropathy. Numerous red blood cell fragments are present in this small Kimmelstiel–Wilson nodule. Red blood cell fragmentation has been associated with increased plasminogen-activator inhibitor-1 (PAI-1), and is associated with more severe disease. This is postulated to reflect local more severe microvascular injury (H&E, ×1000).

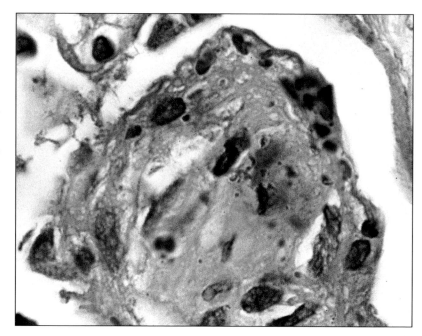

Fig. 2.12 Diabetic nephropathy. Insudation of plasma proteins may occur in any state where there is vascular injury, and is often a prominent component of diabetic nephropathy. The term 'fibrin cap' is often used for the presence of hyalinosis within the diabetic glomerulus. The glassy, smooth hyalin appearance of the insudated protein is evident, along with clear areas due to foam cells and lipid. The expanded mesangial matrix and thick glomerular basement membrane of diabetic nephropathy are evident (Jones' silver stain, ×1000).

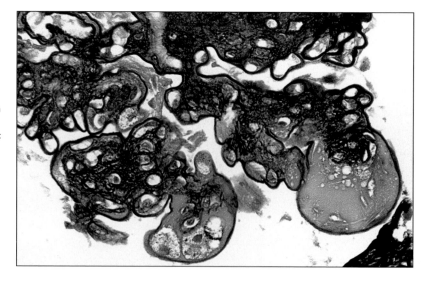

Diabetic nephropathy is invariably accompanied by lesions of arterioles and arteries. Both afferent and efferent arterioles show hyalinosis in DN (Fig. 2.13). In contrast, arterionephrosclerosis affects the afferent, but not the efferent arteriole. Interlobular and larger arteries show arteriosclerosis in DN.

There is proportional tubulointerstitial fibrosis in diabetic nephropathy. Recent studies have shown that increase in the cellular

Fig. 2.13 Diabetic nephropathy. Insudation of plasma proteins within Bowman's capsule is a fairly rare, but characteristic, although not pathogno-monic, lesion of diabetic nephropathy. This lesion, termed the 'capsular drop,' is associated in this case with thick basement membrane and a well-organized, lamellated Kimmelstiel–Wilson nodule on the right (Jones' silver stain, ×400).

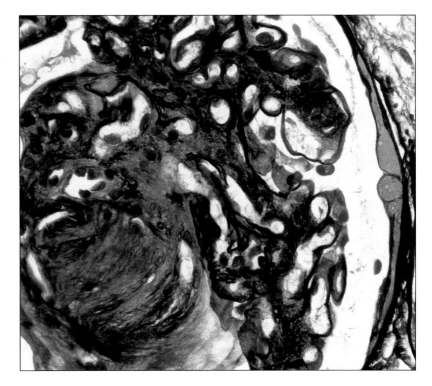

component of the interstitium precedes increase in matrix. Tubular basement membranes are thickened, and tubular atrophy and inter-stitial fibrosis occur in proportion to glomerulosclerosis (Fig. 2.7).

By immunofluorescence microscopy, there may be linear accen-tuation of glomerular basement membranes, typically strongest for IgG (Fig. 2.14). Both kappa and lambda light chain usually stain, thus ruling out possible light chain deposition disease or light and heavy chain deposition disease which has monoclonal light chain staining. Absence of accompanying C3 staining or crescents, and the clinical history also aid in differentiating this staining from anti-GBM antibody mediated glomerulonephritis. There may also be linear accentuation of Bowman's capsule and tubular basement membranes.

Electron microscopy confirms the diffuse glomerular basement membrane thickening due to widened lamina densa without immune complexes (Figs 2.15, 2.16). The GBM may be several fold normal thickness, up to 1200–1500 nm (normal in adult ~325 nm). Glomerular visceral epithelial cells show effacement of foot processes. The mesangial matrix is expanded with increased mesangial cells without immune complexes. Areas of hyalinosis appear electron dense, are often present in sclerotic areas, often contain lipid and

Fig. 2.14 Diabetic nephropathy. By immunofluorescence, there may be linear accentuation of the glomerular basement membrane in diabetic nephropathy. Differentiation from anti-GBM antibody-mediated glomerulonephritis is usually easy by correlation with clinical history, and light microscopic findings of nodular glomerulosclerosis in diabetic nephropathy versus crescents in anti-GBM antibody-mediated glomerulonephritis. In addition, C3 is often positive in a segmental, linear fashion in anti-GBM antibody-mediated glomerulonephritis, but not in diabetic nephropathy (anti-IgG immunofluorescence, ×200).

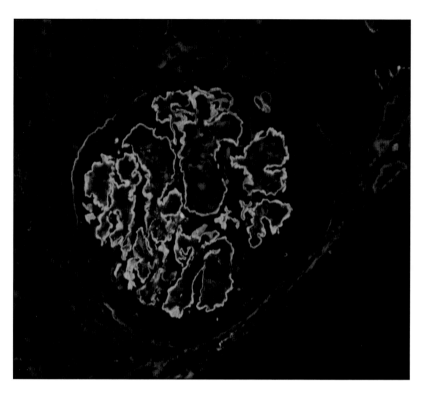

Fig. 2.15 Diabetic nephropathy. The mesangial matrix is expanded with increased mesangial cells without immune deposits. The glomerular basement membrane is usually several times normal in thickness, due to a thickened lamina densa without deposits (TEM, ×5000).

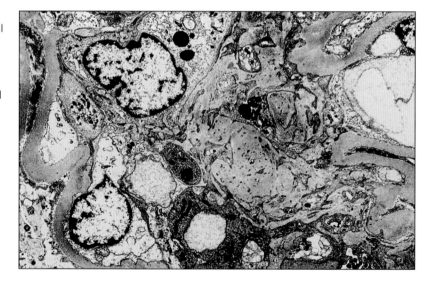

should not be confused with immune complex-type deposits. Correlation with immunofluorescence and light microscopic findings is helpful in this regard. Superimposed, nondiabetic lesions are not uncommon and complete examination by IF and EM should be done to investigate this possibility (Fig. 2.17).

Fig. 2.16 Diabetic nephropathy. The markedly thickened glomerular basement membrane is illustrated here. Even without precise morphometric measurements, the increased thickness is apparent by examining the proportion of the glomerular basement membrane to the base of intact foot processes (TEM, ×6000).

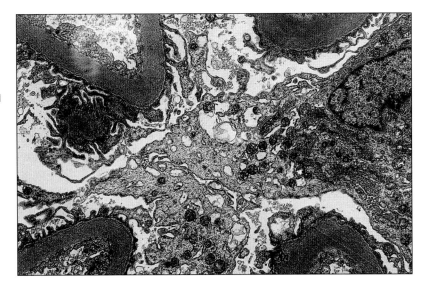

Fig. 2.17 Diabetic nephropathy. Patients with diabetic nephropathy who are biopsied typically have an unusual course of diabetic nephropathy and may occasionally have superimposed disease, as in this patient who had membranous glomerulo-nephritis with small subepithelial and intra-membranous deposits, in addition to mesangial matrix expansion, lamina densa thickening and arteriolar hyalinization related to their underlying diabetes mellitus. IgA nephropathy may also often be associated with diabetic nephropathy in biopsied diabetic patients (TEM, ×3000).

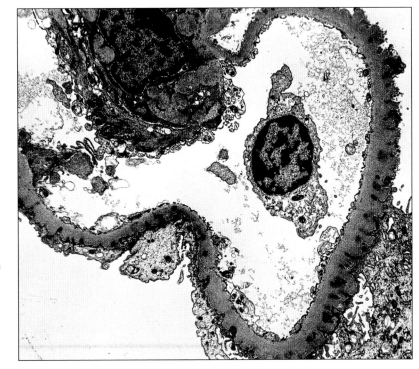

Etiology/pathogenesis

Diabetic nephropathy (DN) occurs in only 30–40% of patients with diabetic nephropathy. Further, not all patients with DM who receive a kidney transplant develop recurrent DN in the transplant. Thus, multiple complex factors are involved with the pathogenesis of DN and are discussed in detail in 'The Kidney'.

In patients with type II DM who are carefully screened by clinical criteria to have DN as a cause of their proteinuria, renal biopsy indeed demonstrated lesions of DN similar to those in type I diabetes. In unscreened patients with type II DM with proteinuria, varying renal lesions, including various immune complex and other diseases were present in one-third of patients. Regression of mild DN lesions occurred in nondiabetic patients who inadvertently received kidney transplants with early DN lesions. In recent studies of patients who had their diabetes mellitus cured by pancreas transplant, regression of existing mild to moderate DN lesions was proven by repeat biopsies over a 10-year period. These important observations show the potential for modifying the course of diabetic nephropathy. Current research is focused on the roles of intraglomerular hemodynamics and permselectivity defects, the renin angiotensin system, advanced glycation end products, growth factors such as transforming growth factor-β, the plasmin/plasminogen activator system and matrix turnover, and cell proliferation.

Selected reading

Bhalla V, Nast C C, Stollenwerk N et al 2003 Recurrent and de novo diabetic nephropathy in renal allografts. Transplantation 75(1):66–71.

Chavers B M, Bilous R W, Ellis E N et al 1989 Glomerular lesions and urinary albumin excretion in type I diabetes without overt proteinuria. New England Journal of Medicine 320:966–970.

Drummond K, Mauer M 2002 The early natural history of nephropathy in type 1 diabetes: II. Early renal structural changes in type I diabetes. Diabetes 51(5):1580–1587.

Fioretto P, Steffes M W, Sutherland D E et al 1998 Reversal of lesions of diabetic nephropathy after pancreas transplantation. New England Journal of Medicine 339:69–75.

Gambara V, Mecca G, Remuzzi G et al 1993 Heterogeneous nature of renal lesions in type II diabetes. Journal of the American Society of Nephrology 3:1458–1466.

Katz A, Caramori M L, Sisson-Ross S et al 2002 An increase in the cell component of the cortical interstitium antedates interstitial fibrosis in type 1 diabetic patients. Kidney International 61(6):2058–2066.

Kimmelstiel P, Wilson C 1936 Intercapillary lesions in glomeruli of kidney. American Journal of Pathology 12:83–97.

Mauer S M, Staffes M V, Ellis E N et al 1984 Structural-functional relationships in diabetic nephropathy. Journal of Clinical Investigation 74:1143–1155.

Østerby R, Gundersen H J, Horlyck A et al 1983 Diabetic glomerulopathy: structural characteristics of the early and advanced stages. Diabetes 2:79–82.

Schwartz M M, Lewis E J, Leonard-Martin T et al 1998 Renal pathology patterns in type II diabetes mellitus: relationship with retinopathy. The Collaborative Study Group. Nephrology, Dialysis, Transplantation 13(10):2547–2552.

Thrombotic microangiopathy/thrombotic thrombocytopenic purpura

The thrombotic microangiopathies (TMA) (Fig. 2.18) which involve the kidney consist of a heterogeneous group of disorders of different etiologies. Clinically, they are characterized by the triad of microangiopathic hemolytic anemia, thrombocytopenia and acute renal failure. They may or may not have associated systemic involvement. Evidence of involvement of multiple organs may be present including manifestations such as petechia, purpura, intestinal bleeding and neurological symptoms such as aphasia, dysphasia, parasthenia and visual problems and even seizures and coma. Evidence of renal involvement is present in a majority of patients with thrombotic microangiopathies, which are described under the general rubric of hemolytic uremic syndrome. Predominant central nervous system involvement with similar peripheral blood manifestations is seen in thrombotic thrombocytopenic purpura (TTP). Glomerular capillary and large vessel thrombosis identical to that seen in hemolytic uremic syndrome (HUS) or TTP also occurs in lupus patients with circulating antiphospholipid antibodies.

The pathological findings can be divided into those which affect the glomeruli and those which affect the arteries and arterioles. Furthermore, they can be analyzed as the lesions seen early after the onset of the disease and those which are prominent after the disease progresses. The lesions of the thrombotic microangiopathies can show a wide range of changes according both to the severity and duration of disease. The basic morphologic changes are similar in most cases regardless of the cause and relate to the presence of endothelial injury and the subsequent activation of the coagulation system.

In the early stages, glomeruli show thickening of the capillary walls caused by endothelial cell swelling and the accumulation of material between the endothelial cell and the underlying basement membrane (Fig. 2.19). By light microscopy the capillary walls show a double contour on silver stains (Fig. 2.20), and by electron microscopy this is demonstrated to correspond to acellular fibrillar material in the subendothelial region (Fig. 2.21). The term 'blood-less glomeruli' has been used to characterize glomeruli in which the capillary loops are collapsed and which may contain fragmented red blood cells, fibrin and platelet thrombi (Fig. 2.22). Fibrinoid necrosis in the afferent arteriole as it enters the glomerulus, associated with thrombosis, is also characteristic of the early phase (Fig. 2.23). Generally no increase in cellularity is seen. The mesangium may demonstrate loss of its architecture with apoptosis of mesangial cells, a process which has been termed mesangiolysis (Figs 2.24, 2.25). Partial or complete dissolution of the mesangial matrix and cells results in the development of an aneurysmatic

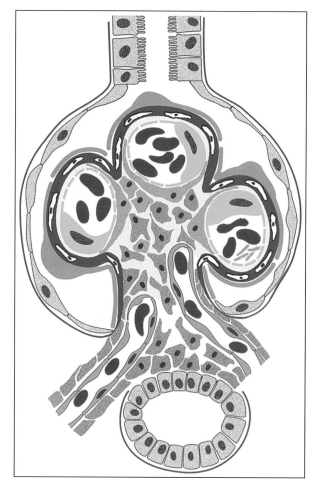

Fig. 2.18 Chronic thrombotic microangiopathy shows a split GBM by light microscopy, due to increased lamina rara interna, often with flocculent fibrin degradation products. Occasional fibrin tactoids may still be seen by EM.

Fig. 2.19 TMA. Glomerulus demonstrates thickening of the capillary walls caused by endothelial cell swelling and accumulation of material between the endothelial cell and the basement membrane. Microthrombi are also present (H&E, ×400).

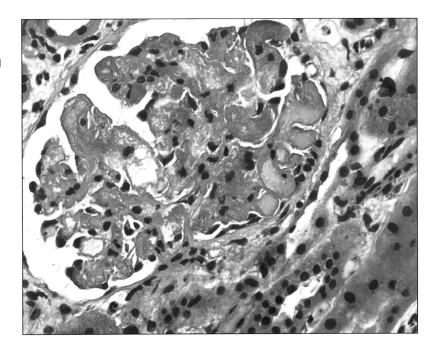

Fig. 2.20 TMA. There is mesangiolysis and focal double contours of the peripheral capillary loops (Jones' Trichrome, ×400).

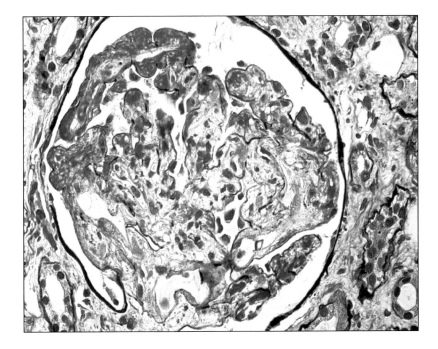

Fig. 2.21   TMA. Electron microscopy demonstrates electron lucent material separating the swollen endothelial cells from the basement membrane (TEM, ×5000).

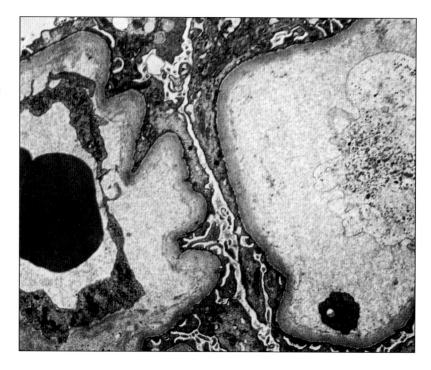

Fig. 2.22   TMA. Trichrome stain demonstrates a 'bloodless glomerulus' in which capillary loops are collapsed and occasionally contain fragmented red blood cells (Trichrome, ×400).

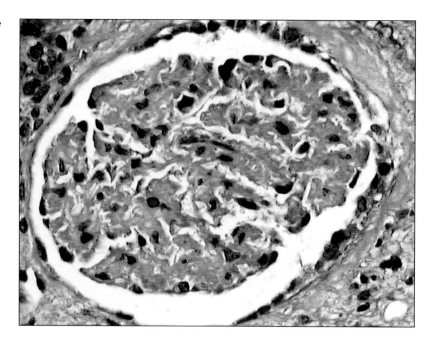

Fig. 2.23 TMA. Fibrinoid necrosis of the afferent arteriole accompanies the characteristic collapsed and bloodless glomerulus (H&E, ×400).

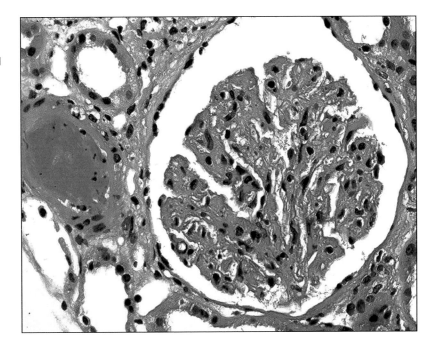

Fig. 2.24 TMA. Glomerulus demonstrating loss of the normal architecture with apoptosis of mesangial cells, a process termed mesangiolysis (H&E, ×400).

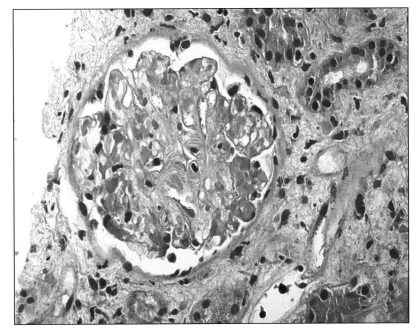

dilatation of the capillaries (Fig. 2.26). Ischemic glomerular injury characterized by collapse of capillary loops and thickening and wrinkling of the capillary walls is prominent when there are severe acute vascular lesions including thrombosis of arterioles and arteries

Fig. 2.25 TMA. Trichrome silver stain demonstrates the lack of internal mesangial core with thrombosis of the peripheral capillaries (Jones Trichrome, ×400).

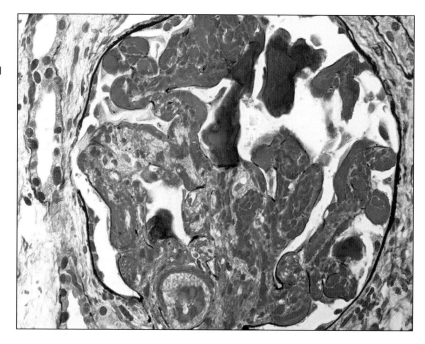

Fig. 2.26 TMA. Glomerulus demonstrates aneurysmatic dilatation of the capillaries following mesangiolysis (H&E, ×400).

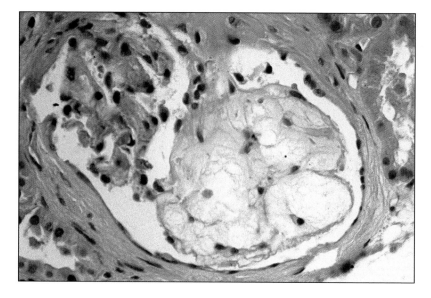

(Figs 2.27, 2.28). When necrosis of the glomerular capillaries occurs, small crescents may also be seen. As the lesion progresses, both a proliferative and sclerotic response can be seen individually and combined within the glomeruli (Fig. 2.29). Areas of mesangiolysis progress into sclerotic changes, proliferation of intrinsic glomerular cells can yield a membranoproliferative pattern which in some cases

Fig. 2.27 TMA. The afferent arterioles are also affected with evidence of fibrinoid necrosis and thrombosis (Trichrome, ×400).

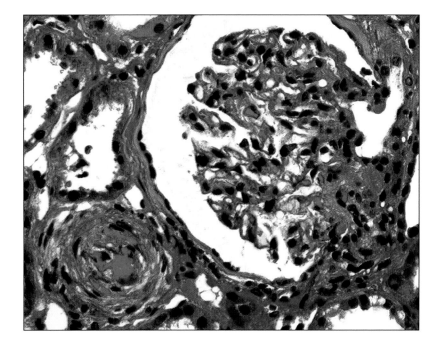

Fig. 2.28 TMA. Thrombosis extends into the glomerular capillary loops from the afferent arteriole at the vascular pole (Trichrome, ×400),

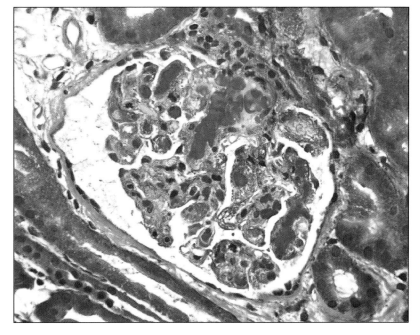

is indistinguishable by light microscopy from membranoproliferative glomerulonephritis Type I (Fig. 2.30). Examination by IF and EM allow correct classification as to the cause of the glomerular basement membrane (GBM) splitting.

Fig. 2.29 TMA. The later stage of the disease demonstrates interstitial fibrosis, tubular atrophy and beginning glomerulosclerosis (Trichrome, ×400).

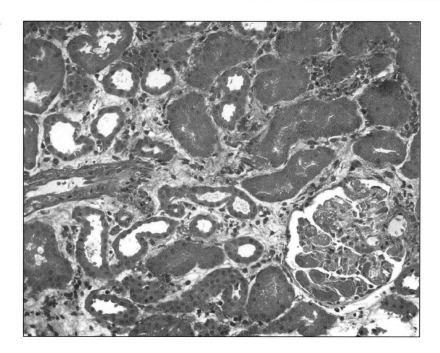

Fig. 2.30 TMA. There is advanced glomerulosclerosis with nodularity mimicking lobular glomerulonephritis (Jones silver stain, ×400).

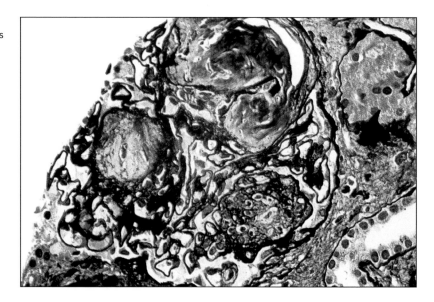

The acute arterial changes can range from mild with swelling of the endothelium to severe with evidence of fibrinoid necrosis of the media and thrombosis of the lumen (Fig. 2.31). As the disease progresses, there is myointimal proliferation with narrowing of the lumen, which involves the interlobular and arcuate arteries (Fig. 2.32). Myointimal cells have a swollen appearance. This lesion has been

Fig. 2.31 TMA. Arterial changes are present in more advanced cases with evidence of fibrinoid necrosis of the media and extravasation of red blood cells with mild intimal proliferation (Trichrome, ×400).

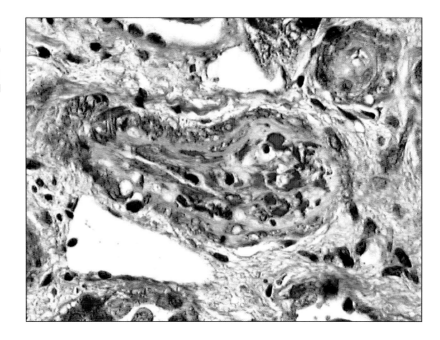

Fig. 2.32 TMA. Cross section of the vessel demonstrating marked myointimal proliferation and narrowing of the lumen with foci of fibrinoid necrosis (H&E, ×400).

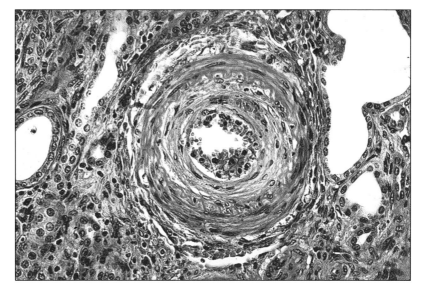

termed mucoid intimal hyperplasia and is highly characteristic for thrombotic microangiopathies. As the lesion advances, duplication of the internal elastic lamella occurs with permanent compromise of the vascular lumen. This phase is often associated with severe hypertension.

Tubular and interstitial changes are secondary to the glomerular and vascular lesions. There is often tubular collapse occasionally associated with focal tubular necrosis. Patchy necrosis and true infarcts are also occasionally present in severe cases.

Immunofluorescence microscopy demonstrates the deposition of fibrin or fibrinogen in the glomeruli and in the mesangium as well as within the vessel walls (Fig. 2.33). Occasionally, non-specific deposition of other immunoglobulins and complement may be seen.

Electron microscopic findings are consistent with those seen by light microscopy and immunofluorescence. Early lesions demonstrate the separation of the endothelium from the basement membrane and the accumulation of subendothelial fibrillar material which corresponds to the presence of fibrinogen (Figs 2.34–2.37). Thrombosis of the capillary lumina with fibrin tactoids is also occasionally seen as are accumulations of platelets. Endothelial cells in the glomeruli, arteries, and arterioles show swelling and separation from the underlying structures and evidence of apoptosis.

Etiology/pathogenesis

Hemolytic uremic syndrome can be divided into individuals who present with diarrhea or those in which diarrhea is not associated. Non-diarrhea-associated disease can be further classified as sporadic or familial. Diarrhea-associated disease is secondary to infection

Fig. 2.33 TMA. Immuno-fluorescence studies reveal diffuse deposition of fibrin throughout glomerular capillary loops (anti-fibrin immunofluorescence, ×200).

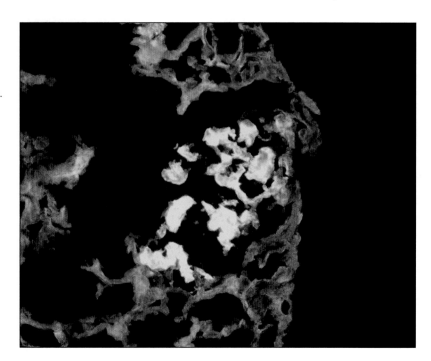

Fig. 2.34 TMA. Electron micrograph demonstrates evidence of mesangiolysis with denudation of the endothelium from the basement membrane and loss of the mesangial architecture (TEM, ×3000).

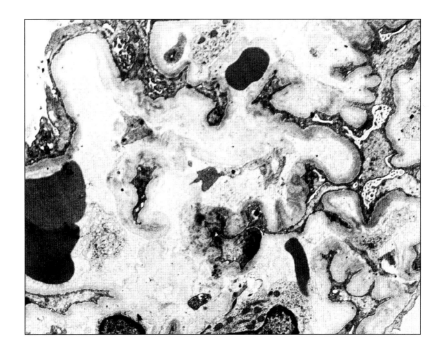

Fig. 2.35 TMA. Electron micrograph demonstrates the presence of fibrin deposition within the capillary lumen and separating the endothelial cell from the basement membrane (TEM, ×5000).

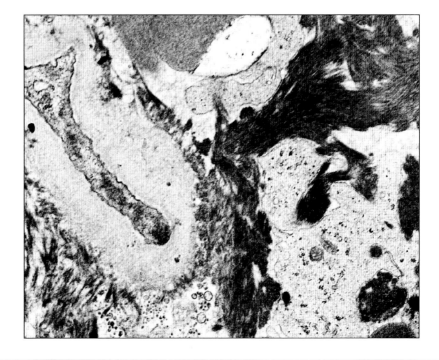

Fig. 2.36 TMA. Electron micrograph demonstrates the presence of fragmented red blood cells within the capillary lumen and endothelial cell swelling and subendothelial fibrillar material (TEM, ×5000).

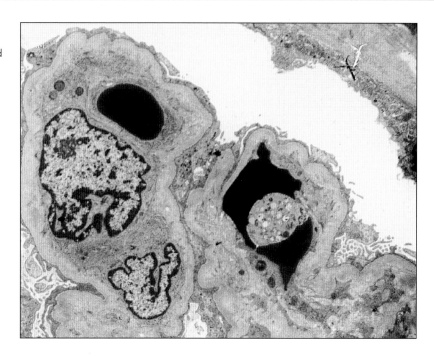

Fig. 2.37 TMA. Electron micrograph demonstrates evidence of glomerular capillary thrombosis with fragmented red blood cells bound in a fibrin matrix (TEM, ×3000).

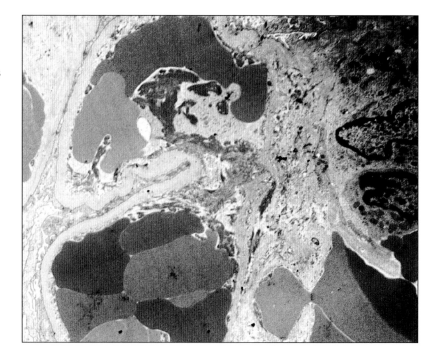

with *Escherichia coli* 0157. Pathogenic factors for *E. coli* 0157 are the production of verotoxins and adhesion molecules, which facilitate the binding of the bacteria tightly to colonocytes facilitating the transfer of the toxins. The sporadic form of the disease can be associated with pregnancy, systemic lupus erythematosus, HIV infection and a variety of drugs including oral contraceptives and cyclosporin or tacrolimus. The sporadic form has been linked to mutations in complement regulatory protein factor H. The form which has been given the name thrombotic thrombocytopenic purpura has been linked to abnormalities of the metalloproteinase which is responsible for the breakdown of large Von Willebrand factor aggregates or multimeres into smaller less active multimeres (now called ADAMTS-13). There may be a deficiency or an inhibitor of this protease. The absence of the protease results in an excess of VWF multimeres, which are pro-thrombotic. Familial HUS is due to a deficiency in ADAMTS-13.

Selected reading

Boyce T G, Swerdlow D L, Griffin P M 1995 *Escherichia coli* O157:H7 and the hemolytic uremic syndrome. New England Journal of Medicine 333:364–8.

Churg J, Strauss L 1985 Renal involvement in thrombotic microangiopathies. Seminars in Nephrology 5:46–56.

Moake J L 2002 Thrombotic microangiopathies. New England Journal of Medicine 347:589–600.

Scleroderma (progressive systemic sclerosis)

Progressive systemic sclerosis (PSS) is a multisystem disease that affects the skin, the gastrointestinal tract, the lung, the heart and the kidney. Kidney involvement occurs in approximately 60–70% of PSS patients. Age at onset of systemic sclerosis is 30–50 years and females are affected more than males, with slight predominance of African Americans vs. Caucasians. Survival over 5 years in PSS ranges from 34% to 73%, with scleroderma renal crisis the most common cause of death. In the cutaneous limited form (CREST; calcinosis, Raynaud's phenomenon, esophageal hypomotility, sclerodactyly, telangiectasia), visceral involvement typically takes much longer to become manifest. Kidney involvement in CREST is rare, occurring in ~1%.

Scleroderma renal crisis develops in approximately 20% of patients with systemic sclerosis. Patients present with malignant hypertension and acute renal failure. Grossly, petechial hemorrhages or even renal infarcts may be present in patients with scleroderma renal crisis, similar to HUS or malignant hypertension. Microscopically, there is fibrinoid necrosis of afferent arterioles. Fibrin can extend to glomeruli (Figs 2.38, 2.39). Glomeruli may show ischemic collapse or fibrinoid necrosis (Figs 2.38–2.41). Interlobular arteries show

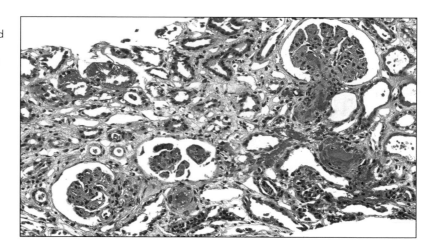

Fig. 2.38 PSS. In scleroderma crisis there is fibrinoid necrosis of interlobular arteries and arterioles, with fibrin thrombi sometimes extending to glomeruli. There is ischemic tubular injury, and early interstitial edema and fibrosis (H&E, ×100).

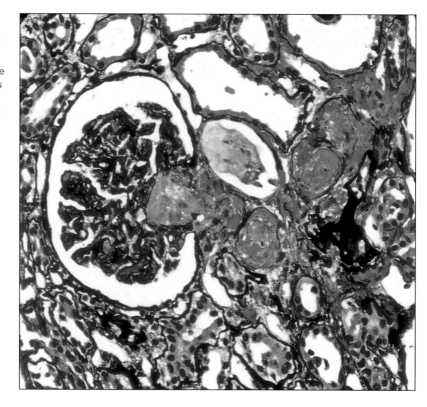

Fig. 2.39 PSS. Fibrinoid necrosis of the arteriole is present, with fibrin thrombi occluding the lumen and extending to the hilus of the glomerulus. The glomerulus itself shows only ischemic change with corrugation of the GBM and retraction of the tuft (Jones' silver stain, ×200).

Fig. 2.40 PSS. Even in glomeruli without demonstrable arteriolar injury or fibrin thrombi, there may be segmental corrugation and re-duplication of the glomerular basement membrane, related to subacute endothelial injury (Jones' silver stain, ×400).

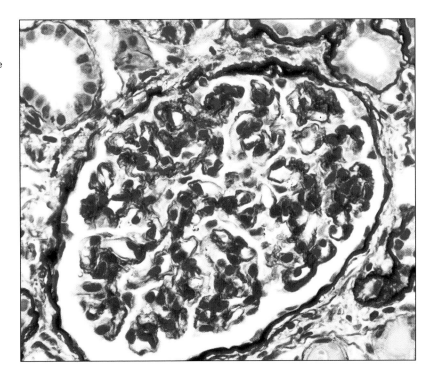

Fig. 2.41 PSS. There is fibrinoid necrosis of the wall of this arteriole, with red blood cell fragments trapped within the wall and disruption of the internal elastic lamina (Jones' silver stain, ×400).

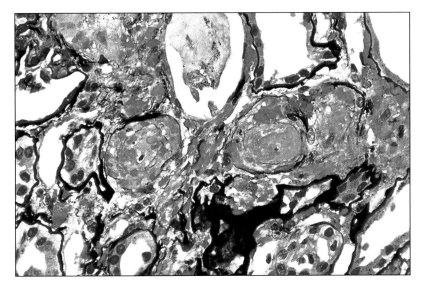

intimal thickening, proliferation of endothelial cells, and edema with mucoid change, while arterioles more often show fibrinoid necrosis (Figs 2.42–2.44). RBC fragments are often present within the injured vessel wall, and there may be vessel wall necrosis and/or fibrin thrombi within vessels. Glomeruli may show ischemic collapse,

Fig. 2.42 PSS. There is extensive injury of these medium-sized interlobular arteries, with mucoid change, necrosis and numerous red blood cell fragments, leading to occlusion of the lumens. There is surrounding acute tubular necrosis with flattening and regeneration injury of the epithelium, and ischemic corrugation of the GBM (Jones' silver stain, ×200).

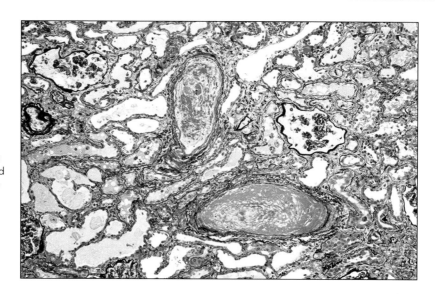

Fig. 2.43 PSS. The mucoid expansion of the intima, with fibrin occluding the lumen and numerous red blood cell fragments within the vessel wall are shown (Jones' silver stain, ×400).

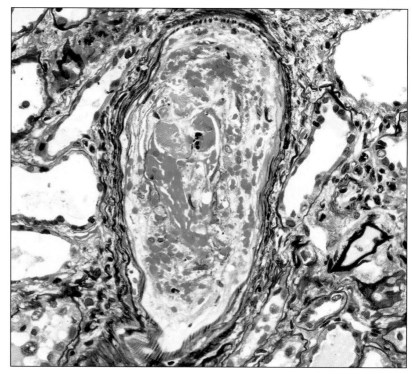

or fibrinoid necrosis. In chronic injury, there is reduplication of the elastic internal lamina, so-called onionskin pattern (Figs 2.45–2.48). Tubules may show degeneration and even necrosis, especially in scleroderma crisis (Fig. 2.42). Tubulointerstitial fibrosis develops with chronic injury. There are no immune complexes, and EM

Fig. 2.44 PSS. A less severely affected arteriole shows intimal re-duplication and mucoid change of the intima, with swelling of the endothelium (PAS, ×200).

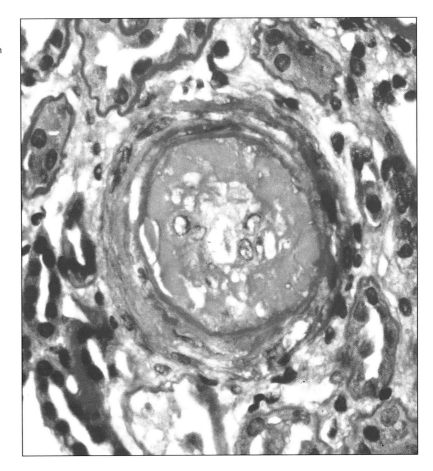

Fig. 2.45 PSS. With more chronic injury, there is early intimal fibroplasia developing from the mucoid change, with small areas of fibrin and red blood cells. The lumen is virtually occluded (Jones' silver stain, ×200).

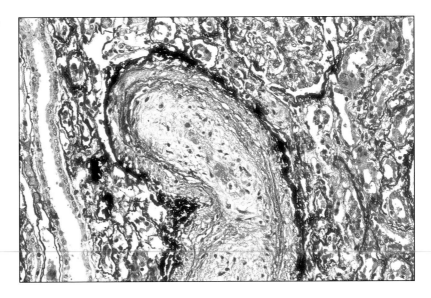

Fig. 2.46 PSS. There is remarkable mucoid change and early concentric intimal fibroplasia of these arterioles in the more chronic phase of injury (Jones' silver stain, ×200).

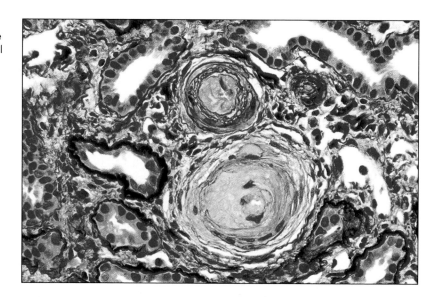

Fig. 2.47 PSS. Intimal fibroplasia is occluding the lumen of the interlobular artery, with early so-called 'onion-skinning' change, without any inflammation (Jones' silver stain, ×400).

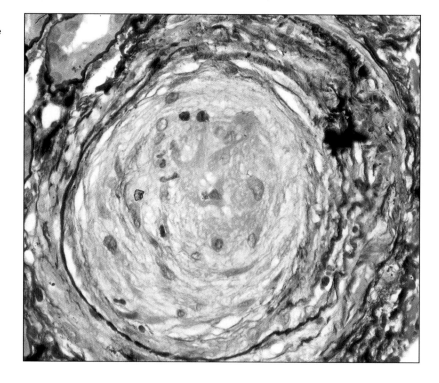

shows only increased lucency of the lamina rara interna, similar to thrombotic microangiopathy (TMA) (Fig. 2.49).

The pathologic appearance overlaps with malignant hypertension and thrombotic microangiopathy. Idiopathic malignant hypertension tends to involve smaller vessels, i.e. afferent arterioles, whereas PSS

Fig. 2.48   PSS. The well-established intimal fibroplasia following the acute injury is evident, with concentric intimal fibroplasia, the so-called 'onion-skinning' appearance (Jones' silver stain, ×400).

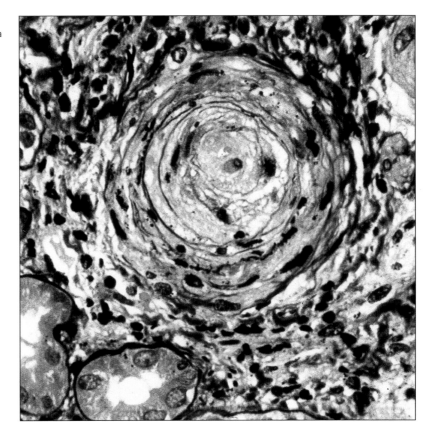

renal crisis may extend to interlobular size and larger vessels, and TMA typically involves primarily glomeruli. However, distinction of PSS and malignant hypertension solely on morphological grounds is not feasible, and clinicopathologic correlation is required for specific diagnosis.

Etiology/pathogenesis

The pathogenesis is unknown, but probably involves immune mechanisms, endothelial injury with unknown inciting events, associated with excess collagen accumulation. Endothelial injury is thought to play a key role in renal PSS, but whether it is primary or initiated by immune injury has not been elucidated.

Autoantibodies are often present, including anti-topoisomerase I, anti-centromere, anti-RNA polymerase, each present in 25% of patients with PSS. Some studies have demonstrated cytotoxic anti-endothelial factors in serum from PSS patients. Imbalance of

Fig. 2.49   There is corrugation of the GBM, with expansion of the lamina rara interna, related to chronic endothelial injury. There are no immune complexes. Overlying foot processes show extensive effacement with occasional vacuoles and lipid droplets (TEM, ×8000).

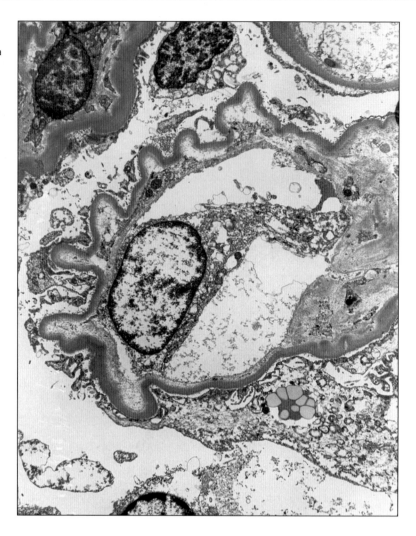

vasodilators (e.g. nitric oxide, vasodilatory neuropeptides such as calcitonin gene-related peptide, substance P) and vasoconstrictors (e.g. endothelin-1, serotonin, thromboxane A2) has been described in PSS patients. A deficiency of circulating endothelial progenitor cells, postulated to result in less vasculogenesis to contribute to repair of injured vessels, has recently been described. Prolonged vasoconstriction could contribute to structural changes and fibrosis in the kidney.

Selected reading

Cannon P J, Hassar M, Case D B et al 1974 The relationship of hypertension and renal failure in scleroderma (progressive systemic sclerosis) to structural and functional abnormalities of the renal cortical circulation. Medicine (Baltimore) 53(1):1–46.

Donohoe J F 1992 Scleroderma and the kidney. Kidney International 41:462–477.

Kuwana M, Okazaki Y, Yasuoka H et al 2004 Defective vasculogenesis in systemic sclerosis. Lancet 364(9434):603–610.

Leinwand I, Duryee A W, Richter M N 1954 Scleroderma (based on study of over 150 cases). Annals of Internal Medicine 41:1003–1041.

Steen V D, Medsger T A Jr 2000 Long-term outcomes of scleroderma renal crisis. Annals of Internal Medicine 133:600–603.

Anti-phospholipid antibody disease

Anti-phospholipid antibody disease (APL) disease may occur in conjunction with systemic lupus erythematosus (SLE) or without other underlying systemic disease. Clinical manifestations are due to thrombosis. Women may have a history of repeated miscarriages.

Patients with APL antibodies may have systemic hypertension. The kidney may be involved by thrombotic microangiopathy with acute renal failure, or symptoms may be more insidious. The involved kidney acutely shows thrombi in arterioles and interlobular arteries and also may involve glomeruli as in TMA of any cause (see detailed description of these lesions above). Chronically, the vascular lesions organize and there is fibrous intimal hyperplasia of interlobular arteries with associated focal cortical atrophy.

Etiology/pathogenesis

APL antibodies may be lupus anticoagulant or anticardiolipin antibodies and may occur as primary APL antibody syndrome or in association with SLE or other mixed connective tissue disease. These antibodies are prothrombotic, and often result in thrombosis both systemically and occasionally in the kidney, with consequent tissue ischemia and injury, similar to that seen with TMA of any cause. The involvement of larger vessels does typically in primary APL antibody syndrome result in sharply defined areas of cortical atrophy chronically.

Selected reading

Daugas E, Nochy D, Huong du L T et al 2002 Antiphospholipid syndrome nephropathy in systemic lupus erythematosus. Journal of the American Society of Nephrology 13:42–52.

Nochy D, Daugas E, Droz D et al 1999 The intrarenal vascular lesions associated with primary antiphospholipid syndrome. Journal of the American Society of Nephrology 10:507–518.

Pre-eclampsia and eclampsia

Toxemia of pregnancy includes both pre-eclampsia and eclampsia and can occur with or without an underlying primary renal disease. Pre-eclampsia is primarily a disease of nulliparas and manifests after the 20th week of gestation. It is characterized by hypertension, proteinuria and edema. Pre-eclampsia occasionally progresses to a convulsive phase that is called eclampsia. This is often life threatening and clinically is manifested by a greater degree of hypertension and proteinuria. The pathology is similar to that seen in thrombotic microangiopathies. However, it is likely that the pathogenesis is different. The clinical manifestations may also extend to include hemolysis and red blood cell fragmentation, low platelet count and elevated liver enzymes, due to endothelial activation of the hepatic sinusoids in addition to that of the glomeruli (HELLP syndrome).

Pathology

Light microscopy shows a lesion characterized by enlarged glomeruli which appear bloodless and have swollen endothelial cells, coined the endotheliosis lesion (Figs 2.50–2.54). More severe cases demon-

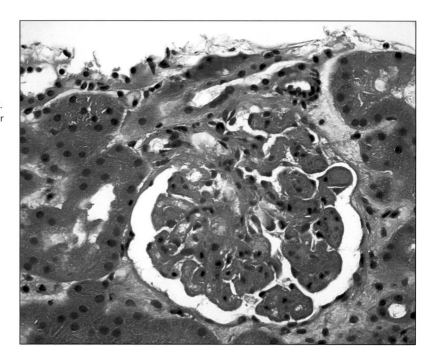

Fig. 2.50 Pre-eclampsia. Glomerulus demonstrates lobular accentuation with mesangial proliferation. The glomerular capillaries are collapsed. Occasional capillaries show microthrombi. The endothelial cells appear swollen (H&E, ×400).

Fig. 2.51 Pre-eclampsia. The glomerulus demonstrates a bloodless appearance. The capillary loops are collapsed and appear to be thickened largely as a result of endothelial cell swelling (H&E, ×400).

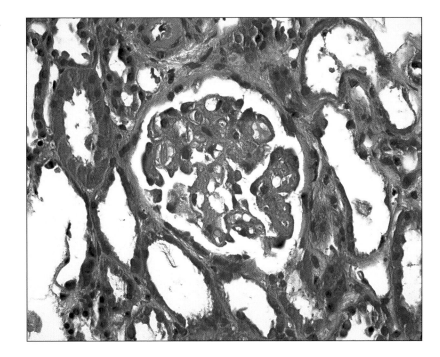

Fig. 2.52 Pre-eclampsia. The glomerulus demonstrates the same findings as in Fig. 2.51 with evidence of capillary thrombosis, thickening of the capillary walls and endothelial cell swelling (Trichrome, ×400).

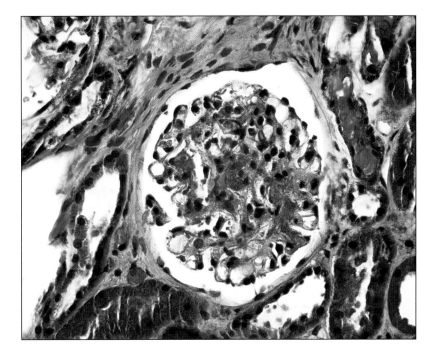

Fig. 2.53 Pre-eclampsia. Some glomerular capillaries are markedly dilated and there is evidence of mesangiolysis and focal necrosis (Trichrome, ×400).

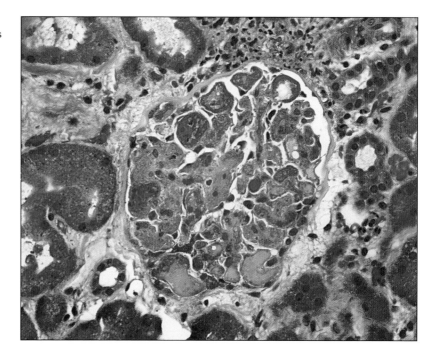

Fig. 2.54 Pre-eclampsia. In glomeruli not as severely involved, there is an increase in mesangial matrix and thickening of the capillary walls as a result of endothelial cell swelling (Trichrome, ×400).

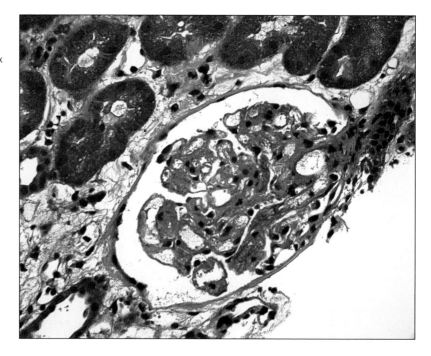

Fig. 2.55 Pre-eclampsia. Immunofluorescence demonstrates the presence of fibrinogen diffusely throughout the glomerulus (anti-fibrinogen immunofluorescence, ×200).

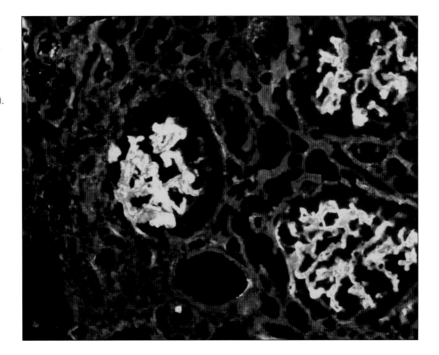

strate the presence of fibrin both on light and immunofluorescence (IF) microscopy, particularly if HELLP syndrome is present. IF confirms the presence of fibrin and only rarely are trapped immunoglobulins found (Figs 2.55, 2.56). In patients with pre-eclampsia and acute renal failure, the important findings are primarily ultrastructural with evidence of endothelial cell swelling. Electron microscopy shows endothelial swelling with separation of the endothelium from the basement membrane by lucent material consistent with fibrinogen and foci of necrosis (Figs 2.57–2.59).

Etiology/pathogenesis

Placental vascular abnormalities often accompany the presence of pre-eclampsia. There is abnormal differentiation of the cyto-trophoblasts and altered expression of adhesion molecules. These lesions lead to thrombosis of placental vasculature and infarction. It has been hypothesized that the placental injuries release a factor into the systemic circulation that induces endothelial cell activation and initiation of intravascular coagulation. Genetic links have also

Fig. 2.56 Pre-eclampsia. Higher power demonstrates fibrinogen deposition in the glomerulus and surrounding peritubular capillaries (anti-fibrinogen immunofluorescence, ×400).

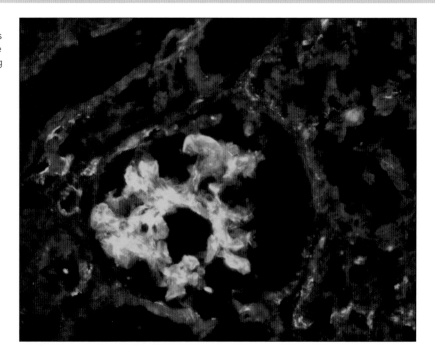

Fig. 2.57 Pre-eclampsia. Electron micrograph demonstrates the capillary lumina to be patent, the endothelial cells have lost fenestration and are swollen and separated from the basement membrane by electron lucent material (TEM, ×2000).

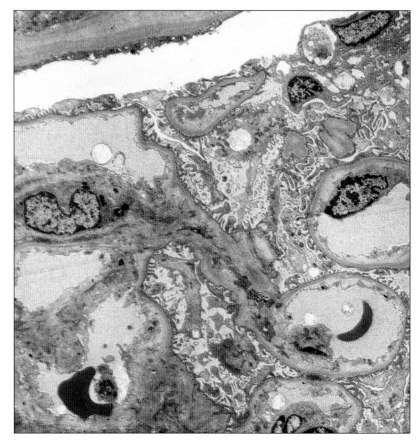

Fig. 2.58 Pre-eclampsia. Electron microscopy demonstrates the separation of the endothelium from the basement membrane with accumulation of lucent material. There is extensive effacement of the foot processes (TEM, ×3000).

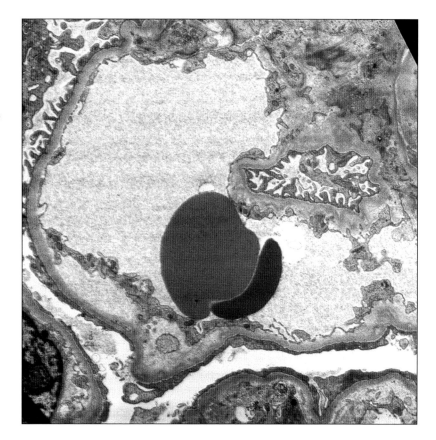

been implicated as a result of familial aggregation of the syndrome between mother and daughters. Recent studies point to a primary importance of vascular endothelial-derived growth factor (VEGF) in pre-eclampsia. Increased placental soluble fms-like tyrosine kinase 1 (sFlt1) inhibits VEGF and placental growth factor (PlGF), which in turn appear to cause endothelial dysfunction and the classic endotheliosis lesion.

Selected reading

Gaber L W, Spargo B H, Lindheimer M D 1994 Renal pathology in pre-eclampsia. Baillières Clinical Obstetrics and Gynaecology 8:443–468.

Maynard S E, Min J Y, Merchan J et al 2003 Excess placental soluble fms-like tyrosine kinase 1 (sFlt1) may contribute to endothelial dysfunction, hypertension, and proteinuria in preeclampsia. Journal of Clinical Investigation 111:649–658.

Fig. 2.59 Pre-eclampsia. Remodeling of the basement membrane is present with focal lamination and folding as a process of repair (TEM, ×5000).

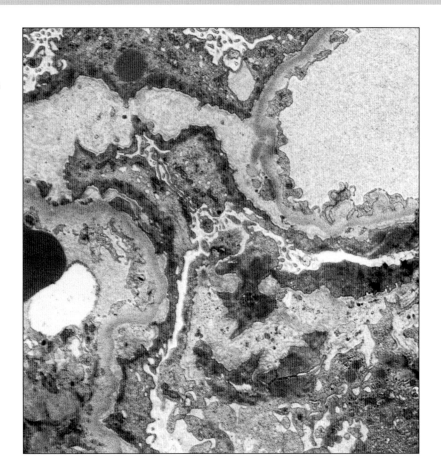

Fibromuscular dysplasia

A clinically important group of lesions of the renal artery are the so-called dysplastic lesions of the renal artery. These lesions may involve vessels outside of the renal artery but become clinically important when they cause obstruction initiating severe hypertension by creating a Goldblatt kidney. The lesions can be subdivided into six separate groups including intimal fibroplasias, medial fibroplasias, medial hyperplasia, perimedial fibroplasias, medial dissection and periarterial fibroplasias. The term fibromuscular dysplasia has been used to encompass several of these separate categories but it appears useful to sub-classify them because they may affect different patient populations (Table 2.1).

TABLE 2.1   Dysplastic lesions of the renal artery

	Age (years) and sex incidence	Relative frequency[a] (%)	Lesion
Intimal fibroplasia	1–50 M = F	1–2	Narrowing by intimal proliferation without lipid
Medial fibroplasia with aneurysms	30–60 F > M	60–70	"String of beads"; alternating stenosis and mural thinning
Medial hyperplasia	30–60 F > M	5–15	Smooth muscle hyperplasia and thickening
Perimedial fibroplasia	30–60 F > M	15–24	Fibrosis of outer media; occasionally aneurysms
Medial dissection	30–60 F > M	5–15	Fibrosis of media with dissecting aneurysms
Periarterial fibroplasia	15–50 F > M	1	Perivascular fibrosis & inflammation

M, male, F, female. [a]Relative to all forms of dysplastic lesions, ie. Medial fibroplasia is the most common form of renal arterial dysplasia.

Etiology/pathogenesis

Little is known relative to the pathogenesis but it is thought to be related to a potential defect in matrix synthesis and regulation.

Pathology

The most common of the dysplastic lesions is medial fibroplasia. This usually results in a multi-focal stenotic lesion alternating with micro aneurysms. This pattern of disease leads to the characteristic string of beads appearance seen on arteriography (Figs 2.60, 2.61). Histopathologically, there is atrophy of the muscle and fibrosis of the wall in the region of the small aneurysms alternating with the stenotic lesions where there is medial muscular hypertrophy with an increase of interstitial collagen (Fig. 2.62). The second most frequently encountered variation of fibromuscular hyperplasia is perimedial fibroplasias. In contrast to medial fibroplasias, segmental aneurysmal dilatation is not present but focal aneurysms occasionally occur (Fig. 2.63). The lesions consist of thickening of the outer half of the

Fig. 2.60 Medial fibroplasias. Radiograph from a
patient with fibromuscular
dysplasia demonstrating the
'string of beads' appearance
of the renal arteries.

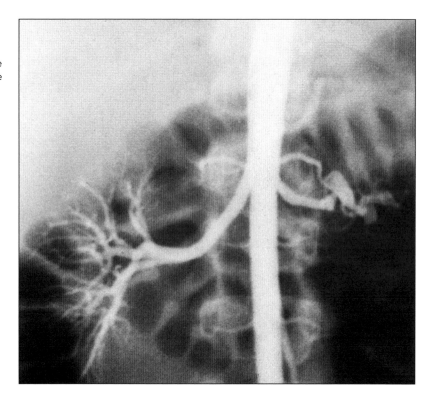

Fig. 2.61 Medial fibroplasias. Fibromuscular dysplasia. The artery shows
irregular saccular dilatations
with bands of narrowing
between the aneurysmal
dilatations. These correspond
to the 'string of beads'
findings on the radiograph.

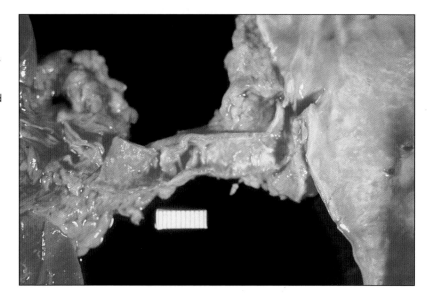

Fig. 2.62 Medial fibroplasias. Elastic stain of the vessel shows focal areas of atrophy of the smooth muscle and fibrosis in the region of the aneurysmal dilatations (elastic stain, ×200).

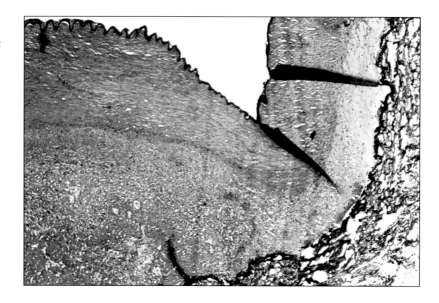

Fig. 2.63 Perimedial fibroplasia. Radiograph showing area of constriction and a focal aneurysmal dilatation distal to the constriction.

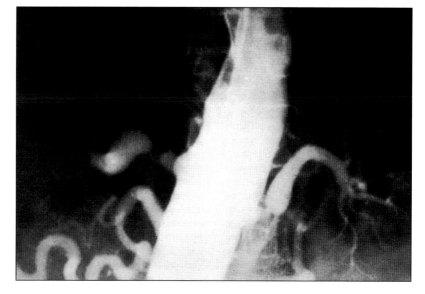

media with an increase in fibrous tissue (Fig. 2.64). The muscle is disoriented and there is generalized thickening of the wall although the elastic and intima as well as the inner portion of the media retain a normal architecture. Far less common is medial hyperplasia. Here there is hyperplasia of the muscle, which results in uniform thickening of the vessel wall and results in generalized narrowing of the lumen (Fig. 2.65). Periarterial fibroplasias is a rare lesion in which fibrosis of the adventia extends into the surrounding adipose

Fig. 2.64 Perimedial fibroplasia. Elastic stain demonstrates thickening of the outer half of the media and an increase in fibrous tissue (elastic stain, ×200).

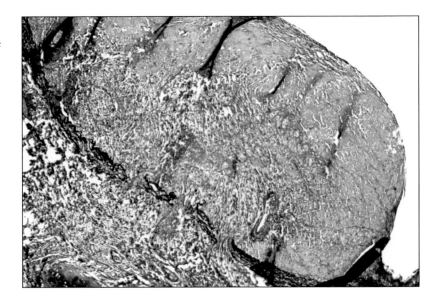

Fig. 2.65 Medial hyperplasia. Hyperplasia of the muscular layers of the wall results in uniform thickening of the vessel wall with generalized narrowing of lumen without aneurysmal dilation (H&E, ×400).

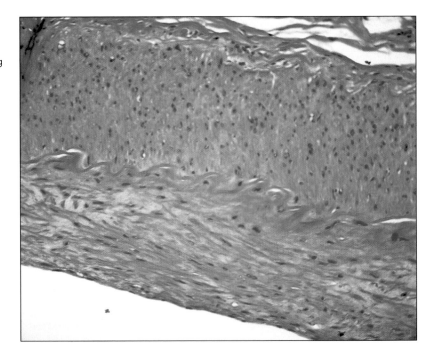

and connective tissue resulting in constriction of the vessel from without rather than from within the vessel wall. In intimal fibroplasias, the fibrotic lesion involves only the intima of the vessel with the elastica and media maintaining a normal structure (Fig. 2.66). There is hyperplasia of the intima, which is essentially indistin-

Fig. 2.66 Periarterial fibroplasias. Fibrosis is predominantly present in the adventitia with irregular changes within the muscular media (H&E, ×400).

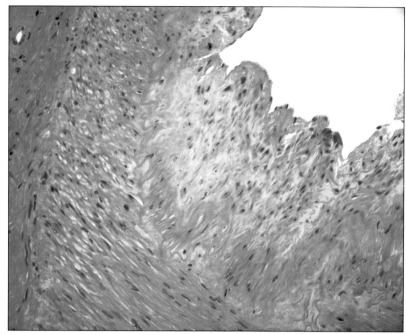

guishable from the proliferative stage of arteriosclerosis, but is not associated with an increased deposition of lipid. The lesion has been reported in an individual as young as one year of age but most commonly seen in the third and fourth decades.

Selected reading

Kashgarian M 1995 Hypertensive disease and kidney structure. In: Laragh J H and Brenner B M (eds) Hypertension. Raven, New York pp. 433–444.

Arterionephrosclerosis

Patients usually have a history of hypertension and may have renal insufficiency and varying proteinuria. Proteinuria can be nephrotic range, particularly if hypertension is severe. Arterionephrosclerosis (ANS) is associated with renal insufficiency in African-Americans more commonly than in Caucasians.

'Benign' nephrosclerosis results in small kidneys with finely granular surface and thinned cortex in late stages (Fig. 2.67). Microscopically, there is vascular wall medial thickening with frequent afferent arteriolar hyaline deposits (Figs 2.68, 2.69). The hyalinization is due to endothelial injury and increased pressure, leading to an insudate

Fig. 2.67 The kidney shows a finely granular surface, related to arteriolar sclerosis with associated glomerular obsolescence and tubulointerstitial fibrosis. The broad-based scars are due to disease in slightly larger, interlobular arteries with depressed cortical areas of scarring.

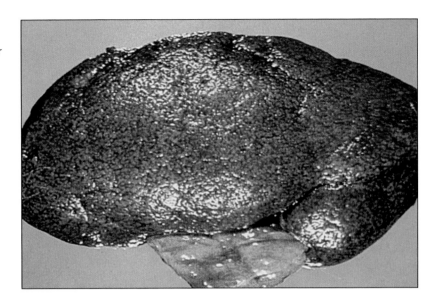

Fig. 2.68 ANS. Endothelial injury is frequently accompanied by hyalinosis, a lesion due to an insudation of plasma proteins. The material is glassy smooth and PAS-positive (PAS, ×200).

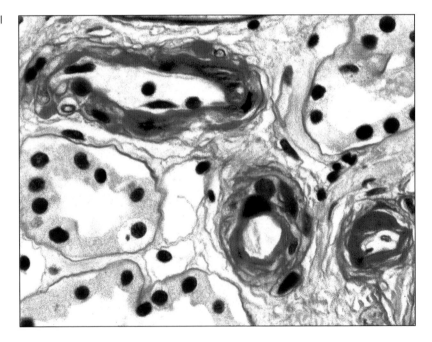

of plasma macromolecules. With accelerated hypertension, endothelial cells are swollen and RBC fragments can be trapped within the vessel wall (Fig. 2.70). Interlobular and larger arteries show varying medial hypertrophy and intimal fibrosis with reduplication of the internal elastic lamina (Figs 2.71–2.73). There are associated focal glomerular ischemic changes with variable thickening and wrinkling

Fig. 2.69 ANS. Moderate to severe hyalinosis is present in this arteriole. It is cut multiple times in this section, because of its tortuosity. The hyalinosis is eccentric (H&E, ×200).

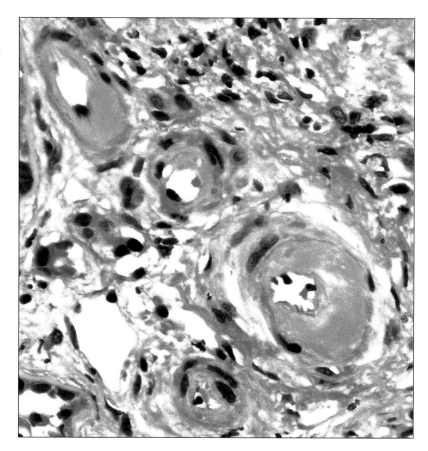

Fig. 2.70 ANS. There is severe hyalinosis of this interlobular artery, with swollen endothelial cells and a few red blood cell fragments, indicative of early, accelerated endothelial injury (Jones' silver stain, ×200).

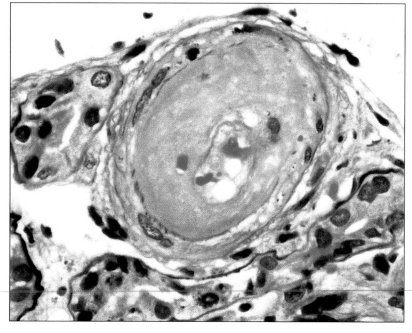

Fig. 2.71 ANS. There is re-duplication of the intima, with intimal fibroplasia, resulting in a thicker, less compliant wall of this inter-lobular artery (PAS, ×200).

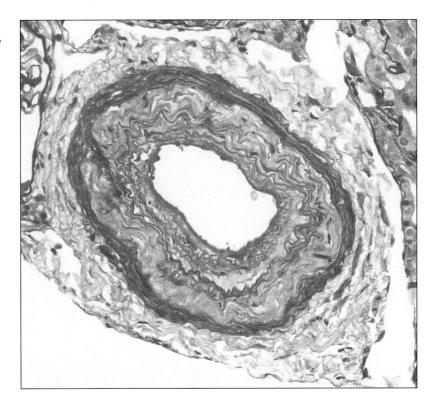

Fig. 2.72 ANS. There is intimal fibrosis, thickening of the media, and increased thickness of the adventitia (PAS, ×100).

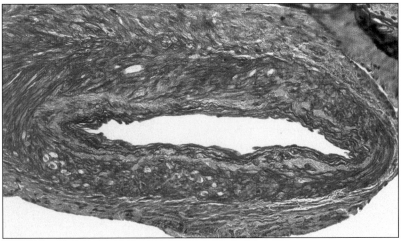

of the basement membrane, and/or global sclerosis, tubular atrophy and interstitial fibrosis. Global sclerosis can be either of the obsolescent type (i.e. glomerular tuft sclerosed and Bowman's space filled with collagenous material) or of the solidified type (global solidification of the tuft without collagenous material within Bowman's space) (Figs 2.74–2.78). Globally sclerosed glomeruli can

Fig. 2.73 ANS. A large artery shows marked intimal fibroplasia. Adjacent arterioles show severe hyalinosis (Jones' silver stain, ×200).

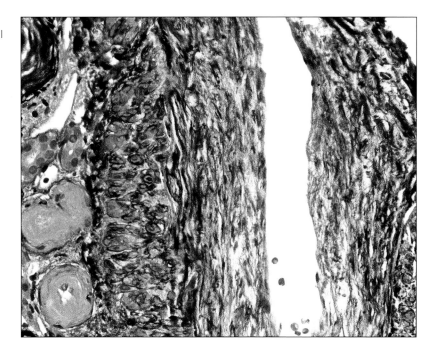

Fig. 2.74 ANS. The solidified type of global sclerosis is characterized by solidification of the entire glomerular tuft (PAS, ×200).

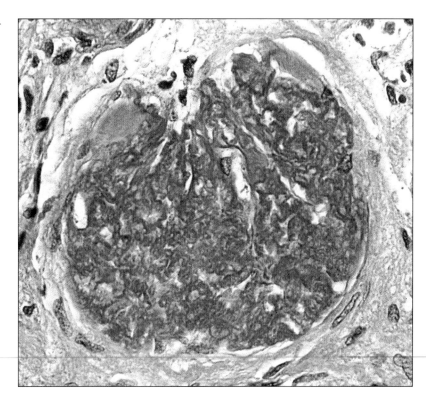

Fig. 2.75 ANS. The solidified glomerulus is completely solidified, with wrinkled glomerular basement membrane clearly discernible on silver stain (Jones' silver stain, ×200).

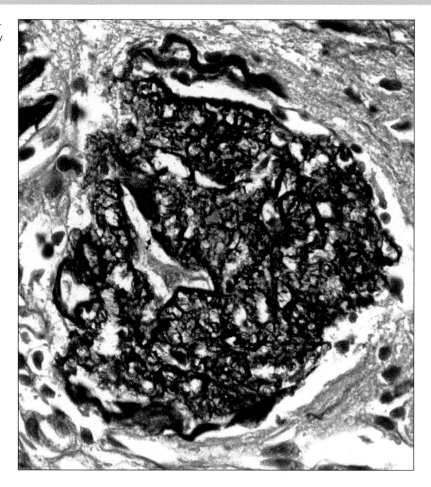

Fig. 2.76 ANS. Two solidified glomeruli are shown, along with an artery with intimal fibroplasia. The glomerulus on the far right is becoming resorbed, with dissolution of Bowman's capsule, becoming continuous with the surrounding interstitial fibrosis. The adjacent glomerulus is still easily recognizable by silver stain, but Bowman's capsule is no longer intact. The remnant of another glomerulus is evident on the left, with small area of contours of GBM still visible on silver stain. There is severe associated tubular atrophy, so-called 'thyroidization' with interstitial fibrosis (Jones' silver stain, ×200).

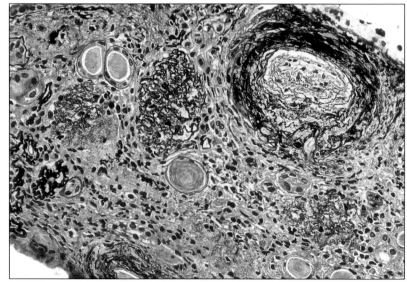

Fig. 2.77 ANS. Glomeruli may also become globally sclerosed by becoming obsolescent. The obsolescent glomerulus has a totally sclerosed glomerular tuft with fibrous material filling in and obliterating Bowman's capsule. The adjacent artery shows intimal re-duplication, and there is surrounding tubulointerstitial fibrosis (PAS, ×200).

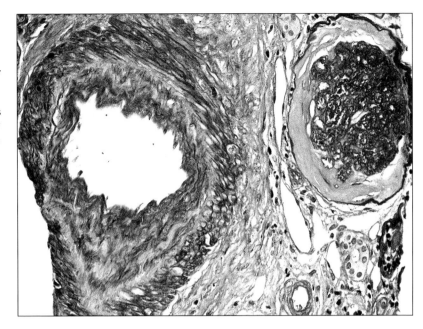

Fig. 2.78 ANS. The obsolescent glomerulus is easily differentiated from the soliditied type by silver stain, highlighting the retracted, globally sclerosed glomerular tuft and the collagenous material filling in Bowman's space. There is surrounding tubulointerstitial fibrosis (Jones' silver stain, ×200).

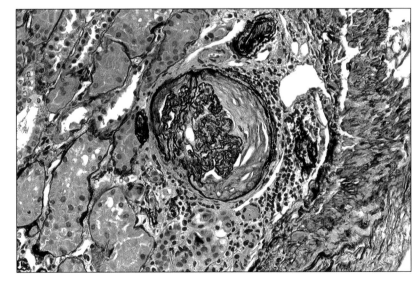

even become continuous with the surrounding interstitial fibrosis as Bowman's capsule is resorbed. The globally sclerosed glomerulus may then be difficult to discern and may even disappear as a recognizable structure (Fig. 2.76). Secondary focal segmental glomerulosclerosis (FSGS) may also occur, often with associated GBM corrugation and periglomerular fibrosis and subtotal foot process

Fig. 2.79 Arterionephro-sclerosis may also show glomerular lesions, with secondary segmental glomerulosclerosis, often characterized by hilar location of segmental sclerosis with associated hyalin, vascular sclerosis, and periglomerular fibrosis.

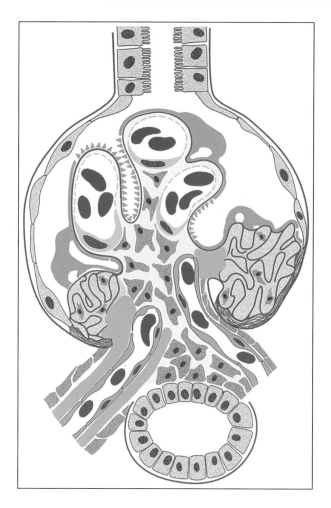

effacement (Figs 2.79–2.81). In addition, the associated vascular lesions and the clinical history, with hypertension preceding other manifestations of renal disease, are useful in favoring a secondary etiology of the segmental sclerosis rather than primary FSGS. Immunofluorescence may show trapping of IgM and C3 in glomeruli. Electron microscopy confirms the corrugated, wrinkled GBM and ischemic changes with increased lucency of the lamina rara interna without immune deposits (Fig. 2.82). Some foot process effacement may also be present, but it is usually not as extensive as in primary FSGS. Hyaline deposits are often present in arterioles as well as in sclerosed segments of glomeruli (Fig. 2.83).

Although none of these lesions is pathognomonic, the constellation of these changes in the absence of other lesions of primary glomerular disease is indicative of arterionephrosclerosis.

Fig. 2.80 ANS. There may be associated secondary segmental glomerulosclerosis, as shown on the left, associated with globally sclerotic glomeruli, arteriolo- and arteriosclerosis. There is proportional tubulointerstitial fibrosis (Jones' silver stain, ×100).

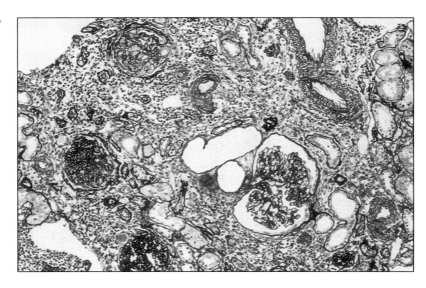

Fig. 2.81 ANS. Segmental sclerosis in ANS typically has associated periglomerular fibrosis, obsolescent glomeruli, vascular disease out of proportion to segmental sclerosis, and subtotal foot process effacement (PAS, ×200).

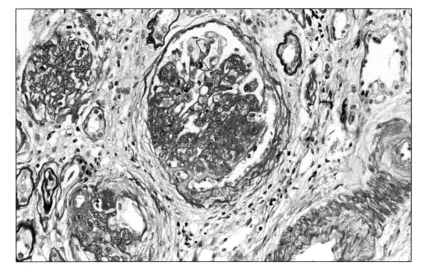

Etiology/pathogenesis

Hypertension has been presumed to cause end organ damage in the kidney. In a large series of renal biopsies in patients with essential hypertension, arteriolar nephrosclerosis was present in 81.2%, and the severity of arteriolar sclerosis correlated significantly with level of diastolic blood pressure. However, in several large autopsy series

Fig. 2.82 ANS. Although segmental sclerosis was present in this patient with ANS, there is only minimal foot process effacement, segmental increase in lamina rara interna lucent material, and segmental corrugation of the GBM (TEM, ×11,250).

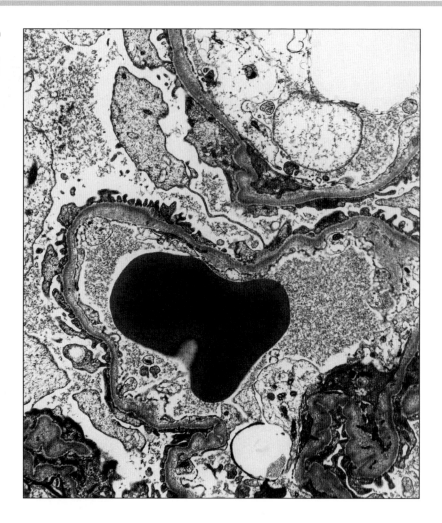

of patients with presumed benign hypertension, significant renal lesions were rare. Further, the level of blood pressure does not directly predict degree of end organ damage: African Americans have higher risk for more severe end organ damage at any level of blood pressure. It is possible that underlying microvascular disease causes the hypertension and the renal disease in susceptible patients. Underlying causes include possible genetic and structural components, such as low-term birth weight, linked to increased risk of cardiovascular disease and hypertension in adulthood. Low birth weight is also associated with fewer nephrons at birth, and enlarged glomeruli. Low birth weight occurs more commonly in African Americans than in Caucasians, and healthy African Americans have larger glomeruli than age- and body mass-matched Caucasians. The fewer nephrons

Fig. 2.83 ANS. An arteriole with hyalinosis is shown (TEM, ×11 250).

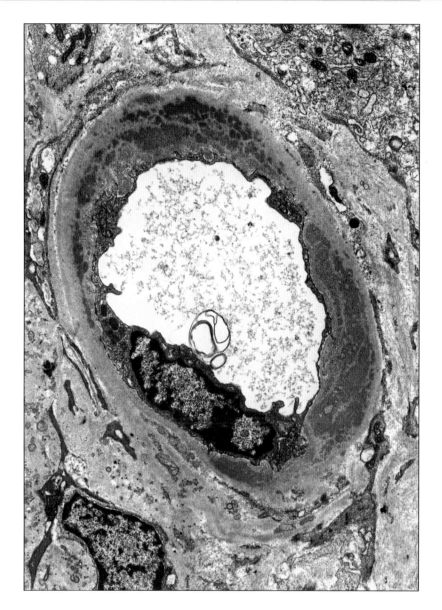

are postulated to be exposed to greater hemodynamic stress. In addition, genetic polymorphisms contributing to retarded intrauterine development might also play a role in augmented fibrotic responses to injuries later in life.

Our recent data suggest a different phenotype of scarring in arterionephrosclerosis in African Americans vs. Caucasians. The solidified type of global glomerulosclerosis was more frequent in African Americans, contrasting the predominance of the obsolescent type of global sclerosis in Caucasians. The solidified type was also associated with more severe disease clinically, echoing its original description as 'decompensated benign nephrosclerosis'.

Selected reading

Barker D J, Osmond C, Golding J et al 1989 Growth in utero, blood pressure in childhood and adult life, and mortality from cardiovascular disease. British Medical Journal 298(6673):564–567.

Böhle A, Ratschek M 1982 The compensated and decompensated form of benign nephrosclerosis. Pathology, Research and Practice 174:357–367.

Brenner B M, Garcia D L, Anderson S 1988 Glomeruli and blood pressure. Less of one, more the other? American Journal of Hypertension 1:335–347.

Fogo A, Breyer J A, Smith M C et al 1997 Accuracy of the diagnosis of hypertensive nephrosclerosis in African Americans: a report from the African American Study of Kidney Disease (AASK) Trial. AASK Pilot Study Investigators. Kidney International 51:244–252.

Freedman B I, Iskandar S S, Buckalew V M et al 1994 Renal biopsy findings in presumed hypertensive nephrosclerosis. American Journal of Nephrology 14:90–94.

Innes A, Johnston P A, Morgan A G et al 1993 Clinical features of benign hypertensive nephrosclerosis at time of renal biopsy. Quarterly Journal of Medicine 86:271–275.

Katz S M, Lavin L, Swartz C 1979 Glomerular lesions in benign essential hypertension. Archives of Pathology Laboratory Medicine 103:199–203.

Keller G, Zimmer G, Mall G et al 2003 Nephron number in patients with primary hypertension. New England Journal of Medicine 348(2):101–108.

Marcantoni C, Ma L-J, Federspiel C et al 2002 Hypertensive nephrosclerosis in African-Americans vs. Caucasians. Kidney International 62:172–180.

McManus J F A, Lupton C H Jr 1960 Ischemic obsolescence of renal glomeruli: the natural history of the lesions and their relation to hypertension. Laboratory Investigations 9:413–434.

Sommers S C, Relman A S, Smithwick R H 1958 Histologic studies of kidney biopsy specimens from patients with hypertension. American Journal of Pathology 34:685–713.

Accelerated/malignant hypertension

Malignant or accelerated hypertension is more rare than previously in the USA. However, in other countries, malignant hypertension at initial presentation is still not uncommon. The average age is 40 years and men are affected more commonly than women. Patients may have a history of 'benign' hypertension, or present *de novo* with malignant hypertension, defined as blood pressure usually higher than 200/130 mmHg. Fewer than 1% of patients with hypertension, either primary or secondary, develop the malignant phase. Patients usually present with severe headaches, vomiting, visual disturbances, stupor, coma, convulsions, congestive heart failure, oliguria or renal failure. Any one or all of the above may be present. Patients may have proteinuria, even nephrotic range, which decreases with control of blood pressure. Hematuria may also be present in some patients. Severe retinopathy is present with hemorrhage and exudates, with papilledema being present only in malignant, but not accelerated hypertension. If left untreated, survival is poor, while long-term survival is >90% if blood pressure is controlled.

Malignant (accelerated) nephrosclerosis grossly shows petechial hemorrhage of the subcapsular surface, with mottling and occasional areas of infarct (Fig. 2.84). Microscopically, arterioles show mucoid change and endothelial cell swelling with RBC fragments in accelerated hypertensive injury (Fig. 2.85). In malignant hypertension, there is fibrinoid necrosis of arterioles, and interlobular arteries have a concentric onion-skin pattern of intimal fibrosis, overlapping with the appearance of progressive systemic sclerosis and thrombotic microangiopathy (Figs 2.86–2.88). Larger arteries do not usually show specific lesions in primary malignant hypertension. In secondary hypertension, there may be underlying intimal fibrosis and reduplication of the elastica. Glomeruli may be normal, or show focal segmental necrosis or severe congestion. With more chronic, ongoing injury, there is corrugation of the GBM with occasional reduplication

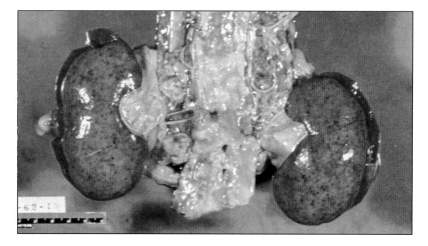

Fig. 2.84 Malignant hypertension. Grossly, there are petechial hemorrhages, secondary to the arteriolar necrosis, giving rise to a 'flea-bitten' appearance.

Fig. 2.85 Accelerated hypertension. There is endothelial swelling and mucoid change with red blood cell fragments within the wall, but without frank fibrinoid necrosis, associated with accelerated hypertension (Jones' silver stain, ×200).

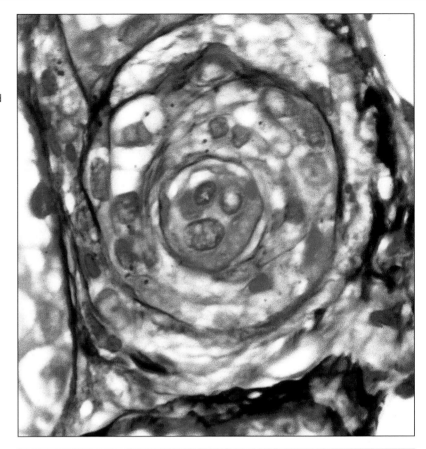

Fig. 2.86 Malignant hypertension. There is frank fibrinoid necrosis of the arteriole, which has led to obliteration of the glomerulus. There is surrounding tubulointerstitial fibrosis. This appearance cannot be distinguished morphologically from the acute injury in progressive systemic sclerosis, and clinicopathological correlation is needed (H&E, ×200).

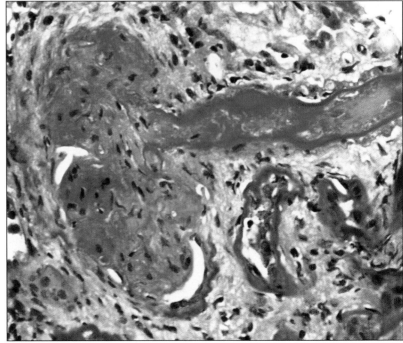

Fig. 2.87 Malignant hypertension. An inter-lobular artery is occluded by swollen endothelial cells with karyorrhectic debris, occasional PMNs and chunks of fibrin within the swollen endothelium. The media is still intact (Jones' silver stain, ×200).

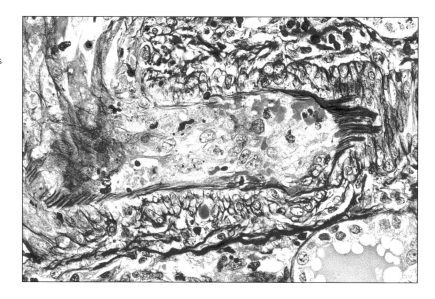

Fig. 2.88 Malignant hypertension. There is extensive injury of the interlobular artery, with occlusion by endothelial swelling with mucoid change and fibrin thrombi, with fibrinoid necrosis extending into the media (Masson trichrome stain, ×400).

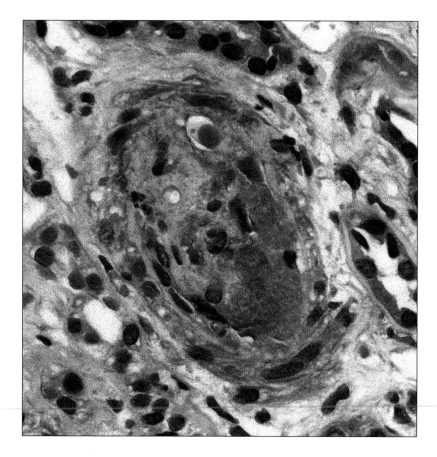

Fig. 2.89 Malignant hypertension. There is endothelial swelling and fibrin occluding the arteriole at the glomerular hilus, with ischemic retraction of the glomerular tuft (Jones' silver stain, ×400).

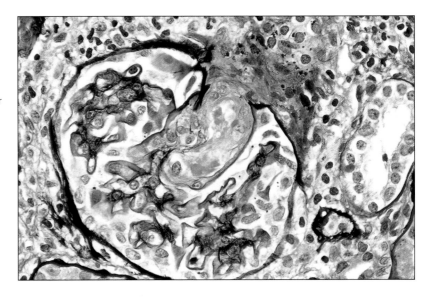

Fig. 2.90 Malignant hypertension. Even glomeruli without thrombotic occlusion may show ischemic injury with corrugation of the GBM and segmental re-duplication (Jones' silver stain, ×400).

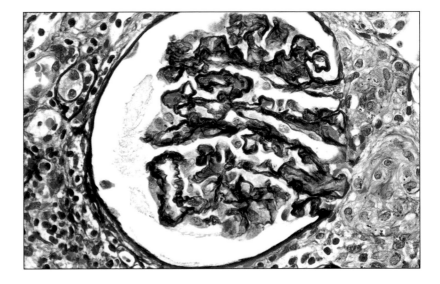

(Figs 2.89, 2.90). These changes typically are superimposed on lesions of benign arterionephrosclerosis, such as medial hypertrophy, arteriolar hyaline, intimal fibrosis and global glomerulosclerosis with proportional tubulointerstitial fibrosis. By IF, there may be trapping of IgM and C3 in sclerotic areas. Necrotic vessels and glomeruli may stain for fibrinogen. Electron microscopy shows corrugation of the GBM, and expansion of the lamina rara interna (Fig. 2.91). Foot processes may show segmental effacement. Fibrin tactoids may be visualized by EM. There are no immune complexes.

Fig. 2.91 Malignant hypertension. There is expansion of the lamina rara interna and corrugation of the glomerular basement membrane, with segmental effacement of the overlying foot processes (TEM, ×9750).

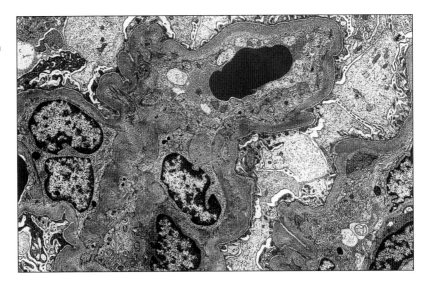

Etiology/pathogenesis

Fibrinoid necrosis of the arterioles plays a key role in development of the signs and symptoms. However, the etiology is unknown. Abnormalities in the renin angiotensin system have been postulated to play a role. An animal model with rats transgenic for renin mirrors many aspects of malignant hypertension.

Selected reading

Bohle A, Helmchen U, Grund K E et al 1977 Malignant nephrosclerosis in patients with hemolytic uremic syndrome (primary malignant nephrosclerosis). Current Topics in Pathology 65:81–113.

Caetano E R, Zatz R, Saldanha L B et al 2001 Hypertensive nephrosclerosis as a relevant cause of chronic renal failure. Hypertension 38(2):171–176.

Hsu H, Churg J 1980 The ultrastructure of mucoid 'onionskin' intimal lesions in malignant nephrosclerosis. American Journal of Pathology 99(1):67–80.

Lip G Y, Beevers M, Beevers G 1994 The failure of malignant hypertension to decline: a survey of 24 years' experience in a multiracial population in England. Journal of Hypertension 12(11):1297–1305.

Murphy C 1995 Hypertensive emergencies. Emerg Clin N Am 13:973–1001.

Atheroemboli

Atheroembolic disease occurs in older patients who have underlying atherosclerosis. Men are more frequently affected than women, reflecting higher incidence of atherosclerotic disease. Cholesterol emboli most often involve multiple organs, and have been reported

Fig. 2.92 Atheroemboli. Atheroemboli typically lodge in arterioles and interlobular arteries. Multiple cleft-shaped spaces, reflecting the empty space left after dissolution of the cholesterol by standard processing, are present in the artery in the middle, with surrounding inflammatory cell reaction. In the early weeks, this infiltrate consists primarily of mononuclear cells. An older lesion, more organized and with more subtle cholesterol emboli is seen in the arteriole on the right, with a single cleft-like space and surrounding hyperplasia and fibrosis of the arteriole (H&E, ×100).

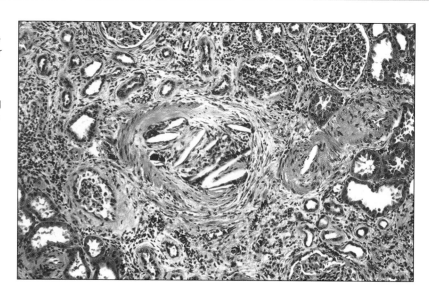

Fig. 2.93 Atheroemboli. The acute phase of cholesterol emboli is shown, with multiple stacks of varying shapes of cleft-like spaces in an artery with surrounding giant cell and mononuclear cell reaction. There is minimal fibrosis (Masson trichrome stain, ×200).

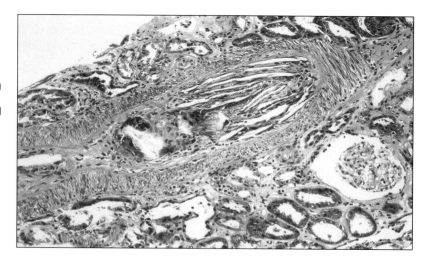

in virtually all tissues. The kidney is the most commonly involved organ at autopsy (75%), followed by spleen (55%), pancreas (52%), gastrointestinal tract (31%) and the adrenals (20%).

The histological diagnosis of cholesterol emboli is based on the finding of the characteristic needle-shaped slits of dissolved cholesterol crystals in the lumina of blood vessels (Figs 2.92–2.96). The crystals are dissolved by routine tissue processing, but are birefringent and stain positive for fat on frozen section. The cholesterol

Fig. 2.94 Atheroemboli. Immediately after cholesterol emboli showering, there are only rare inflammatory cells with a mix of PMNs and monocytes, with red blood cell fragments, fibrin and platelets surrounding the cleft-like spaces occluding this interlobular artery (H&E, ×200).

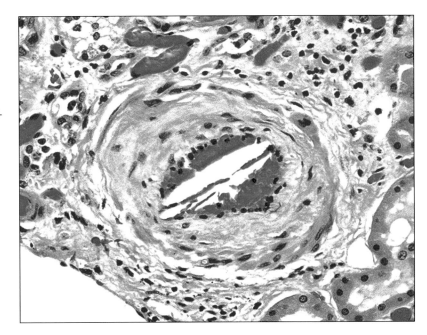

Fig. 2.95 Atheroemboli. Intimal fibrosis and mild cell proliferation with occasional mononuclear cells are seen in this artery with a single cleft-like space, representing a dissolved cholesterol embolus. When these cleft-like spaces are oriented at an angle parallel to the lumen of the artery, they may easily be overlooked (H&E, ×200).

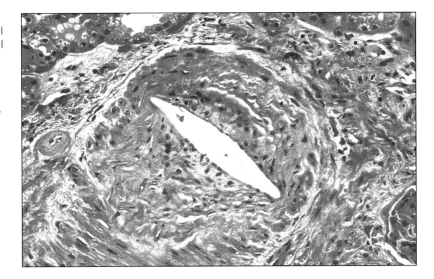

emboli usually lodge in vessels of 150–300 μm diameter. In the kidney, therefore, the lesions are most common in arcuate and interlobular arteries, although glomeruli may also be involved (Fig. 2.97). When there is massive showering of cholesterol emboli, there may be patchy cortical necrosis and tubular necrosis and injury secondary to ischemia. If the process is more gradual, there may be a mixture of necrosis due to acute local ischemia from occluded vessels, and more chronic ischemic changes, such as glomerular scarring, tubular atrophy and interstitial fibrosis. The early response, based on animal models, consists of mononuclear cell infiltration in the vessel and foreign body giant cell reaction surrounding the crystals (Fig. 2.93).

Fig. 2.96 Atheroemboli. A single, small inconspicuous cholesterol embolus was present in this patient, who presented with acute worsening of hypertension and acute decline in renal function. There is surrounding mononuclear cell reaction and underlying arteriosclerosis (Jones' silver stain, ×200).

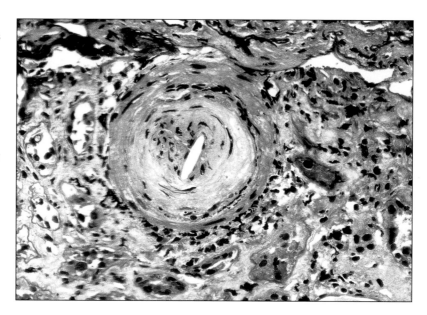

Fig. 2.97 Atheroemboli. Cholesterol emboli may rarely enter the glomerulus. Here there is focal surrounding mononuclear cell reaction. Numerous cholesterol emboli were found in other arterioles and arteries in this patient (PAS, ×400).

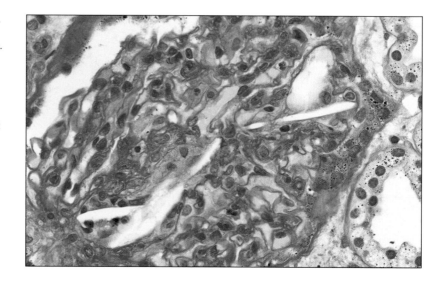

Fig. 2.98 Atheroemboli. Occasionally the only cholesterol embolus in the sample may be present in the sample dedicated for electron microscopy. The clear needle-shaped space left by the cholesterol crystal is illustrated, with surrounding foamy macrophage reaction (TEM, ×6000).

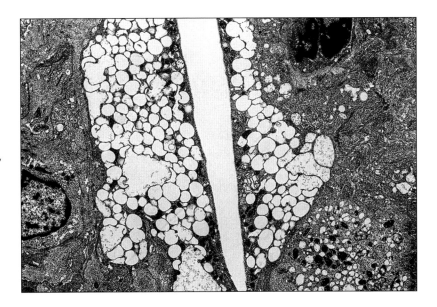

Polymorphonuclear leukocytes and eosinophils may also be seen transiently in the vessel lumen in the first 24 h after embolization (Fig. 2.94). The vessel may then become thrombosed in the sub-acute stage from 24–72 h. After the initial acute phase of injury, there is endothelial cell proliferation and intravascular fibrosis (Fig. 2.95). Cholesterol crystals may remain detectable for as long as 9 months after the acute event.

Immunofluorescence and electron microscopy show no specific changes, but occasionally the tissue submitted for these studies may contain the only cholesterol emboli in the biopsy (Figs 2.98, 2.99). Diagnostic cholesterol emboli are very localized, and multiple step sections and examination of all tissue is necessary to ensure optimal detection. Cholesterol emboli are typically present superimposed on changes of arterionephrosclerosis, i.e. sclerosis of arterioles and arteries and global glomerulosclerosis (Fig. 2.96). Rarely, there may be associated focal segmental glomerulosclerosis, likely secondary, and significant proteinuria.

Etiology/pathogenesis

Atherosclerosis is the requisite underlying condition for occurrence of atheroemboli. Cholesterol emboli may happen spontaneously, or more commonly following invasive procedures or vascular surgery.

Fig. 2.99 Atheroemboli. The needle-shaped space left by the cholesterol crystal is seen distorting and pushing the endothelium in this small arteriole (TEM, ×3000).

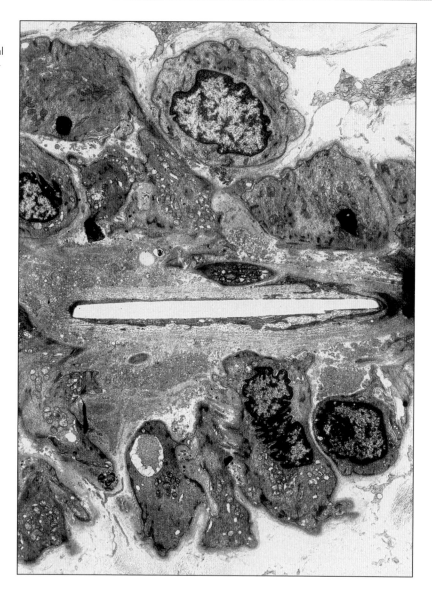

In autopsies of patients with mild atherosclerosis of the aorta, cholesterol emboli were rare (1.7%–4%), rising to 7%–30% in patients with severe disease or abdominal aortic aneurysms. Some 25% of patients who had undergone aortography had cholesterol emboli, and in patients who had undergone resection of an abdominal aneurysm, cholesterol emboli were present in 77%.

The surface of the atheromatous plaque is covered by endothelial cells with an underlying fibrous cap, consisting of smooth muscle cells, macrophages and extracellular matrix proteins. The center of the plaque contains necrotic cellular debris, cholesterol bound to proteins and cholesteryl esters, macrophages and foam cells. When the plaque ruptures, grumous fluid extrudes (*athere*, Greek for gruel), including the cholesterol crystals, which shower the organs below the site of plaque rupture. Atherosclerotic plaques are much more common in the abdominal aorta than in the thoracic aorta, and have a particular propensity for the areas adjacent to or surrounding the ostia of branch vessels. Thus, the distribution of cholesterol emboli is largely to organs below the diaphragm.

Suggested reading

Fine M J, Kapoor W, Falanga V 1987 Cholesterol crystal embolization: a review of 221 cases in the English literature. Angiology 38(10):769–784.

Flory C M 1945 Arterial occlusions produced by emboli from eroded aortic atheromatous plaques. American Journal of Pathology 21:549–565.

Fogo A, Stone W J 1992 Atheroembolic renal disease. In: Martinez-Maldonado M (ed.) Hypertension and Renal Disease in the Elderly. Blackwell Scientific, Cambridge, MA, p 261–271.

Gore I, McCombs H L, Lindquist R L 1964 Observations on the fate of cholesterol emboli. Journal of Atherosclerosis Research 4:527–535.

Greenberg A, Bastacky S I, Iqbal A et al 1997 Focal segmental glomerulosclerosis associated with nephrotic syndrome in cholesterol atheroembolism: clinicopathological correlations. American Journal of Kidney Disease 29(3):334–344.

Ramirez G, O'Neill W M, Lambert R et al 1978 Cholesterol embolization. A complication of angiography. Archives of Internal Medicine 138:1430–1432.

Tubulointerstitial diseases

References to **Brenner & Rector's** *The Kidney* 7th edition are given in parentheses below.

Introduction

The tubulointerstitial compartment is affected in all forms of renal disease with changes that include tubular epithelial injury, atrophy, hypertrophy and fibrosis. These changes can be primary with the tubule and interstitium as the target of damage, but are often secondary to primary glomerular or vascular disease where tubular atrophy and interstitial scarring accompany primary glomerular or vascular disease. This chapter will focus on those tubular and interstitial diseases where the tubules and interstitium are the primary target of the pathogenic process and which results in structural and functional alterations.

Primary tubular and interstitial diseases are a group of diverse renal diseases with involvement of the renal tubules and interstitium resulting from a variety of different etiologies and pathogenic mechanisms. The various etiologies and mechanisms include infection, obstruction, immune mediated, ischemic and toxic tubular and interstitial injury (Table 3.1). Despite the diverse etiology, the clinical presentations usually have great similarities. In acute cases, the clinical presentation may be so severe as to result in acute renal failure. In less severe and chronic cases, the functional manifestations usually include impaired urinary concentrating ability, impaired ability to secrete acid into the urine, diminished reabsorption of sodium, hyperkalemia, and azotemia. In advanced cases, the presentation may be that of chronic renal failure or end stage kidney. In cases of moderate renal failure a sudden worsening of renal failure may herald an activation of a new tubulointerstitial nephritis. It is under circumstances such as these that renal biopsy is often performed to identify the underlying process.

TABLE 3.1	Etiologies of tubular and interstitial diseases
Infections	Bacterial Viral Parasitic
Toxins	Drug-induced 　Direct toxic-mediated 　Hypersensitivity-mediated Environmental toxins 　Heavy metals 　Hydrocarbons 　Fungal toxins
Metabolic diseases	Diabetes Hypercalcemia Urate nephropathy Oxalate nephropathy
Physical	Obstruction Radiation
Vascular disease	Acute tubular necrosis Hypertensive nephropathy
Neoplasms	Lymphoma Myeloma

The World Health Organization Collaborating Center for Histologic Classification of Renal Diseases proposed a new classification that takes into account the etiologic pathogenetic and clinical features in addition to the histology (Table 3.2). This chapter will focus on morphology as applied to renal biopsy diagnosis.

Infection is a major cause of tubulointerstitial nephritis. In the WHO classification, four different forms of renal involvement are described:

1   Acute infectious tubulointerstitial nephritis, which is the result of the direct invasion of the renal parenchyma by microorganisms and subsequent proliferation of bacteria,

---

TABLE 3.2   WHO classification of tubulointerstitial diseases

Infection
    Acute infectious tubulointerstitial nephritis
    Acute tubulointerstitial nephritis associated with systemic infection
    Chronic infectious tubulointerstitial nephritis (chronic pyelonephritis)
    Specific renal infection

Drug-induced tubulointerstitial nephritis
    Acute drug-induced tubulotoxic injury
    Drug-induced hypersensitivity tubulointerstitial nephritis
    Chronic drug-induced tubulointerstitial nephritis

Tubulointerstitial nephritis associated with immune disorders
    Induced by antibodies reacting with tubular antigens
    Induced by autologous or exogenous antigen–antibody complexes
    Induced by, or associated with, cell-mediated hypersensitivity
    Induced by immediate (IgE-type) hypersensitivity

Obstructive uropathy

Vesicoureteral reflux associated nephropathy (reflux nephropathy)

Tubulointerstitial nephritis associated with papillary necrosis

Heavy metal-induced tubular and tubulointerstitial lesions

Acute tubular injury/necrosis
    Toxic
    Ischemic

Tubular and tubulointerstitial nephropathy caused by metabolic disturbances

Hereditary renal tubulointerstitial disorders

Tubulointerstitial nephritis associated with neoplastic disorders

Tubulointerstitial lesions in glomerular and vascular diseases

Miscellaneous disorders
    Balkan endemic nephropathy

fungi or viruses. Classical acute bacterial pyelonephritis is the paradigm of this form.

2   Acute tubulointerstitial nephritis associated with systemic infection but not caused by direct renal infection which may be due to a hypersensitivity reaction. The histologic picture is often similar to that of drug induced tubulointerstitial nephritis. The interstitial nephritis associated with Legionnaires' disease is an example of this type of involvement.

3   Chronic infectious tubulointerstitial nephritis, in which bacteria have an important role but renal injury may persist and occur in the absence of continued bacterial infection. Xanthogranulomatous pyelonephritis and malakoplakia are examples.

4   Specific renal infections such as tuberculosis and leprosy, which have distinctive histologic manifestations similar to involvement by these organisms in other organ systems.

Acute pyelonephritis

In acute bacterial pyelonephritis associated with ascending infection, the inflammatory infiltrate is predominately polymorphonuclear involving both medullary and cortical portions of the kidney. Polymorphonuclear leukocytes are present within the tubular lumina as well as invading the tubular epithelium and being abundantly present in the interstitium (Fig. 3.1). Areas of necrosis and abscess formation may be seen as well. Hematogenous infection of the kidney results in the presence of numerous small cortical abscesses without significant medullary involvement (Fig. 3.2). The abscesses are frequently glomerulocentric and tubular involvement may not be prominent (Fig. 3.3). While the presence of a neutrophilic invasion of the tubular lumina or of abscesses is characteristic of acute bacterial tubulointerstitial nephritis (Figs 3.4–3.6), it should be remembered that the cellular infiltrate frequently includes some lymphocytes, plasma cells, macrophages, and occasionally eosinophils and the differential diagnosis should include consideration of the possibility of idiopathic or drug-induced tubulointerstitial nephritis which is not infectious. In addition in viral renal infections such as with adenovirus and Hanta virus the infiltrate is often hemorrhagic and mononuclear cells tend to predominate (Fig. 3.7).

Fig. 3.1 Acute pyelo-nephritis. Low power image of a renal biopsy showing diffuse interstitial infiltrate which is predominately polymorphonuclear leukocytic. There is inter-stitial edema, some tubular atrophy and leukocytes can be seen in the lumen of the tubules (H&E, ×100).

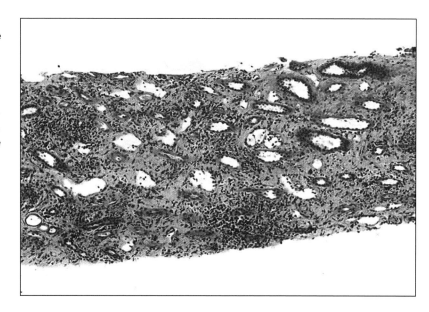

Fig. 3.2 Acute pyelo-nephritis. There is a diffuse interstitial infiltrate with polymorphonuclear leukocytes (H&E, ×200).

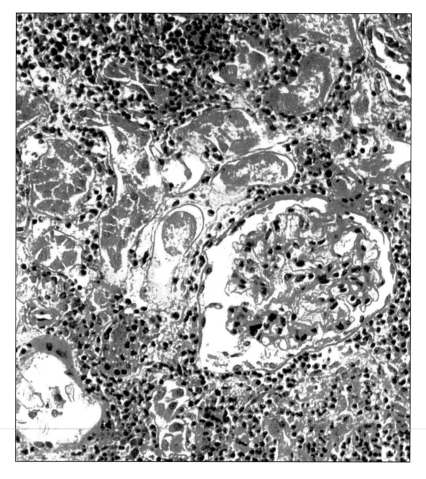

Fig. 3.3 Acute pyelo-
nephritis with abscess
formation. The abscesses
are frequently glomerulo-
centric and are destructive
of the renal parenchyma
(H&E, ×200).

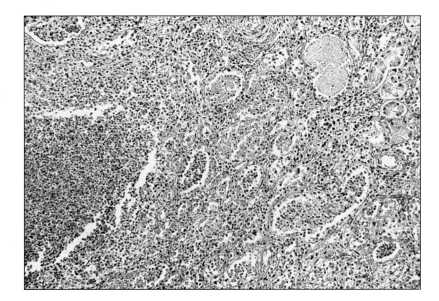

Fig. 3.4 Acute pyelo-
nephritis. The infectious
nature of an active interstitial nephritis is best identified by the presence of
polymorphonuclear leuko-
cytes within the lumen
(H&E, ×400).

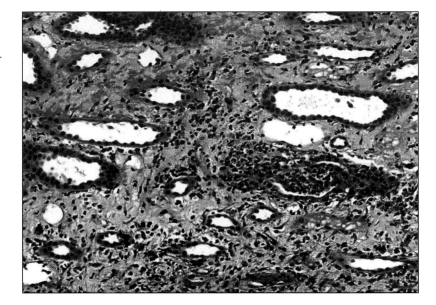

Etiology/pathogenesis

Infectious tubulointerstitial nephritis is generally designated as
pyelonephritis, implying that there is involvement of the collecting
system as well as the renal parenchyma by the inflammatory
process. Both acute and chronic pyelonephritis are frequently associated with congenital or acquired obstructive lesions of the lower

Fig. 3.5 Acute pyelo-nephritis. The infiltrate of polymorphonuclear leukocytes is not only present within the interstitium and in the lumen but also evidence of tubulitis is seen (H&E, ×400).

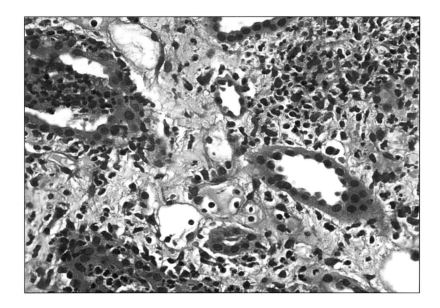

Fig. 3.6 Acute pyelo-nephritis. Electron microscopy demonstrates coliform organisms within the lumen of a tubule (TEM, ×10,000).

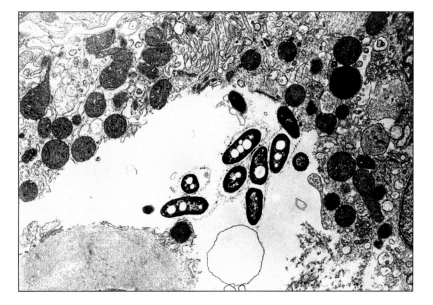

urinary tract or are associated with conditions resulting in retention of residual urine in the bladder. A variety of pathogens can be identified using staining techniques for microorganism identification, which include Brown-Brenn, PAS and Grocott Silver stains. Generally speaking, ascending infections are usually associated with gram negative organisms, in particular *Escherichia coli*. Hematogenous infections are most frequently caused by *Staphylococcus aureus* or

Fig. 3.7 Acute pyelo-
nephritis. Viral infections
may mimic acute pyelo-
nephritis but can be often
distinguished by the
presence of atypical tubular
epithelial cells. Viral
infection is described
separately later (H&E,
×400).

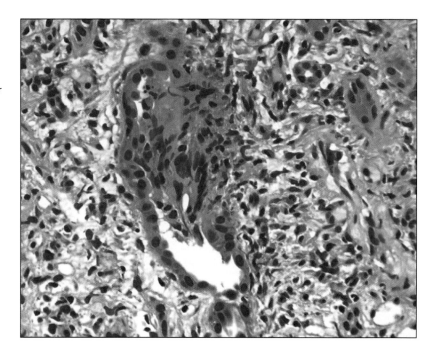

fungal organisms including Candida and Aspergillus. These are
especially important in immunosuppressed individuals. Although
renal biopsy rarely gives a sampling of the renal papilla and pelvis,
it is important to remember that these structures are involved in
infection.

Selected reading

Tolkoff-Rubin N E R R 1983 Urinary tract infection. Tubulo-interstitial
    nephropathies. Contemporary issues in nephrology, Vol. 10. Churchill
    Livingstone, New York, p 49–82.

Chronic pyelonephritis and reflux nephropathy

Chronic pyelonephritis is a controversial term. It is often difficult to
separate chronic infectious tubulointerstitial nephritis or true chronic
pyelonephritis from many other chronic interstitial diseases, as the
histologic changes are relatively non-specific. Chronic interstitial
scarring, tubular atrophy and the presence of an infiltrate of lymphocytes and plasma cells are common to many disorders. Similar
changes can be seen in hypertensive nephrosclerosis, chronic urinary
tract obstruction, chronic glomerular diseases, diabetic nephro-

pathy and numerous other causes. For this reason, chronic infectious tubular interstitial nephritis cannot be diagnosed with any degree of certainty on the limited sampling usually achieved by renal biopsy. A better diagnosis can be made when information concerning the renal papilla, calyces and pelvis is available from radiologic examination as well as the gross morphology of the kidney obtained with sophisticated imaging techniques such as ultrasonography or magnetic resonance imaging (MRI).

Chronic pyelonephritis results in a coarse renal scarring which is characteristically focal in its distribution. Microscopically the findings consist of tubular atrophy, interstitial scarring and a chronic inflammatory infiltrate (Figs 3.8, 3.9). The tubules are either collapsed or dilated and lined by a flattened epithelium and sometimes filled with colloid casts (Fig. 3.10). This latter pattern has been termed thyroidization. The inflammatory infiltrate is quite variable but consists predominately of lymphocytes as well as plasma cells and to a lesser extent mononuclear cells, but may contain neutrophils.

In chronic pyelonephritis associated with reflux or obstruction, Tamm-Horsfall protein can be identified in the interstitium by the presence of strongly PAS positive amorphous or finely fibrillar material. In instances where reflux has contributed to the development of chronic pyelonephritis, focal and segmental glomerulosclerosis

Fig. 3.8 Chronic pyelonephritis is a non-specific interstitial infiltrate predominately with lymphocytes. There is evidence of destruction of the renal parenchyma with atrophy of tubules (H&E, ×200).

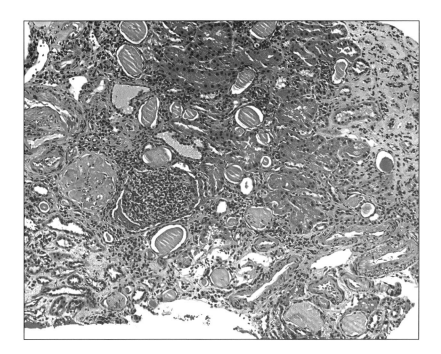

Fig. 3.9 Chronic pyelo-nephritis. Tubules are filled with proteinaceous casts associated with a diffuse interstitial infiltrate of lymphocytes and interstitial scarring (H&E, ×200).

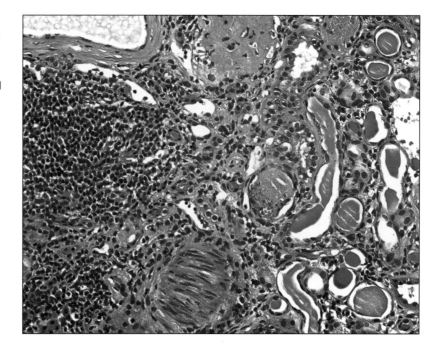

Fig. 3.10 Chronic pyelo-nephritis. Scarring may be extensive with marked destruction of the normal architecture leading to end stage renal disease. The dilatation of the tubules filled with proteinaceous material has often been termed thyroidization (H&E, ×200).

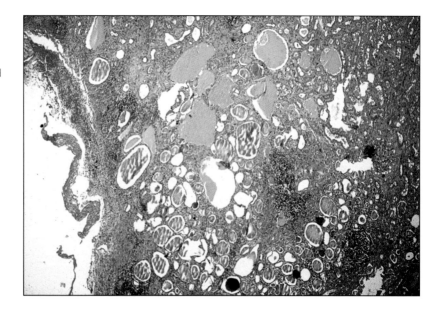

may be extremely prominent and may suggest the possibility of a primary glomerular lesion. The histopathologic changes of chronic pyelonephritis have also been described with so called reflux nephropathy associated with vesicoureteral reflux.

Etiology/pathogenesis

Chronic pyelonephritis is the consequence of persistence of untreated and incompletely resolved acute pyelonephritis and thus has many of the same risk factors and pathogeneses. In addition, structural abnormalities promoting reflux contribute to the lesions of chronic pyelonephritis and reflux nephropathy.

Selected reading

Tolkoff-Rubin N E R R 1983 Urinary tract infection. Tubulo-interstitial nephropathies. Contemporary issues in nephrology, Vol. 10. Churchill Livingstone, New York, p 49–82.

Xanthogranulomatous pyelonephritis

Xanthogranulomatous pyelonephritis is a distinct type of infectious pyelonephritis. Microscopically, there is a diffuse granulomatous inflammatory infiltrate, which includes large numbers of foamy histiocytes and occasional multi-nucleated giant cells in addition to lymphocytes, plasma cells and neutrophils (Figs 3.11, 3.12). The lesion is destructive and renal parenchyma may not be easily identified within affected areas.

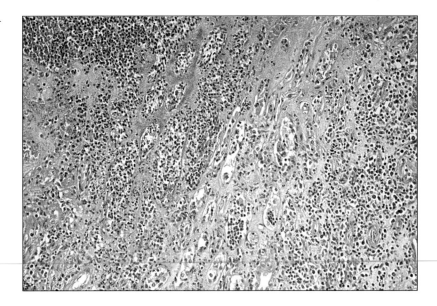

Fig. 3.11 Xanthogranulomatous pyelonephritis is a distinct type of infectious pyelonephritis. There is a diffuse granulomatous infiltrate, which includes macrophages as well as polymorphonuclear leukocytes (H&E, ×200).

Fig. 3.12 Xanthogranulomatory pyelonephritis. Granulomatous structures can be seen involving both cortex and medulla as seen here. Microabscesses' containing eosinophilic homogenous material are also present (H&E, ×100).

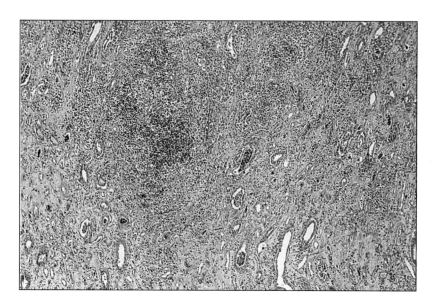

Etiology/pathogenesis

Escherichia coli is the most frequently associated etiologic agent but *Proteus mirabilis* and *Staphylococcus aureus* have also been reported as causative agents. Occasionally, microabscesses containing basophilic bacterial colonies surrounded by eosinophilic homogenous material (Botryomycosis) can be identified.

Selected reading

Hill G S, Droz D, Nochy D 2001 The woman who loved well but not too wisely, or the vicissitudes of immunosuppression. American Journal of Kidney Disease 37:1324–1329.

Mignon F, Mery J P, Mougenot B et al 1984 Granulomatous interstitial nephritis. Advances in Nephrology from the Necker Hospital 13:219–245.

Malakoplakia

Malakoplakia has a similar gross and microscopic appearance to xanthogranulomatous pyelonephritis. Confluent nodules of the homogenous yellow–tan tissue are seen to replace large areas of renal parenchyma grossly. Microscopically, there is an inflammatory infiltrate, which consists of histiocytes with relatively few lymphocytes and plasma cells. Characteristic Michaelis–Gutmann bodies are found both within cells and extracellularly in the stroma. The calcospherites stain positively with Von Kossa (calcium) PAS and fibroblastic proliferation and scarring are extremely prominent.

Etiology/pathogenesis

Malakoplakia is an unusual consequence of an inflammatory reaction most frequently secondary to infection by *E. coli*. It is similar to xanthogranulomatous pyelonephritis and may represent a chronic sequelae in this process.

Selected reading

Hill GS, Droz D, Nochy D 2001 The woman who loved well but not too wisely, or the vicissitudes of immunosuppression. American Journal of Kidney Disease 37:1324–1329.

Mignon F, Mery J P, Mougenot B et al 1984 Granulomatous interstitial nephritis. Advances in Nephrology from the Necker Hospital 1984; 13:219–245.

Acute interstitial nephritis – drug related

Although the clinical manifestations of acute interstitial nephritis (AIN) may be variable, they are usually heralded by fever and hematuria, as well as azotemia. Eosinophilia occurs in a majority of cases. Urinalysis reveals hematuria, sterile pyuria and moderate proteinuria. Eosinophils may be detected in the urinary sediment. A skin rash is seen in some patients lending support to the concept that the disease may be immunologically mediated. The azotemia may be severe and patients may present with acute renal failure leading to the use of the renal biopsy as a diagnostic procedure.

One of the most distinguishing features of acute drug-induced tubulointerstitial nephritis AIN is the nature of the interstitial infiltrate. The interstitium is edematous with tubules separated by a pale staining interstitium (in contrast to the dense staining of fibrosis) and infiltrated with a significant number of eosinophils and mononuclear cells (Figs 3.13–3.15). The infiltrate is characteristically focal and most prominent at the corticomedullary junction and often surrounds individual tubules. The mononuclear portion of the infiltrate is predominately lymphocytes with some plasma cells and macrophages, which sometimes form granulomas (Figs 3.16, 3.17). The eosinophils tend to concentrate in small foci and may form eosinophilic microabscesses (Figs 3.18, 3.19). Neutrophils can

Fig. 3.13 AIN. There is a diffuse interstitial infiltrate with evidence of interstitial edema. Glomeruli are relatively well preserved (H&E, ×100).

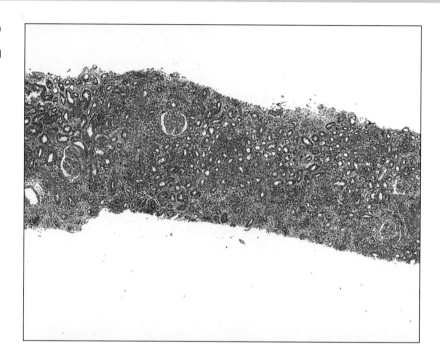

Fig. 3.14 AIN. Higher power demonstrates the presence of mononuclear cells throughout the interstitium, the tubule lumina are relatively free of leukocytic infiltrate (H&E, ×200).

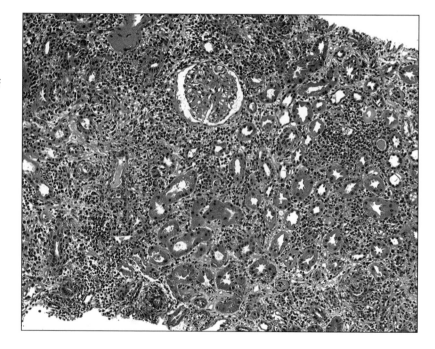

Fig. 3.15   AIN. There is evidence of infiltration of the tubules by the interstitial infiltrate, which is distinctive of tubulitis (H&E, ×400).

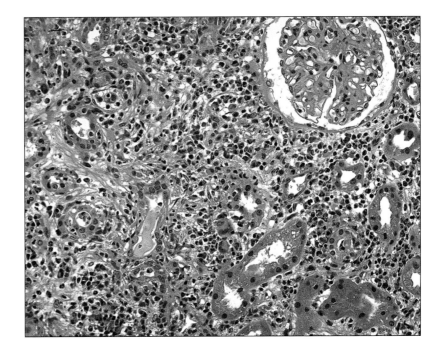

Fig. 3.16   AIN. The mononuclear infiltrate is accompanying by abundant eosinophils and may have a granulomatous appearance. (H&E, ×400).

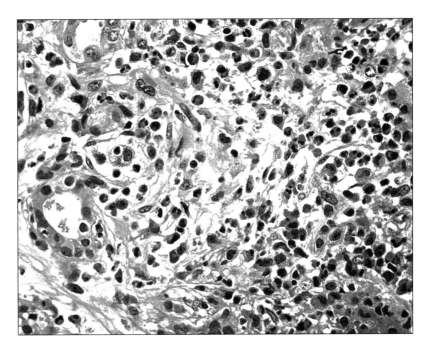

Fig. 3.17   AIN. The granulomata often involve the tubules in a destructive fashion (H&E, ×400).

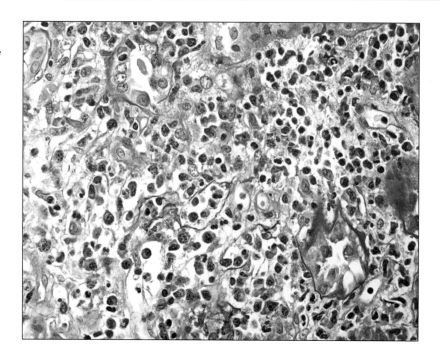

Fig. 3.18   AIN. The eosinophilic infiltrate can sometimes be dense and form small eosinophilic abscesses (H&E, ×200).

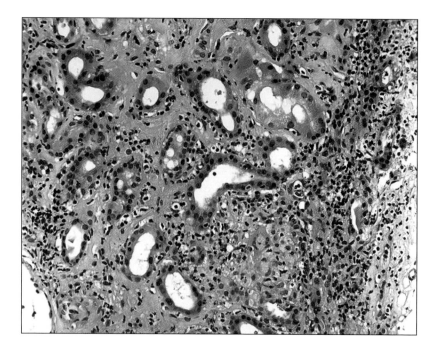

be present, but are uncommon (Fig. 3.20). A second distinguishing characteristic is the presence of tubulitis (Fig. 3.21, 3.22). Particularly with PAS stains, lymphocytes can be seen invading the tubules beneath the tubular basement membrane. Variable degrees of

Fig. 3.19 AIN. There is destruction of the tubular epithelium with relative preservation of the basement membrane (PAS, ×400).

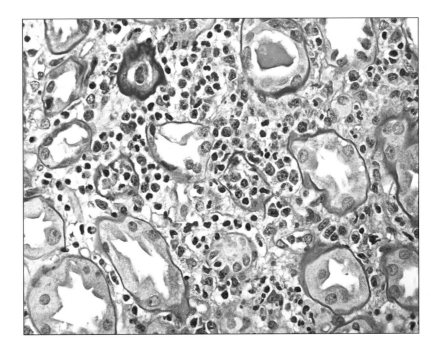

Fig. 3.20 AIN. Neutrophils may be present but are relatively uncommon (H&E, ×400).

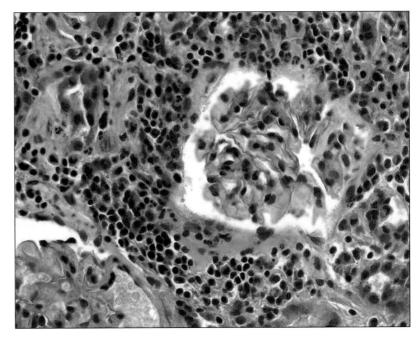

Fig. 3.21 AIN. Higher power of tubulitis demonstrating interstitial edema and invasion of the tubular epithelium by lymphocytes (H&E, ×400).

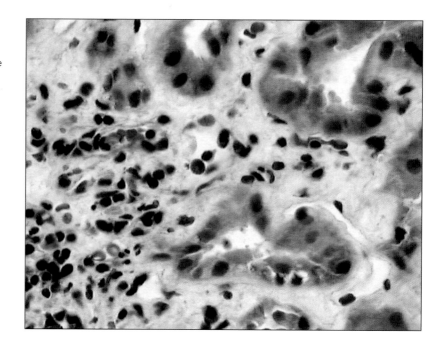

Fig. 3.22 AIN. Electron micrograph demonstrates the mononuclear infiltrate with the eosinophils, plasma cells and activated lymphocytes (TEM, ×2000).

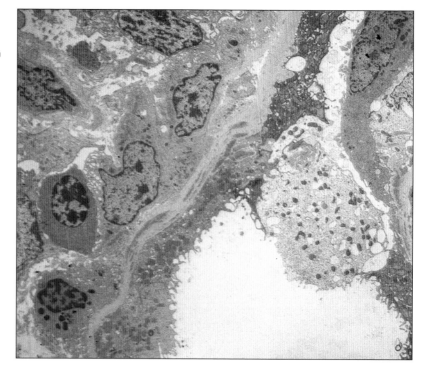

tubular epithelial cell damage (Figs 3.23–3.25) with evidence of regener-ation as identified by the presence of mitotic figures and pleomor-phic nuclei are almost always found but extensive necrosis of the epithelium is rare.

Etiology/pathogenesis

It is now widely recognized that a large variety of drugs including β-lactam antibiotics, non-steroidal anti-inflammatory drugs, diuretics, anticonvulsants and an increasingly diverse group of other drugs can be associated with an allergic acute tubular interstitial nephritis. Although drugs have been implicated in most cases of allergic

Fig. 3.23 AIN. Mono-nuclear cells traversing the endothelium of a peritubular capillary are shown (TEM, ×3000).

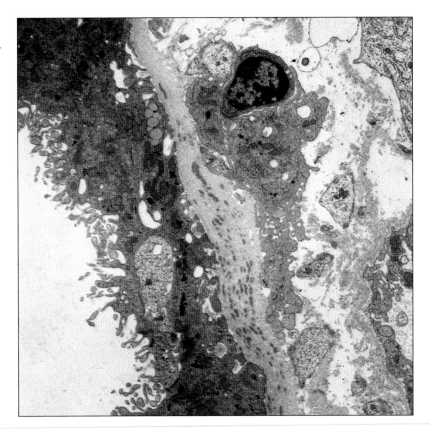

Fig. 3.24 AIN. Varying degrees of epithelial damage are present demonstrated here by loss of the apical membrane and swelling of the cells (TEM, ×3000).

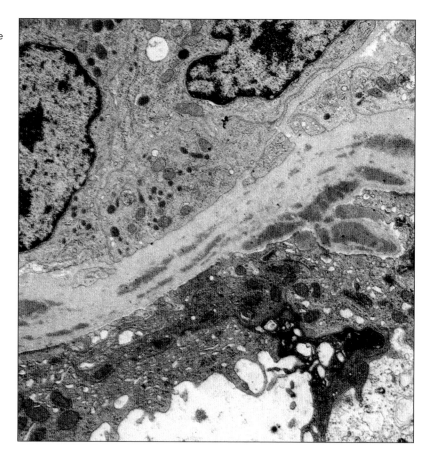

interstitial nephritis, a similar picture can be found in patients with lupus nephritis and rarely in association with anti-tubular basement membrane antibodies. Biopsy-proven instances of acute oliguric tubular interstitial nephritis with a similar histologic picture but without any known drug exposure have also been reported.

One special group includes the association of acute tubulointerstitial nephritis with uveitis (TINU syndrome) and bone marrow and lymph node granulomata. This syndrome occurs predominately in adolescent girls and young women, and is presumed to have an autoimmune etiology. This entity must be distinguished from renal sarcoid involvement, which also characteristically has numerous granulomata in the biopsy.

Fig. 3.25 AIN. More severe damage with evidence of cellular necrosis is also seen (TEM, ×4000).

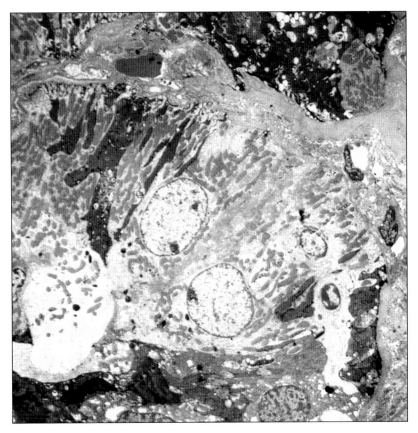

Selected reading

Bender W L, Beschorner W E, Darwish M O et al 1984 Interstitial nephritis, proteinuria and renal failure caused by nonsteroidal anti-inflammatory drugs. Immunologic characterization of the inflammatory infiltrate. American Journal of Medicine 76:1006–1012.

Rastegar A, Kashgarian M 1998 The clinical spectrum of tubulointerstitial nephritis. Kidney International 54:313–327.

Acute interstitial nephritis – viral infection

Bacterial infections result in predominantly intratubular PMNs, characteristic of acute pyelonephritis (see 'Acute pyelonephritis'). Other infections may give rise to a more predominantly interstitial infiltrate, with admixed mononuclear cells and more scarce PMNs. In viral renal infections such as with adenovirus and Hanta virus the interstitium is often hemorrhagic and mononuclear cells tend to predominate (Fig. 3.7). Other viruses may also infect the kidney, notably HIV, BK virus and cytomegalovirus, and are discussed under the Transplantation section and under HIV-associated nephropathy.

Etiology/pathogenesis

Viruses may cause renal injury by direct parenchymal infection (e.g. CMV) and/or by cytokine injury secondary to systemic and/or infiltrating cell/dendritic cell infection. Direct evidence of parenchymal infection may be seen by viral inclusions, or cytopathic changes, with enlarged, smudgy nuclei. Adenovirus infection occurs in immunocompromised hosts. In contrast, Hanta virus infection may occur in immunocompetent patients. The varying clinical syndromes due to Hanta virus in Europe vs. the USA appears to reflect differences in the carrier rodent population. Subclinical Hanta virus infection has been postulated to result in hypertension consequent to parenchymal scarring, based on serological studies, but the causality has not been proven.

Selected reading

Peters C J, Simpson G L, Levy H 1999 Spectrum of hantavirus infection: hemorrhagic fever with renal syndrome and hantavirus pulmonary syndrome. Annual Review of Medicine 50:531–545.

Settergren B, Ahlm C, Alexeyev O et al 1997 Pathogenetic and clinical aspects of the renal involvement in hemorrhagic fever with renal syndrome. Renal Failure 19:1–14.

Teague M W, Glick A D, Fogo A B 1991 Adenovirus infection of the kidney: mass formation in a patient with Hodgkin's disease. American Journal of Kidney Disease 18:499–502.

Sarcoidosis

Considering the potential differential diagnoses, it must be noted that if the interstitial infiltrate is not prominent, it may be difficult to distinguish acute drug-induced tubular interstitial nephritis from nephrotoxic tubular injury or ischemic acute tubular necrosis, since a minimal infiltrate with occasional eosinophils have been described in each of these entities. When the interstitial infiltrate is so intense that it forms granulomas, the differential diagnosis must include sarcoidosis (Figs 3.26–3.28). In general however, sarcoid involvement of the kidney is characterized by the presence of randomly distributed distinct granulomata with or without areas of central

Fig. 3.26 Sarcoidosis may present as a granulomatous interstitial nephritis with well-defined sarcoid granulomata as seen here (H&E, ×200).

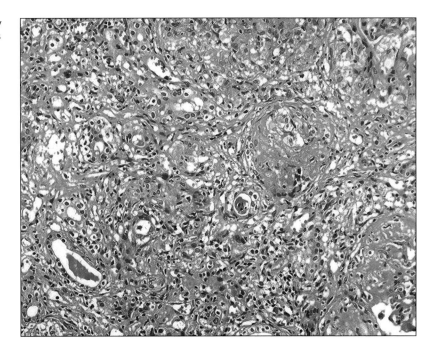

Fig. 3.27 Sarcoidosis. Silver stains demonstrate the architecture of the granulomata with evidence of interstitial fibrosis (Jones, ×200).

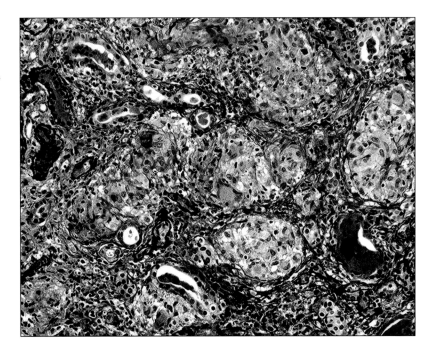

Fig. 3.28 Sarcoidosis. The granulomata consists predominately of mononuclear cells and epithelioid macrophages, and occasional foci of necrosis are seen (Jones, ×200).

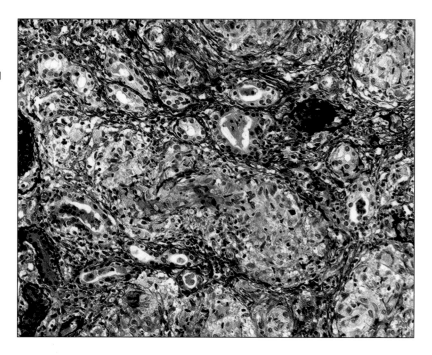

necrosis (Figs 3.29, 3.30). When the granulomata are confluent (Figs 3.31, 3.32) involving the glomeruli or with prominent necrosis, consideration in the differential diagnosis must include Wegener's granulomatosis.

Fig. 3.29 Sarcoidosis. Granulomata may become large with central areas of necrosis. Examination for fungi and tuberculosis is essential when necrosis is present (H&E, ×200).

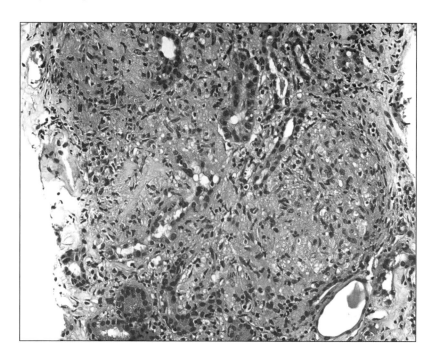

Fig. 3.30   Sarcoidosis. Central areas of necrosis may be present in granulomas (Jones, ×400).

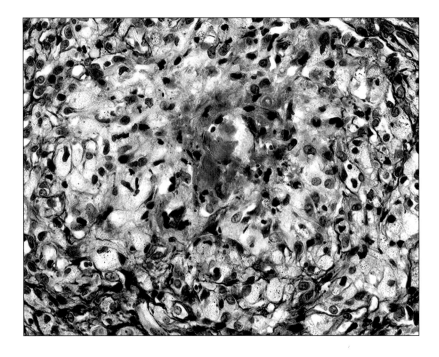

Fig. 3.31   Sarcoidosis. When granulomata are confluent and areas of necrosis are present, the differential diagnosis must include Wegener's granulomatosis (Jones, ×200).

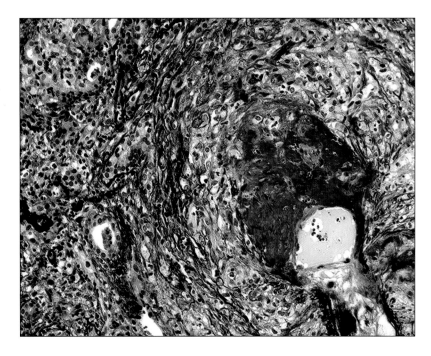

Fig. 3.32 Sarcoidosis. Glomeruli may also be involved in the granulomatous process (Jones, ×400).

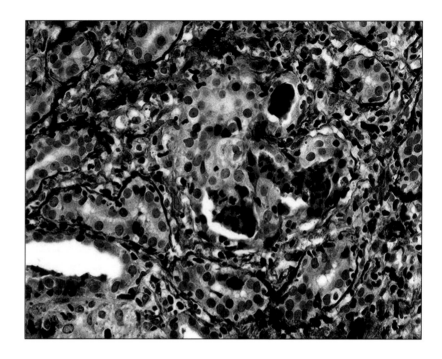

Etiology/pathogenesis

Sarcoid is a diagnosis of exclusion. The presence of necrotizing granulomas should bring up the possibility of tuberculosis or fungal infection of the kidney, and investigated as appropriate by special stains. Sarcoid is presumed to have autoimmune etiology, but the pathogenesis remains unknown.

Selected reading

Hannedouche T, Grateau G, Noel L H et al 1990 Renal granulomatous sarcoidosis: report of six cases. Nephrology, Dialysis, Transplantation 5:18–24.

Acute tubular injury/necrosis

A common indication for renal biopsy is the development of the syndrome of acute renal failure. Acute renal failure is the clinical situation in which there is a sudden loss of renal function. It is usually characterized by oliguria and the rapid development of azotemia. Some forms of acute renal failure however may not exhibit oliguria and may even be polyuric. A rapid cessation in renal function can occur as a result of extra renal events as well as intrinsic renal disease.

Ischemic acute tubular necrosis

The histologic picture of acute tubular necrosis (ATN) varies with the evolution of the lesion in relationship to the onset of the acute renal failure. Individual cell necrosis with denudation of the basement membrane and shedding of epithelial cells and necrotic debris into the tubular lumen is characteristic (Figs 3.33–3.37). Hyaline, granular and pigmented casts are seen in the distal portions of the nephron. These casts consist of Tamm–Horsfall proteins, which stain positively with PAS stains. In the specific instances of acute tubular necrosis following hemolysis or following muscle damage, deeply pigmented hemoglobin and myoglobin casts are also present. In segments of the tubules that do not show significant necrosis, the tubules are often dilated and lined by flattened epithelial cells often called tubular simplification (Figs 3.38, 3.39). In PAS stains, the brush border of proximal tubules is often thinned or absent (Fig. 3.40). The interstitium is markedly edematous. As the lesion progresses following the initial injury, evidence of tubular regeneration with mitotic figures can be seen. There may be a mild interstitial inflam-

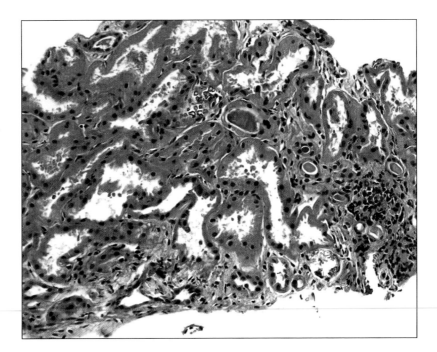

Fig. 3.33 ATN. In acute tubular necrosis, there is dilatation of the tubules and interstitial edema. In addition, the proximal tubules show evidence of loss of the brush border with blebbing of the apical membrane into the tubular lumen (H&E, ×100).

Fig. 3.34 ATN. There are fragments of cells within the tubular lumina. Flattening of the tubular epithelium, loss of nuclei and a marked interstitial infiltrate with occasional inflammatory cells are also present (H&E, ×200).

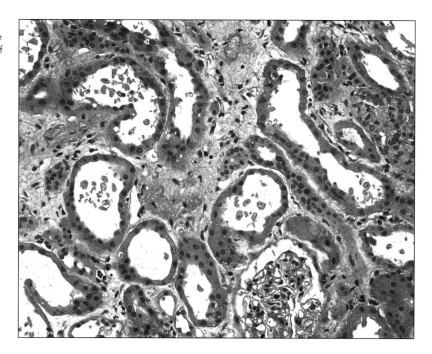

Fig. 3.35 ATN. Focal calcification of the tubular epithelium is also seen with evidence of denudation of the basement membrane (H&E, ×200).

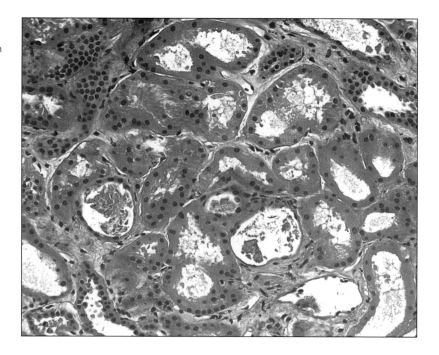

Fig. 3.36 ATN. Foci of calcified epithelial cells can sometimes be present with flattened regenerating epithelium along the basement membrane (H&E, ×400).

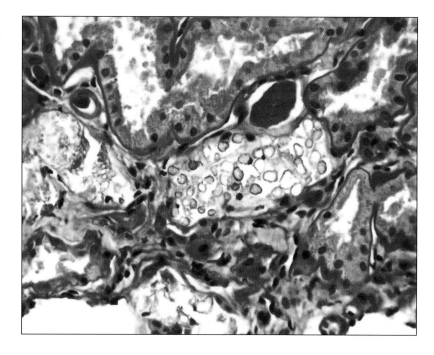

Fig. 3.37 ATN. Proteinaceous casts are present in the distal tubules made up of Tamm–Horsfall protein (H&E, ×400).

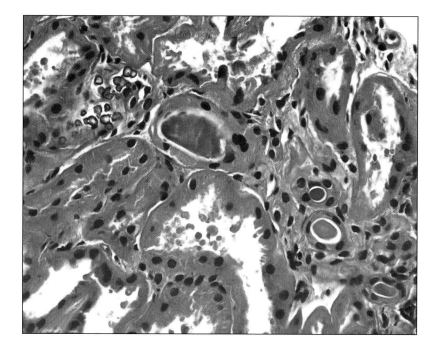

Fig. 3.38 ATN. In cases where there is no evident necrosis, the most prominent finding is loss of the architecture of the proximal tubules with dilatation and flattening of the epithelium (H&E, ×200).

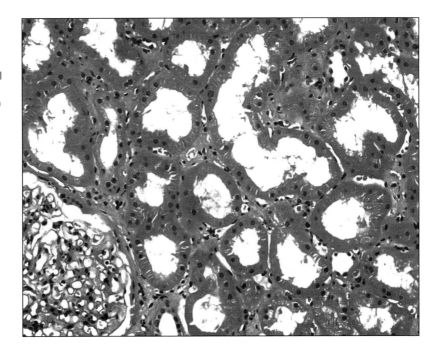

Fig. 3.39 ATN. Higher power demonstrates interstitial edema, flattening of the epithelium and loss of occasional nuclei (H&E, ×400).

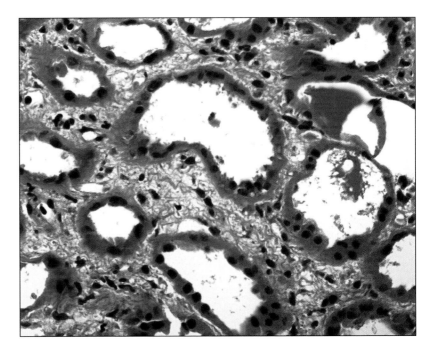

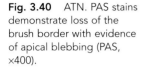

Fig. 3.40 ATN. PAS stains demonstrate loss of the brush border with evidence of apical blebbing (PAS, ×400).

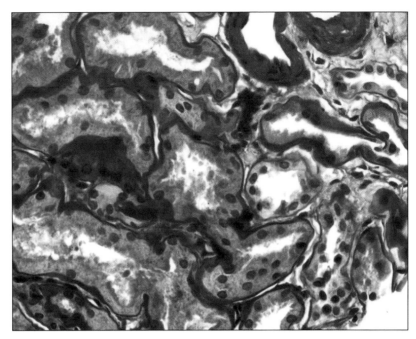

matory infiltrate with small numbers of lymphocytes, macrophages, neutrophils or occasionally eosinophils present. It is in these late stages that distinctions have to be made between ischemic acute tubular necrosis and acute tubulointerstitial nephritis but generally the infiltrate is much less prominent in cases of acute tubular necrosis.

One caveat, which must always be remembered in evaluating the biopsy of a patient with acute renal failure, is not to quickly assign the cause to acute tubular necrosis. Because of the paucity of findings in acute tubular necrosis one must search carefully for other potential causes including glomerular diseases such as minimal change nephrotic syndrome where a patient can present with oliguria due to hypovolemia secondary to shifts in extracellular fluid as a result of the massive proteinuria.

Whereas electron microscopy generally does not add significantly to the evaluation of most tubular interstitial diseases, it is helpful in evaluating the tubular epithelial changes in both forms of acute tubular necrosis (Figs 3.41–3.43). In ischemic acute tubular necrosis scattered epithelial cell changes show a variety of different cytopathic alterations. There is loss of the brush border, blebbing of the apical membrane with shedding of apical membrane blebs into the tubular lumina, high amplitude swelling with condensation of

Fig. 3.41 ATN. Electron microscopy reveals of evidence of fragments of epithelial cells filling the tubular lumen (TEM, ×2000).

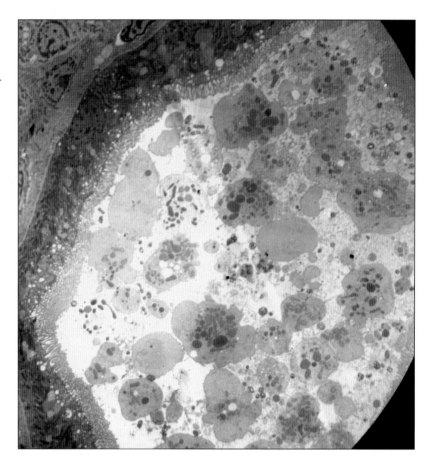

the cristae of the mitochondria, individual cell apoptosis as seen as cell shrinkage with nuclear fragmentation and a variety of other degenerative changes including necrosis. Electron microscopy may therefore be useful in evaluating those instances where the diagnosis is questionable or where other causes are suspected.

Nephrotoxic acute tubular necrosis

The clinical picture may be similar to that of ischemic acute tubular necrosis with a sudden onset of acute renal failure. In many instances however, particularly in industrial exposures, the onset may be insidious and the patient may not have oliguria but present with polyuric renal insufficiency.

Histologically, severe acute toxic tubular necrosis is associated with extensive epithelial necrosis, which tends to involve all nephrons

Fig. 3.42 ATN. Higher power demonstrating focal loss of brush border of the proximal tubules with the development of apical blebs (TEM, ×4000)

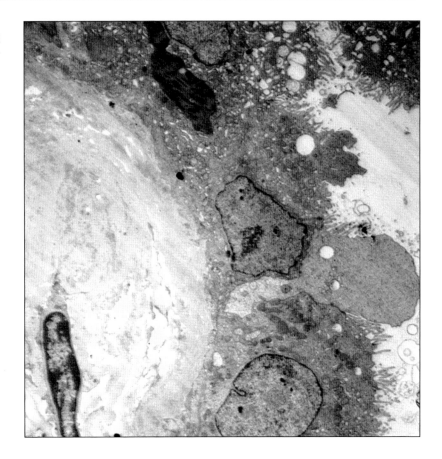

more uniformly than that seen in the ischemic form (Fig. 3.44). The proximal tubule is most severely involved and necrotic cells are dislodged from the basement membrane and the tubular lumens are filled with cellular debris. Focal calcification of the necrotic material occurs very rapidly and can be seen within 1–2 days. As the lesion develops, regeneration of the tubular epithelium can be identified initially by flattened epithelial cells which over several days become cuboidal and then columnar and then finally develop a normal proximal tubule architecture. In addition, specific renal epithelial changes can be seen with different toxins. In acute lead nephropathy for example, dark intranuclear inclusions can be identified (Fig. 3.45) and oxalate crystals are associated with glycol nephrotoxicity. In aminoglycoside nephrotoxicity lysosomal myeloid bodies can be identified by electron microscopy (Fig. 3.46).

Fig. 3.43   Toxic ATN.
Sublethal injury is seen with
marked intracellular edema
and condensation of
adjacent cells (TEM, ×8000).

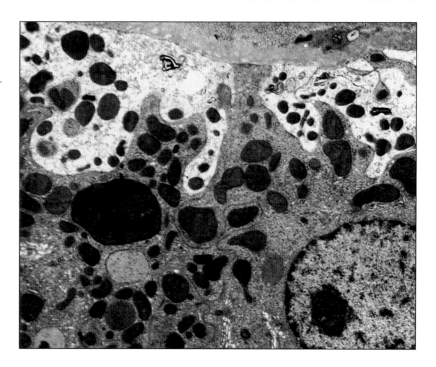

Fig. 3.44   Toxic ATN.
There is evidence of cellular
necrosis with atypical nuclei
representing regenerating
epithelium (H&E, ×400).

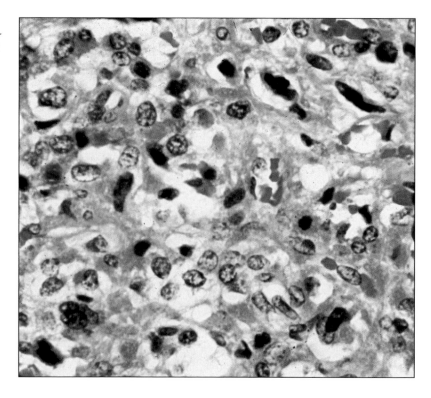

Fig. 3.45 Lead nephropathy. Nuclei of the epithelial cells contain dense bodies consisting of lead metallothyanide complexes (TEM, ×12,000).

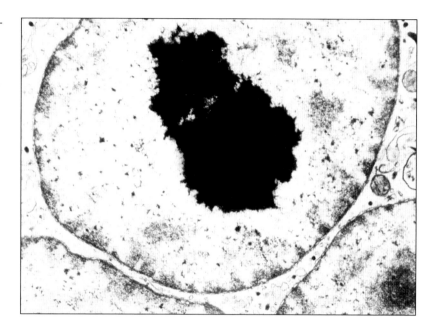

Fig. 3.46 Aminoglycoside nephrotoxicity. Myeloid bodies (arrows) are present in an intracellular localization (TEM, ×12,000).

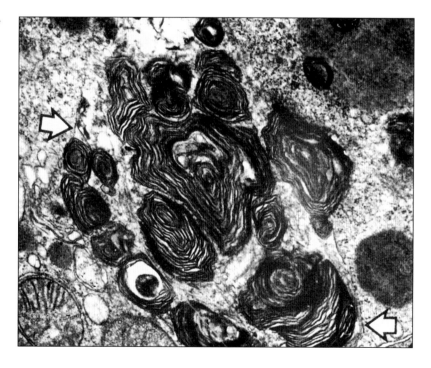

Etiology/pathogenesis

Intrinsic renal causes of acute renal failure include severe acute glomerulonephritis, vasculitis, thrombotic microangiopathies malignant hypertension as well as acute tubulointerstitial nephritis and the entity called acute tubular necrosis. Although 'necrosis' is included in the term to distinguish it from other intrinsic causes of renal disease, tubular epithelial damage is not always readily evident by light microscopy. Acute tubular necrosis is generally divided into two subcategories, post-ischemic acute tubular necrosis and nephrotoxic acute tubular necrosis. Morphologic changes of cellular injury are usually more subtle in the ischemic form and with more obvious cytopathologic changes in the toxic form. In addition, the patterns of tubular damage differ between the two forms. In the ischemic form tubular damage is patchy affecting relatively short length of the straight segments of the proximal tubule and focal areas of the ascending limbs of the loops of Henle. Ischemia plays a major role in its pathogenesis. In the toxic form, the tubular epithelial damage is more extensive along segments of the proximal tubule and the segments involved may vary with the specific toxin. Although distal tubular damage does occur, it is less extensive and more inconsistent than in ischemic acute tubular necrosis. Although most instances of severe nephrotoxic acute tubular necrosis are the result of industrial accidents or accidental or intentional ingestion of toxins, it must be recognized that numerous therapeutic agents such as aminoglycoside antibiotics, anti-neoplastic agents such as cisplatin and plant toxins found in herbal remedies all may be associated with renal epithelial damage and are the most frequently encountered forms of nephrotoxicity in a renal biopsy practice.

Heavy metal nephropathy (lead and cadmium nephropathy)

It has long been recognized that heavy metals can lead to a dose dependent toxic necrosis of renal epithelial cells. Since the kidney is the principal excretory organ of the body and a major route for excretion of toxins absorbed by any route, the kidney and urinary tract are particularly vulnerable to toxic damage. Acute toxicity clinically presents similarly to ischemic tubular necrosis. Chronic nephrotoxicity is more insidious in its onset and in its clinical manifestations. It can mimic other primary renal diseases and may manifest itself by minor functional abnormalities or by the systemic effects of renal damage including hypertension and gradually pro-gressive renal failure. Chronic exposure to lead, mercury, cadmium, platinum, gold, lithium, silver, copper and iron have all been asso-ciated with the development of a chronic nonspecific interstitial nephritis. The histologic findings in heavy metal nephropathy show proximal tubular injury with intranuclear inclusion bodies of metal-metallothionein complexes (Fig. 3.45).

Etiology/pathogenesis

The pathogenesis of the renal disease is related to the proximal tubule reabsorption of filtered lead or cadmium, with subsequent accumulation with metallothioneins in the proximal tubule cells. The renal tubular cells have a considerable capacity to synthesize metallothionein, thereby binding and detoxifying heavy metal ions. When the detoxifying capacity is surpassed, tubular damage results in interstitial inflammation and fibrosis.

Selected reading

Bennett W M 1985 Lead nephropathy. Kidney International 28:212–220.

Bohle A J J, Meyer D, Schubert G E 1976 Morphology of acute renal failure. Comparative data from biopsy and autopsy. Kidney International 10:S9–16.

Humes H 1988 Aminoglycoside nephrotoxicity. Kidney International 33:900–911.

Olsen S, Solez K 1987 Acute renal failure in man: pathogenesis in light of new morphological data. Clinical Nephrology 27:271–277.

Analgesic nephropathy and papillary necrosis

Since the lesion is a chronic progressive one, the clinical presenta-tion is extremely variable, but a common feature is nocturia and polyuria. This is due to the extensive medullary damage frequently associated with renal papillary necrosis resulting in a loss of the concentrating ability. Since renal biopsies rarely give a significant sample of the inner medulla, it is often difficult to assign the rela-tively non-specific cortical changes of interstitial fibrosis and tubular atrophy seen to this entity. Nonetheless, analgesic nephropathy has extensive interstitial scarring which is usually bland with relatively few inflammatory cells which if present, are generally small lym-phocytes (Fig. 3.47–3.51). Extensive tubular atrophy is also seen.

Fig. 3.47 Analgesic nephropathy is associated with marked interstitial fibrosis with a relative paucity of interstitial infiltrate. Tubular atrophy with numerous casts are present. Glomeruli are generally not involved or demonstrate sclerosis (H&E, ×50).

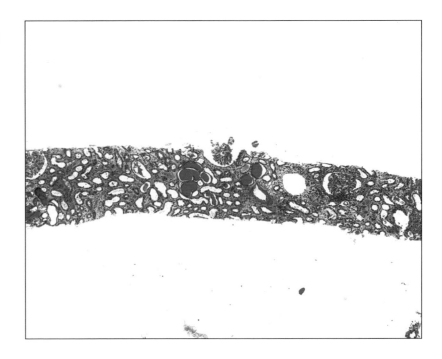

Fig. 3.48. Analgesic nephropathy. The extensive interstitial fibrosis is demonstrated here on trichrome stain associated with marked tubular atrophy (Trichrome, ×100).

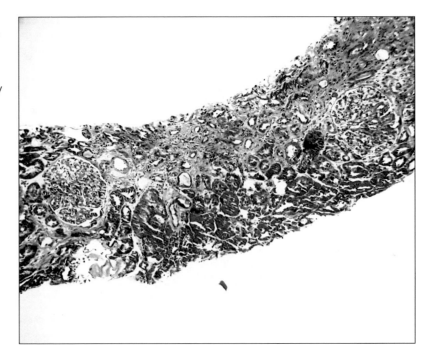

Fig. 3.49 Analgesic nephropathy. Higher power demonstrates a non-specific lymphocytic infiltrate (HPS, ×200).

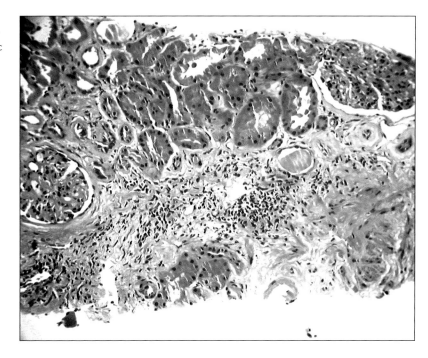

Fig. 3.50 Analgesic nephropathy. There are vascular changes accompanying the chronic interstitial nephritis (PAS, ×200).

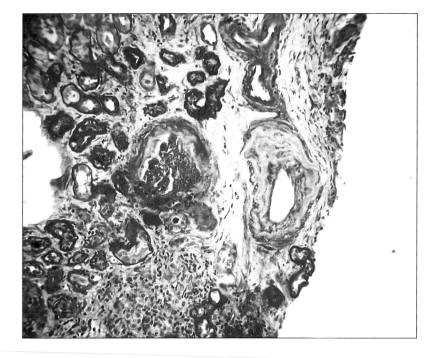

Fig. 3.51 Analgesic nephropathy. There is diffuse fibrosis and trichrome stain with relative preservation of glomeruli (Trichrome, ×100).

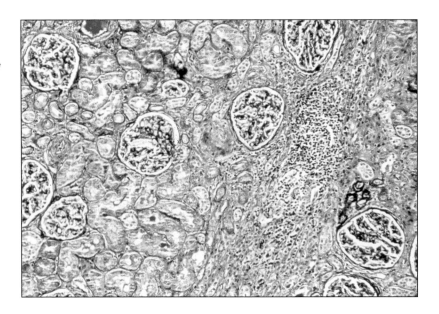

Glomerulosclerosis is also present as a secondary change but more commonly the glomeruli are not damaged and become crowded because of the tubular atrophy. These cortical changes are relatively non-specific but in the presence of radiologic evidence of papillary necrosis are consistent with the diagnosis of analgesic nephropathy. It should be remembered in the differential diagnosis that sickle cell disease and diabetes may also be associated with papillary necrosis.

Etiology/pathogenesis

A particular form of chronic nephrotoxicity, which is of special interest is the lesion associated with analgesic abuse. It has been long recognized that chronic excessive use of analgesic drugs is associated with the development of chronic renal failure due to a chronic tubular interstitial nephritis. Although phenacetin combined with caffeine and codeine, the compound most frequently implicated in the earliest reports, abuse of a number of common analgesics including acetaminophen and non-steroidal anti-inflammatory drugs have more recently also been implicated in the development of this lesion.

Selected reading

Mathew T H 1992 Drug-induced renal disease. Review. Medical Journal of Australia 156:724–728.

Mihatsch M J, Steinmann E et al 1979 The morphologic diagnosis of analgesic (phenacetin) abuse. Pathology, Research and Practice 164:68–79.

Light chain cast nephropathy

Proteinaceous casts are common in all forms of chronic interstitial nephritis. The cast nephropathy associated with myeloma deserves special mention since it has a distinctive histologic appearance and the cast material is involved in the direct pathogenesis of the lesion. Light chain, or so-called myeloma, cast nephropathy is seen in approximately half of patients with multiple myeloma who have renal disease. The remainder of patients with multiple myeloma who have related renal disease have either light chain deposition or amyloid deposition, or rarely combined lesions, as discussed elsewhere. The casts in myeloma cast nephropathy consist of Bence Jones or light chain proteins combined with Tamm–Horsfall protein. Casts can be diffuse or focal involving distal convoluted and collecting tubules and often have a fractured or crystalline appearance (Figs 3.52–3.54). They are frequently surrounded by multi-

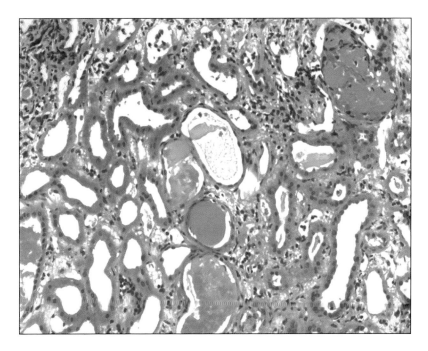

Fig. 3.52 Cast nephropathy. Tubules are dilated and filled with proteinaceous casts completely occluding some tubular lumina (H&E, ×200).

Fig. 3.53 Cast nephropathy. The casts have a fractured appearance and also demonstrate a cellular reaction (H&E, ×400).

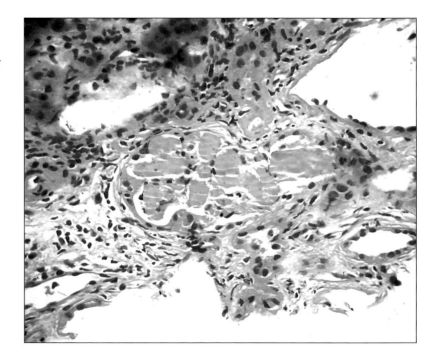

Fig. 3.54 Cast nephropathy. In addition, there is evidence of tubular epithelial damage and interstitial edema (HPS, ×400).

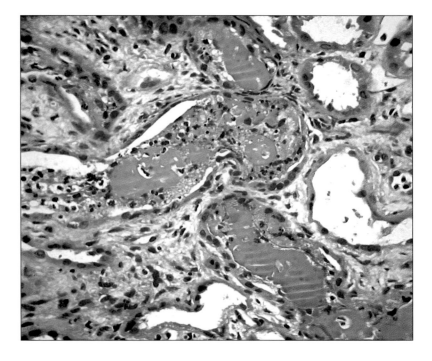

nucleated giant cells formed from infiltrating macrophages (Figs 3.55–3.57). Disruption of the tubules can be seen focally and acute polymorphonuclear or granuloma like inflammation may extend into the adjoining interstitium (Fig. 3.58). The cytoplasm of

Fig. 3.55 Cast nephropathy. The casts are surrounded by multi-nucleated giant cells formed from infiltrating macrophages (Trichrome, ×200).

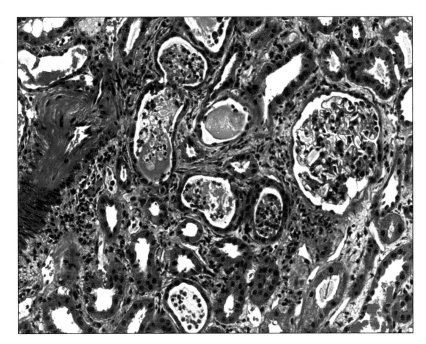

Fig. 3.56 Cast nephropathy. The evidence of tubular necrosis and an inflammatory response is seen involving the interstitium (Trichrome, ×200).

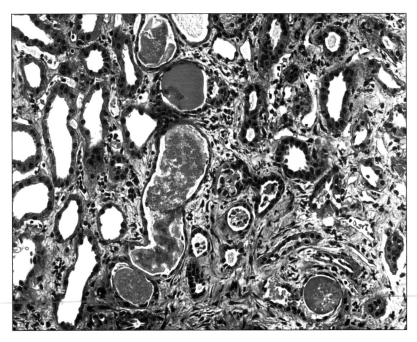

Fig. 3.57 Cast nephropathy. There is Tamm–Horsfall protein intermingled with the light chains (PAS, ×400).

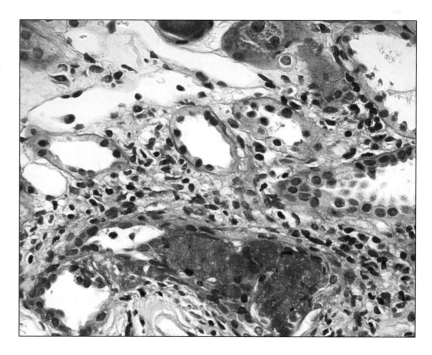

Fig. 3.58 Cast nephropathy. The fractured casts are surrounded by evidence of hyaline material within the epithelial cells (H&E, ×400).

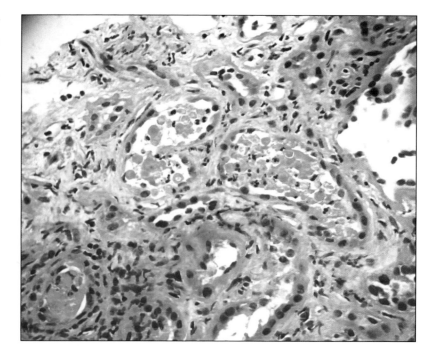

the proximal tubules frequently contains large hyaline protein droplets or needle like inclusion bodies (Figs 3.59, 3.60). There is interstitial fibrosis and a lymphocytic infiltration associated with tubular atrophy. Thus, except for the distinctive nature of the casts and the granulomatous reaction to them, the lesion may mimic other forms of chronic interstitial nephritis. Immunofluorescence microscopy is helpful in cases of suspected light chain cast nephropathy. Monoclonal staining for kappa or lambda light chains helps to confirm the diagnosis, although it should be noted that only about half of casts in proven light chain cast nephropathy stain (Fig. 3.61). Therefore, the absence of monoclonal staining of the casts cannot be taken as definitive evidence ruling out light chain cast nephropathy.

Electron microscopy can also be useful in that the tubular casts have a very distinctive composition of finely granular material of moderate electron density often forming crystal like structures (Figs 3.62–3.64). Because of the distinctive nature of the cast material and the giant cell reaction to it the differential diagnosis is relatively limited but does include other forms of paraproteinemias including Waldenstrom's macroglobulinemia.

Fig. 3.59 Cast nephropathy. Syncytical proliferation of the tubular epithelium surrounding cast material (Trichrome, ×400).

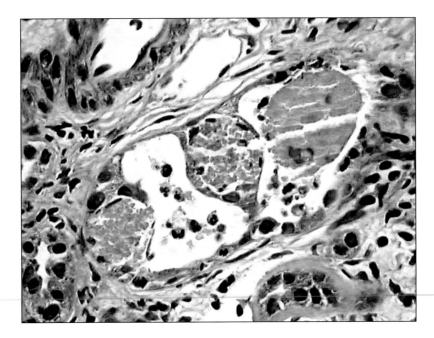

Fig. 3.60 Cast nephropathy. The granulomatous appearance is seen in this tubule with irregular fractured casts and a cellular reaction (Trichrome, ×400).

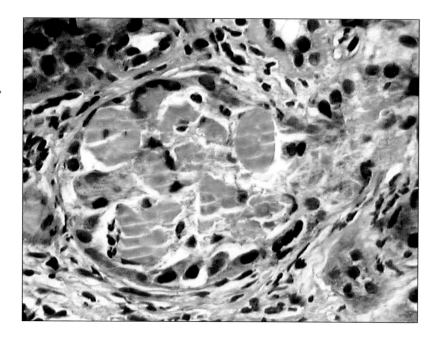

Fig. 3.61 Cast nephropathy. Immunofluorescence reveals the cast material to stain positively with kappa or lambda light chains (anti-kappa, ×200).

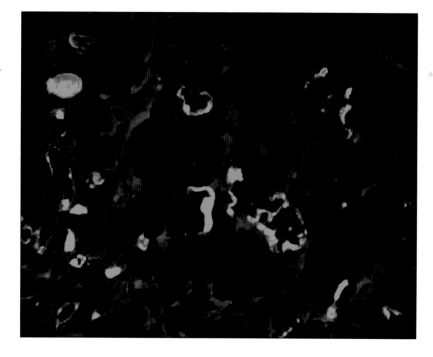

Fig. 3.62 Cast nephropathy. Electron microscopy reveals the tubules to be occluded by a mixture of dense homogenous casts material with fragments of cells and cellular debris (TEM, ×2000).

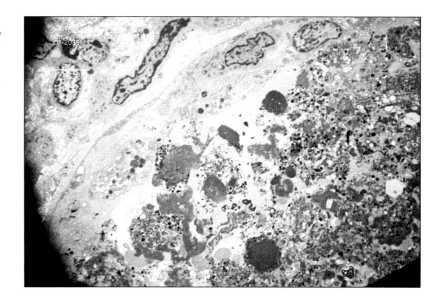

Fig. 3.63 Cast nephropathy. Other casts are more homogenous in appearance and have a dark electron dense appearance (TEM, ×2000).

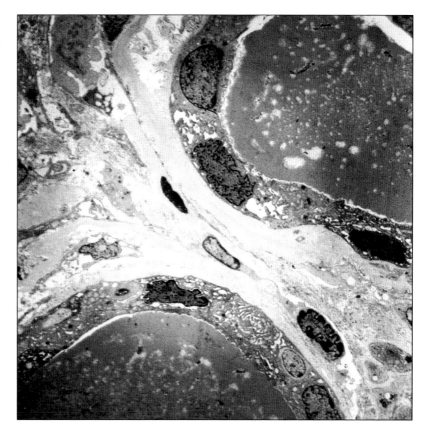

Fig. 3.64 Cast nephropathy. Some casts material also has dense crystalline material surrounded by proteinaceous material (TEM, ×4000).

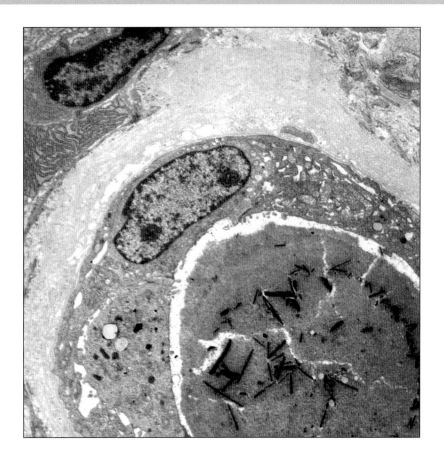

Etiology/pathogenesis

The mechanism by which urinary light chains lead to renal failure is incompletely understood. Light chains precipitate in the tubules, leading to casts in the distal and collecting tubules. These casts contain Tamm-Horsfall mucoprotein, which is a protein normally secreted by the cells of the thick ascending limb of the loop of Henle and constitute the matrix of all urinary casts. The limitation of obstructing casts to the distal nephron reflects the requirement of the excreted light chains to aggregate with Tamm–Horsfall mucoprotein. Experimental studies have shown that light chains are tubulotoxic depending on the potential of an individual light chain to bind Tamm–Horsfall mucoprotein.

Selected reading

Kyle R A 1994 Monoclonal proteins and renal disease. Annual Review of Medicine 45:71–77.

Sanders P W 1993 Renal involvement in plasma cell dyscrasias. Current
Opinion in Nephrology and Hypertension 2:246–252.

Oxalosis

Oxalate crystals within the tubular lumina are frequently present in
end stage kidneys but extensive oxalate crystal deposition is indicative of hyperoxaluric states (Figs 3.65, 3.66). The histological findings are the non-specific findings of tubular atrophy and interstitial
fibrosis with the distinctive feature being crystal deposition. Calcium
oxalate crystals are often fan-shaped and can be seen by light
microscopy, but are more readily visualized by their birefringence
under polarized light. Severe fibrosis and inflammation, even with
giant cell reaction, can occur when crystals break through the tubular lumina into the interstitium. Calcium oxalate tends to precipitate particularly in proximal tubules, although with extensive disease,
all nephron segments may be involved. Calculi are often found in
calyces or the pelvis of the kidney. Glomerulosclerosis is proportional to the degree of interstitial injury. Massive crystal deposition
occurs in primary hyperoxaluria and ethylene glycol ingestion.

Fig. 3.65 Oxalate nephropathy. There is dilatation of the tubules with crystalline material within the lumen. The crystals have a plate like appearance (H&E, ×100).

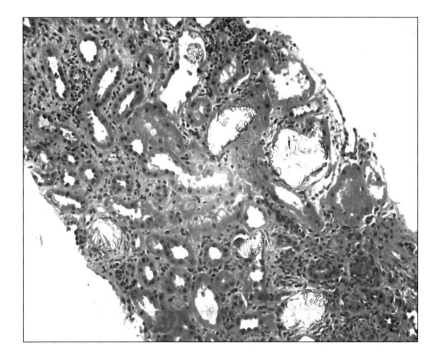

Fig. 3.66 Oxalate nephropathy. Higher power demonstrates the crystals to be fragmented and associated with flattened and necrotic epithelium (H&E, ×100).

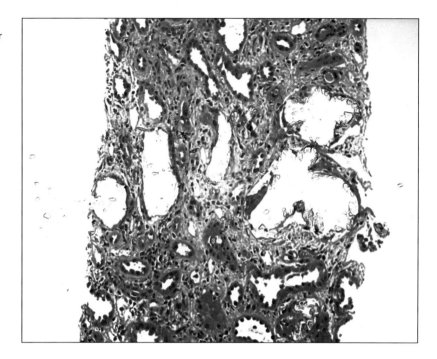

Lesser degree of oxalate crystals can occur secondarily, e.g. ethylene glycol ingestion, after jejunal-intestinal bypass, or in chronic renal disease due to other causes.

Etiology/pathogenesis

There are numerous causes of hyperoxaluria. These include ethylene glycol poisoning, excessive ingestion of oxalate containing foods (cocoa, tea, rhubarb, beet greens, fruit, berries and spinach), chronic intestinal disease (small bowel resections, malabsorptive states) and primary genetic hyperoxaluria. Type I deficiency is the most common, is inherited as an autosomal recessive disease, and is due to lack of hepatic microsomal alanine glyoxylate aminotransferase. Type II deficiency is very rare, and occurs secondary to a defect in hydroxypyruvate metabolism, which has not been defined. Renal disease is less severe than in type I. Type III is due to primary intestinal hyperabsorption of oxalate and appears to be very rare. Treatment with pyridoxine, a co-factor for aminotransferase, has been used with some benefit in primary hyperoxaluria. Kidney transplantation was not successful in early series, with very low graft survival rates due to continued oxalate deposits and mobilization of tissue oxalate pools after surgery. With aggressive supportive therapy with intensive hemodialysis before surgery, pyridoxine and fluid therapy, results have been better. Combined hepatic and kidney transplantation would be necessary to effect a cure for the underlying defect.

Selected reading

Aponte G E, Fetter T R 1954 Familial idiopathic oxalate nephrocalcinosis. American Journal of Clinical Pathology 24:1363–1373.

Morgan S H, Watts R W E 1989 Perspectives in the assessment and management of patients with primary hyperoxaluria Type I. Advances in Nephrology 18:95–106.

Scheinman J 1991 Primary hyperoxaluria: therapeutic strategies for the 90's. Kidney International 40:389–399.

Williams A W, Wilson D M 1990 Dietary intake, absorption, metabolism, and excretion of oxalate. Seminars in Nephrology 10:2.

Urate nephropathy

Urate nephropathy may be difficult to detect since standard histologic procedures result in dissolution of the intratubular deposits of urate (Fig. 3.67). Routine histology reveals distended collecting ducts sometimes containing granular casts and focal calcification. There is interstitial fibrosis and foci of interstitial inflammation with occasional foreign body type giant cells (a tophus reaction).

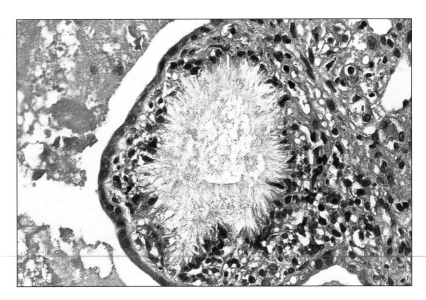

Fig. 3.67 Urate nephropathy. There is an accumulation of needle-like crystals associated with an inflammatory infiltrate in the interstitium typical of a gouty tophus (H&E, ×400).

Urate crystals with their characteristic needle-like configuration can be identified if the tissue is fixed in alcohol instead of aqueous formalin. Nephrosclerosis is a common feature. Thus, a specific diagnosis of urate nephropathy may not be made, unless specialized fixation is used to detect the crystals.

Etiology/pathogenesis

The contribution of serum uric acid levels to chronic kidney disease and the importance of urate nephropathy have been controversial topics. Epidemiological studies show correlations of hyperuricemia with chronic kidney disease and hypertension, but it is not known in humans whether this is causal or merely reflects that serum uric acid may be an excellent marker for glomerular filtration. Certainly, direct tissue injury by urate crystals and surrounding tophus reaction contributes to tubulointerstitial fibrosis. Recent animal studies also have demonstrated that elevated serum uric acid can cause tubulo-interstitial fibrosis and hypertension.

Selected reading

Johnson R J, Kivlighn S D, Kim Y G et al 1999 Reappraisal of the pathogenesis and consequences of hyperuricemia in hypertension, cardiovascular disease, and renal disease. American Journal of Kidney Disease 33(2):225–234.
Mazzali M, Hughes J, Kim Y G et al 2001 Elevated uric acid increases blood pressure in the rat by a novel crystal-independent mechanism. Hypertension 38:1101–1106.

Indinavir nephropathy

The advent of the use of HIV-1 protease inhibitors in the treatment of HIV infection has introduced a new entity of Indinavir nephropathy. This can present clinically as acute renal failure and may be diagnosed clinically by the presence of crystalluria. The crystals are needle-like and obstruct the tubules extensively, with surrounding inflammatory reaction (Figs 3.68, 3.69).

Etiology/pathogenesis

Indinavir is excreted in the urine. Low solubility is exacerbated by elevated pH, dehydration, high drug levels and interactions with

Fig. 3.68 Indinavir nephropathy. Low power view demonstrates the needle-like crystals surrounded by the desquamated tubular epithelium filling the tubular lumina (H&E, ×200).

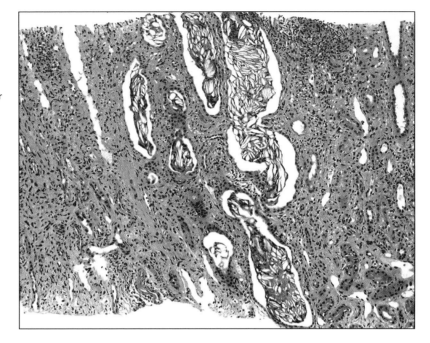

Fig. 3.69 Indinavir nephropathy. Intratubular needle-like crystals are present (H&E, ×200).

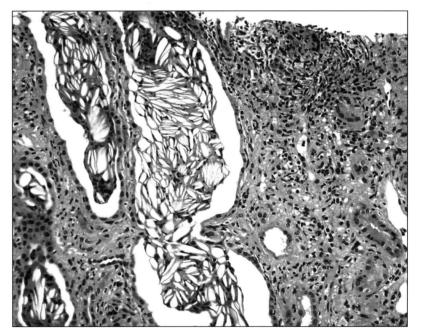

various other drugs. These factors then together cause crystals to form in the tubules, with direct tubular injury. Indinavir crystals have also been observed in biopsies of patients with more insidious renal insufficiency and tubulointerstitial fibrosis.

Selected reading

Famularo G, Di Toro S, Moretti S, De Simone C 2000 Symptomatic crystalluria associated with indinavir. Annals of Pharmacotherapy 34:1414–1418.

Perazella M A, Kashgarian M, Cooney E 1998 Indinavir nephropathy in an AIDS patients with renal insufficiency and pyuria. Clinical Nephrology 50:194–196.

Chronic interstitial nephritis

The group of chronic interstitial nephritides in which the histologic lesion is interstitial fibrosis and tubular atrophy with little or no significant active inflammatory infiltrate can be due to the wide variety of causes described above. It is often difficult to identify a specific etiologic agent and although an association of a particular agent with chronic renal failure or hypertension suggests the possibility of a cause and effect relationship, a strict relationship is often difficult to prove. Even identification of a potential suspect agent may not be sufficient evidence since increased levels could be due to lack of excretion in a patient with renal insufficiency rather than indicative of increased exposure. Chronic interstitial nephritis is therefore often designated as idiopathic. The histologic findings consist of diffuse interstitial fibrosis and tubular atrophy with a variable degree of an interstitial infiltrate of lymphocytes. The findings are nonspecific and are accompanied by vascular changes of arterial and arteriolar sclerosis.

References to **Brenner & Rector's** *The Kidney* **7th edition** are given in parentheses below.

Introduction

Evaluation of the renal morphology in allograft patients is used to answer two major questions. Is the failure of the graft caused by rejection or some other unrelated lesion? And if rejection is present, is the lesion potentially reversible using available therapeutic approaches? In the absence of rejection, it should be ascertained whether the graft failure results from acute tubular necrosis, acute infectious pyelonephritis, obstruction of the vasculature or urinary outflow tract, presence of recurrent or *de novo* glomerular disease or toxicity associated with the therapeutic agents used to modulate the immune response. In assessing whether or not rejection lesions are potentially reversible, it is necessary to evaluate not only the intensity but also the nature of the rejection episode.

The Banff working classification of renal allograft pathology modified in 1997 is now an internationally agreed upon standardized classification of the morphologic changes associated with various types of rejection (Table 4.1). This newer version of the Banff system was influenced by data from several clinical trials using the Banff 94

TABLE 4.1   Banff 97 diagnostic categories for renal allograft biopsies[a]
1. Normal

2. Antibody-mediated rejection
   Rejection demonstrated to be due, at least in part, to anti-donor antibody
   A. Immediate (hyperacute)
   B. Delayed (accelerated acute)

3. Borderline changes: 'Suspicious' for acute rejection   This category is used when no intimal arteritis is present, but there are foci of mild tubulitis (1–4 mononuclear cells/tubular cross section) and at least 1

4. Acute/active rejection	
Type (Grade)	Histopathological findings
IA	Cases with significant interstitial infiltration (>25% of parenchyma affected) and foci of moderate tubulitis (>4 mononuclear cells/tubular cross section or group of 10 tubular cells)
IB	Cases with significant interstitial infiltration (>25% of parenchyma affected) and foci of severe tubulitis (>10 mononuclear cells/tubular cross section or group of 10 tubular cells)
IIA	Cases with mild to moderate intimal arteritis
IIB	Cases with severe intimal arteritis comprising (>25% of the luminal area
III	Cases with 'transmural' arteritis and/or arterial fibrinoid change and necrosis of medial smooth muscle cells (with accompanying lymphocytic inflammation)

5. Chronic/sclerosing allograft nephropathy	
Grade	Histopathological findings
Grade I (mild)	Mild interstitial fibrosis and tubular atrophy without (a) or with (b) specific changes suggesting chronic rejection.
Grade II (moderate)	Moderate interstitial fibrosis and tubular atrophy (a) or (b)
Grade III (severe)	Severe interstitial fibrosis and tubular atrophy and tubular loss (a) or (b)

6. Other changes not considered to be due to rejection

Schema and the results of clinical correlations of the CCTT trials. Interstitial infiltration of activated lymphocytes with tubulitis characteristic of cellular rejection (Type I) and intimal arteritis characteristic of vascular rejection (Type II) are considered the main lesions indicative of acute rejection episodes (Table 4.2). The goal of the use of this classification is to be able to give a diagnostic biopsy

TABLE 4.2   Overview of acute rejection

Banff 97	Banff 93–95	CCTT
Suspicious for acute rejection, borderline	Borderline	Type I[a]
Type 1A (tubulointerstitial with t2 and at least i2)	Grade I	Type I[a]
Type 1B (tubulointerstitial with t3 and at least i2)	Grade IIA	Type I[a]
Type IIA (vascular with v1)	Grade IIB	Type II
Type IIB (vascular with v2)	Grade III	
Type III v3 – (fibrinoid change/transmural arteritis)	Grade III	Type III

[a]A semi quantitative scoring system has been developed to produce an acute or chronic numerical index for purposes of evaluation of severity.

grading which will provide both a prognostic and therapeutic tool (Tables 4.3, 4.4). The standardized classification also promotes international uniformity in reporting of renal allograft pathology and is useful to facilitate the performance of multi-center trials of new therapeutic modalities.

Etiology/pathogenesis

The mechanisms involved in allograft rejection are complex and involve both cellular and humoral immunity. Efforts to reduce the immune response to alloantigens include cross matching HLA antigens as closely as possible and blocking of the presentation and recognition of these antigens. The status of the graft at time of transplant is also important since outcomes are poorer with prolonged cold ischemia times.

TABLE 4.3   Quantitative criteria for tubulitis ('t') score[a]

t0   No mononuclear cells in tubules

t1   Foci with 1 to 4 cells/tubular cross section (or 10 tubular cells)

t2   Foci with 5 to 10 cells/tubular cross section

t3   Foci with >10 cells/tubular cross section, or the presence of at least two areas of tubular basement membrane destruction accompanied by i2/i3 inflammation and t2 tubulitis elsewhere in the biopsy

[a]Applies to tubules no more than mildly atrophic.

TABLE 4.4   Quantitative criteria for intimal arteritis ('v')
v0   No arteritis
v1   Mild-to-moderate intimal arteritis in at least one arterial cross section
v2   Severe intimal arteritis with at least 25% luminal area lost in at least one arterial cross section
v3   Transmural arteritis and/or arterial fibrinoid change and medial smooth muscle necrosis with lymphocytic infiltrate in vessel
Note number of arteries present and number affected. Indicate infarction and/or interstitial hemorrhage by an asterisk (with any level v score).

Hyperacute and accelerated rejection (antibody-mediated rejection)

This category is divided into immediate (hyperacute) and delayed (accelerated acute). Hyperacute rejection refers to allograft failure that occurs within minutes or hours after transplantation. It is thought to be the result of preexisting circulating antibodies of the recipient which are directed against antigens present in the grafted endothelium. Presensitization of the recipient if often related to previous pregnancies, blood transfusions or other previous antigenic stimuli. However, hyperacute rejections may also be related to endothelial damage that is not immunologic in nature. A separate form of acute graft failure that is not immunologic has been termed acute imminent transplant nephropathy and has been related to injury occurring in the graft during the preservation phase. Delayed or accelerated acute rejection refers to situations where sudden graft loss occurs due to the development of antidonor antibodies. Both types have a similar histologic appearance.

Microscopically, fibrin thrombi are seen in all renal vessels (Fig. 4.1) including the glomerular capillaries and peritubular venules. The vascular thrombosis is associated with infarction and tubular necrosis. There is prominent PMN infiltration in peritubular capillaries. Immunofluorescence may show linear staining for immunoglobulins along the capillary walls of the peritubular venules but this is not a constant finding. Electron microscopy demonstrates platelets, fibrin sludged red blood cells and necrosis of glomerular capillaries and other vascular structures.

Fig. 4.1 Hyperacute rejection. The artery is occluded by a fibrin thrombus and there is evidence of congestion in the peritubular capillaries. Focal tubular necrosis is also seen in this silver methenamine Masson stain (×200).

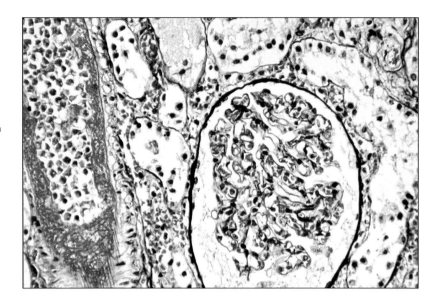

An addition to the Banff 97 classification proposes to replace category 2 described above with a special categorization for antibody mediated rejection (Table 4.5). It takes into account that antibody-mediated rejection is being recognized more frequently and not always in the early posttransplant period. This, combined with the identification of some relatively specific markers such as peritubular capillary staining of C4d, has given rise to a more precise classification (Table 4.5). The criteria for acute antibody-mediated rejection has three cardinal features: evidence of acute renal tissue injury including tubular injury, inflammatory cells in the peritubular capillaries, or vascular necrosis (Fig. 4.2). Immunopathologic evidence of antibody-mediated disease includes C4d staining of peritubular capillaries (Fig. 4.3) or less specifically, immunoglobulin or complement deposition in vessels or serologic evidence of anti-donor antibodies. This classification also recognizes that antibody-mediated rejection may accompany Banff Type I or Type II rejection as described below.

TABLE 4.5 Antibody-mediated rejection (meeting criteria of C4d+ and with circulating anti-donor antibody)

1 ATN-like

2 Capillary-glomerulitis, polymorphonuclear and/or mononuclear leukocytes in peritubular capillaries

3 Arterial–transmural inflammation/fibrinoid change

Fig. 4.2 Acute antibody mediated rejection. Inflammatory cells are present in the peritubular capillaries associated with interstitial edema. Tubulitis and an interstitial infiltrate are not present. These findings are typical of acute antibody mediated rejection (H&E, ×400).

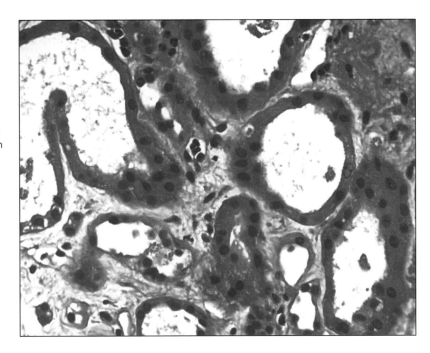

Fig. 4.3 Acute antibody mediated rejection. Immunopathologic evidence of antibody mediated rejection is confirmed by the presence of staining for C4d in peritubular capillaries shown here by indirect immunofluorescence (anti-C4d immunofluorescence, ×400).

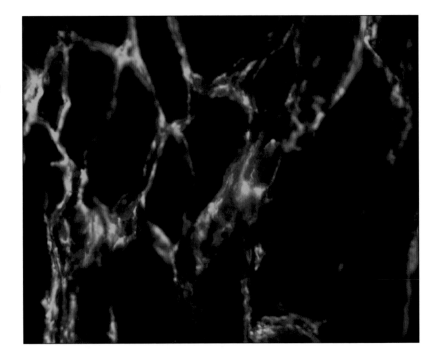

Acute rejection

Acute rejection, despite its terminology, can occur at any time during the course of the life of the allograft. It is most frequently seen during the initial months after grafting but can also be seen later in graft life particularly when disturbances of graft therapy are incurred. In the Banff classification, the severity is determined by the degree of tubulitis and the presence or absence of intimal arteritis.

Borderline changes: 'suspicious for acute rejection'

This category is used to describe very mild, acute interstitial cellular rejection. No intimal arteritis is present and only mild focal mononuclear cell infiltrates with rare foci of mild tubulitis defined as 1–4 mononuclear cells per tubular cross section present (Fig. 4.4). This degree of rejection is frequently encountered and probably does not reflect a degree of rejection that needs modification by additional therapy. Some investigators have suggested that such mild persistent infiltrates may contribute to the progression to chronic rejection.

Banff type I

Type I or acute interstitial cellular rejection is characterized by edema and infiltration of the interstitium by immunoblasts, lymphocytes, plasma cells, macrophages and a scattering of polymorphonuclear

Fig. 4.4 Acute rejection, Banff type, borderline, suspicious for acute rejection. Changes suspicious for acute rejection are seen here as a minimal focal interstitial infiltrate with minimal evidence of tubulitis. Less than four lymphocytes are seen in a single tubule-cross section in this image (H&E, ×200).

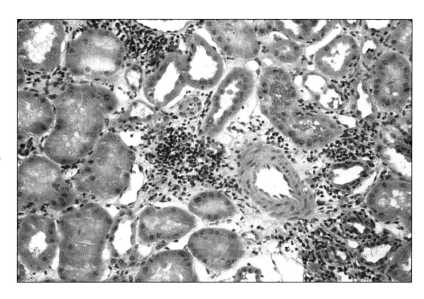

leukocytes in the eosinophils. The infiltrate is generally diffuse but appears somewhat more concentrated around vessels in glomeruli. In Type IA greater than 25% of the parenchyma is affected and foci of moderate tubulitis with greater than four mononuclear cells per tubular cross section or group of ten tubular cells is considered characteristic (Fig. 4.5). In Type IB greater than 25% of the parenchyma is affected and numerous foci of severe tubulitis with greater than ten mononuclear cells per tubular cross section or group of ten tubular cells is considered characteristic (Fig. 4.6).

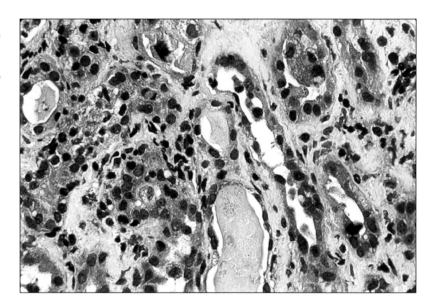

Fig. 4.5   Acute rejection, Banff Type IA. This category is defined by the presence of an interstitial infiltrate of lymphocytes with moderate tubulitis with greater than four mononuclear cells per tubular-cross section. The interstitial infiltrate consists of lymphocytes and is patchy involving less than 25% of the biopsy (H&E, ×400).

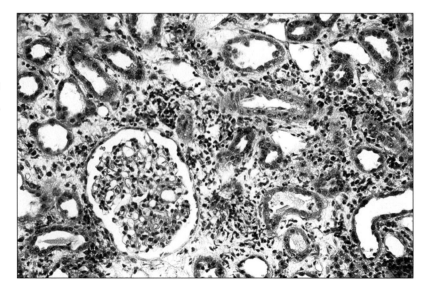

Fig. 4.6   Acute rejection, Banff Type IB. In this category the interstitial infiltrate is more extensive involving greater than 25% of the biopsy with numerous foci of severe tubulitis with greater than 10 mononuclear cells per tubular cross section. The vessels show no evidence of involvement (H&E, ×200).

Identification of the lymphocytes in the infiltrate demonstrates a large population of T cells identifiable by the CD3 antigen (Fig. 4.7) and a greater number of cytotoxic T cells identified by the antigen CD8 than helper inducer T cells identified by the presence of the antigen CD4. The ratio of activation antigens RO and RA are also of use in identifying the activity of the rejection. This degree of rejection generally has a good response to antirejection therapy

Banff type II

Type II or acute rejection with a vascular component consists of cases with mild to moderate intimal arteritis Type IIA in addition to any degree of interstitial cellular rejection. Intimal arteritis is defined as intimal thickening with inflammation of the arterial subendothelial space ranging from rare intimal inflammatory cells to necrosis of the endothelium with deposition of fibrin, platelets and inflammatory cells (Figs 4.8, 4.9). Type IIB describes cases with intimal arteritis compromising greater than 25% of the luminal area. The cellular infiltrate is composed of lymphocytes and monocytes. Severity is determined by the number of vessels affected as well as the intensity of the individual lesions (Fig. 4.10). The

Fig. 4.7   Acute rejection. The interstitial infiltrate consists of a mixed population of T cells. The large population of T cells is identifiable by the presence of the CD3 antigen here shown by immunohistochemistry (anti-C3 immunostaining, ×200).

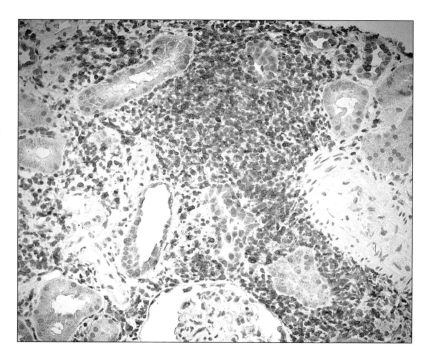

Fig. 4.8 Acute rejection, Banff Type II. In addition to an interstitial infiltrate with tubulitis there is evidence of vascular involvement. The vessel in this low power image demonstrates marked myointimal proliferation associated with lymphocytic infiltration underneath the endothelium (H&E, ×100).

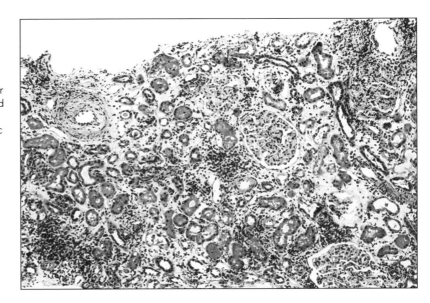

Fig. 4.9 Acute rejection, Banff Type IIA. A higher power of a vessel demonstrates marked endothelial cell swelling and numerous lymphocytes just beneath the endothelium. This is a mild but definite form of endothelial activation (H&E, ×400).

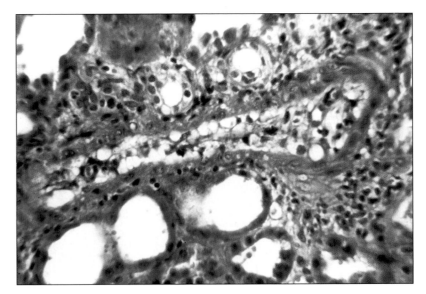

finding of intimal arteritis as seen in these categories is often focal. Response to therapy is more variable in this group.

Banff type III

Grade III consists of severe acute vascular rejection. These are cases with severe intimal arteritis and transmural arteritis as defined by injury and inflammation of the whole arterial wall including the media, necrosis of medial smooth muscles, fibrin deposition and cellular infiltration with mononuclear as well as polymorphonuclear leukocytes (Fig. 4.11). Focal infarction and interstitial hemorrhage without other obvious cause can be assumed to be associated with vascular lesions consistent with this degree of rejection. Rejection episodes of this severity are often associated with graft loss.

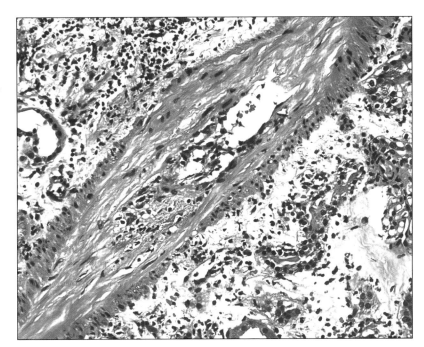

Fig. 4.10 Acute rejection, Banff Type IIB. Severity of Type II is determined by the number of vessels involved as well as the intensity of the individual lesions. In this vessel there is evidence of more severe infiltration with lymphocytes which involves not only the endothelium but also the media. Myointimal proliferation is prominent (H&E, ×200).

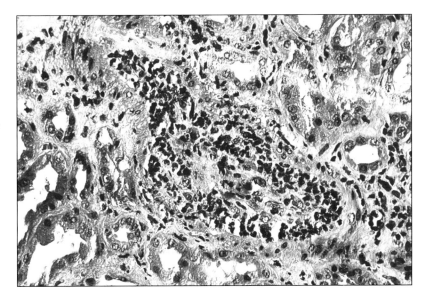

Fig. 4.11 Acute rejection, Banff Type III. This category consists of severe acute vascular rejection, which may be mediated in part by humoral mechanisms. Severe intimal and transmural arteritis with medial necrosis which typify this category are present in this vessel (H&E, ×200).

Chronic allograft nephropathy and transplant glomerulopathy

Chronic allograft nephropathy occurs anywhere from several months to several years after transplantation. Clinically, it is associated with

Fig. 4.12 Chronic/sclerosing allograft nephropathy. An example of Grade II–III is characterized by a diffuse increase in interstitial tissue and marked tubular atrophy as seen on this trichrome stain. Grade I has mild focal interstitial fibrosis and tubular atrophy. Grade II and III are defined as moderate and severe interstitial fibrosis. Microscopically, the picture is relatively non-specific and similar to that seen in nephrosclerosis (Trichrome, ×100).

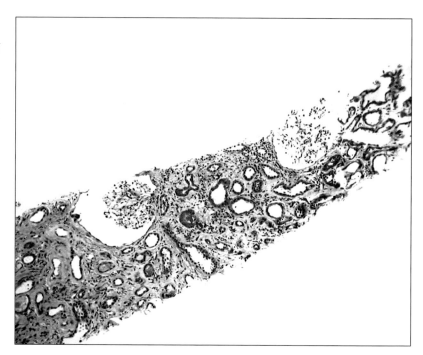

Fig. 4.13 Chronic/sclerosing allograft nephropathy. The classical lesion of chronic transplant vasculopathy is a circum-ferential proliferation of myointimal cells with an intact internal elastic lamina (H&E, ×200).

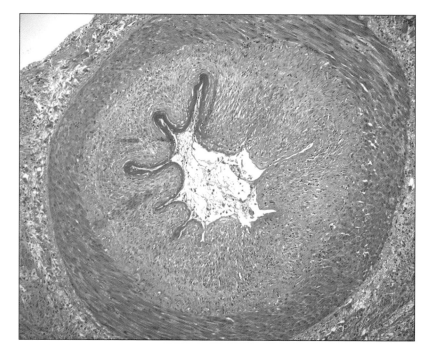

a slow and gradual decrease in renal function in contrast to the more acute explosive loss of renal function seen in acute rejection. Microscopically the picture is similar to that of nephrosclerosis (Fig. 4.12). There is arterial and arteriolar narrowing of the interlobular arcuate and radial arteries by myointimal proliferation and medial hypertrophy (Fig. 4.13). The vascular lesions are associated with a diffuse interstitial fibrosis and tubular atrophy.

The glomerular lesions of chronic rejection consist of ischemic glomerular capillary collapse, thickening of the capillary walls and segmental and global sclerosis (Figs 4.14, 4.15). In so called transplant glomerulopathy, the glomeruli show varying degrees of glomerulosclerosis with an increase in mesangial matrix, mesangial interposition and irregular thickening of basement membrane (Fig. 4.16).

Fig. 4.14   Transplant glomerulopathy. There is segmental sclerosis and splitting of the GBM due to increased lamina rara interna without deposits.

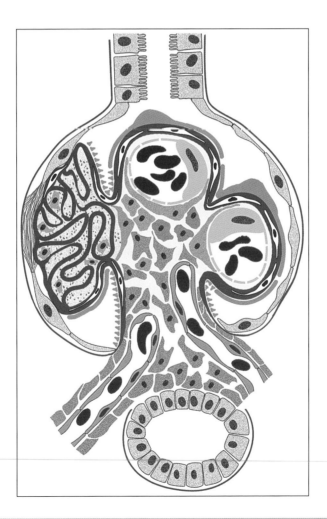

Fig. 4.15 Transplant glomerulopathy shows a split GBM by light microscopy, due to increased lamina rara interna without deposits, which can be seen by EM. There may also frequently be segmental sclerosis, and subtotal foot process effacement (TEM, ×6000).

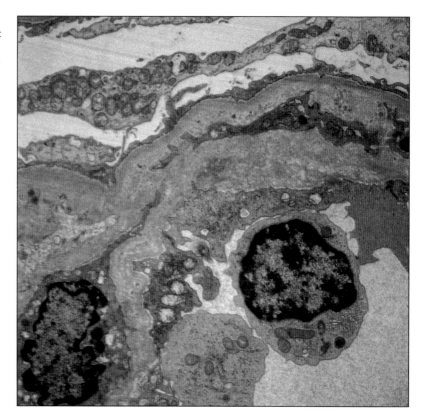

This lesion is associated with significant proteinuria. By electron microscopy, there is separation of the endothelial cells from the basement membrane with the accumulation of a granular material in the subendothelial space.

Chronic allograft nephropathy has also been graded in the Banff schema, Grade I consisting of mild interstitial fibrosis and tubular atrophy, Grade II with moderate degrees and Grade III with severe interstitial tubular atrophy and tubular loss.

Etiology/pathogenesis

The mechanisms involved are still unknown but humoral immunity directed against vascular cellular antigens has been suggested as a likely possibility. In addition, many factors involved with progressive fibrosis in the native kidney may play a role in the transplant, such as hypertension, abnormal lipids, proteinuria, reactive oxygen species.

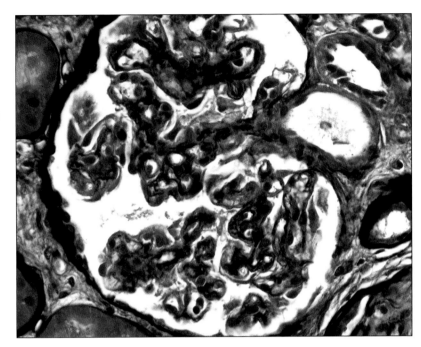

Fig. 4.16 Chronic/sclerosing allograft nephropathy. Glomerular lesions of chronic/sclerosing allograft nephropathy. Consists of an ischemic glomerulopathy with capillary collapse, thickening of the capillary walls and segmental and global sclerosis (Jones, ×400).

Cyclosporin/FK506 nephrotoxicity

The toxic effects of immunosuppressant drugs also are to be considered in the evaluation of the allograft biopsy. The toxic effects of calcineurin inhibitors including both cyclosporin and tacrolimus have fairly characteristic histologic findings. Importantly cyclosporine toxicity on a functional basis, i.e. vasoconstriction-related, should be considered when creatinine has risen quickly and the biopsy is morphologically normal. Characteristic findings include tubular vacuolization, isometric expansion of tubular epithelial cells and evidence of microvascular damage as characterized by the presence of nodular hyaline sclerosis of arterioles (Fig. 4.17). With severe toxic injury, arteriolar myocyte vacuolization can be seen associated with endothelial swelling, mucoid intimal thickening and accumulation of proteins within the vessel wall. Chronic calcineurin inhibitor toxicity is manifested by the ischemic changes that accompany these vascular changes. The most characteristic is that of striped fibrosis (Fig. 4.18). In some instances, thrombotic microangiopathic changes may also be seen and these must be distinguished from acute humoral rejection (Fig. 4.19).

Fig. 4.17 Chronic/
sclerosing allograft
nephropathy. In transplant
glomerulopathy, there is
evidence of marked
widening of the mesangial
areas with reduplication of
the peripheral capillary walls
causing lobular accentuation.
The pattern is similar to that
seen with membranopro-
liferative glomerulonephritis
and must be distinguished
therefore from recurrent
disease (Jones, ×400).

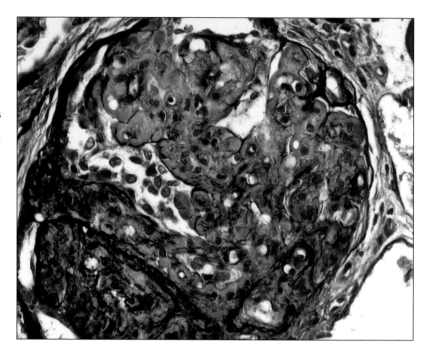

Fig. 4.18 Longitudinal
section of an afferent
arteriole with nodular
hyaline sclerosis typical of
calcineurin toxicity effect
(H&E, ×400).

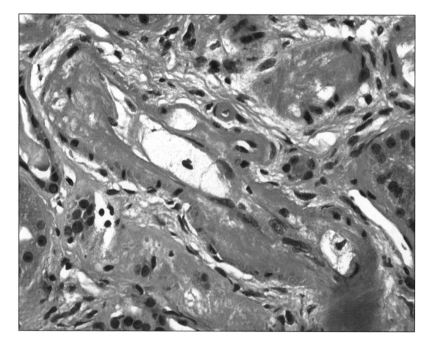

Etiology/pathogenesis

Cyclosporin induces elaboration of several vasoconstrictors, including endothelin, and is also directly toxic to renal parenchymal cells.

Fig. 4.19 Chronic calcineurin inhibitor toxicity is characterized by the presence of stripes of fibrosis as seen here in this low power micrograph (H&E, ×100).

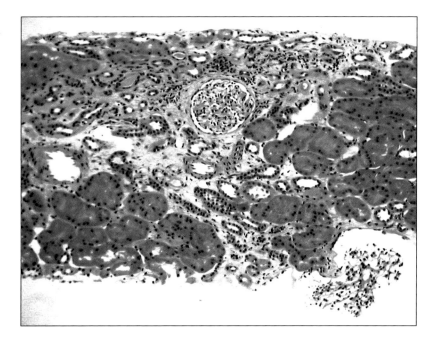

Post-transplant lymphoproliferative disease

Patients typically show systemic signs of hematopoietic illness when disease is more advanced, with hepatosplenomegaly and lymphadenopathy. However, early in the course, these findings may not be present. Renal biopsies show a uniform dense plasma cell infiltrate, which appears to expand between tubules. Cells may have an atypical immunoblastic appearance, or there may be serpiginous necrosis, in which case the diagnosis of post-transplant lympho-proliferative disease (PTLD) may be obvious (Figs 4.20–4.22). More often, the findings by LM are more subtle. Use of immunohisto-chemical staining for the presence of monoclonal B or T cells in the infiltrate is a helpful adjunct in the evaluation of such biopsies. If PTLD is seriously considered, the presence of EB virus can be determined by *in situ* hybridization. The differential diagnosis includes plasma-cell rich acute rejection.

Etiology/pathogenesis

PTLD arises in the setting of abnormal T cell regulation of B cells. Epstein–Barr virus infection is present in nearly all cases, but may

Fig. 4.20 Chronic calcineurin inhibitor toxicity. In some instances of calcineurin inhibitor toxicity, endothelial activation results in a thrombotic microangiopathy seen here by the presence of intracapillary thrombi (HPS, ×400).

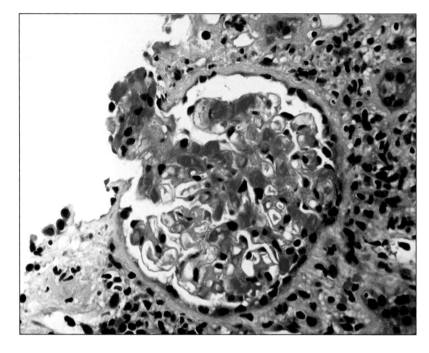

Fig. 4.21 PTLD. Most transplant lymphoproliferative disorders may also mimic the findings of acute allograft rejection. The major difference is the absence of tubulitis and the presence of a space occupying infiltrate without damage to the tubular epithelial cells (H&E, ×200).

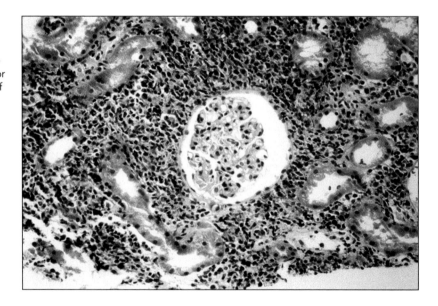

not be detected in all cases. Some PTLD are polyclonal. Typically, the process regresses when immunosuppression is decreased or removed.

Fig. 4.22 PTLD. *In situ* hybridization for Epstein–Barr virus confirms the presence of post-transplant lymphopro-liferative disease (*in situ* hybridization, ×200).

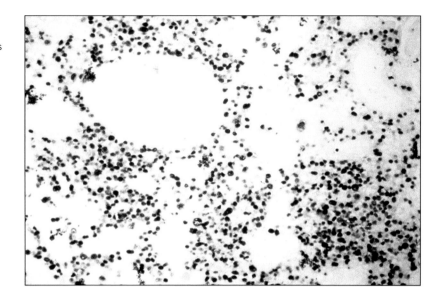

Selected reading

Hanto, D W 1995 Classification of Epstein–Barr virus-associated posttransplant lymphoproliferative diseases: implications for understanding their pathogenesis and developing rational treatment strategies. Annual Review of Medicine 46:381.

Viral infections

It must be remembered that a variety of different processes can involve the allograft other than those associated with an acute or chronic rejection. These processes may present as graft failure and biopsy diagnosis must differentiate these disease entities from those related to rejection. An important example is acute bacterial infection (Fig. 4.23). This entity can be distinguished by the presence of polymorphonuclear leukocytes in tubular lumens and in the interstitium (Fig. 4.24). Viral infections must also be considered Cytomegalovirus, polyomavirus and adenovirus all may infect the allograft.

The biopsy must be examined for the signs of viral infection including nuclear and cytoplasmic inclusions (Fig. 4.25), the presence of cytomegalic cells (Figs 4.26–4.28), and stratification of the epithelium (Figs 4.29–4.31). Viral infections may be particularly difficult to differentiate from acute rejection as they are frequently

Fig. 4.23 PTLD. Another charac-teristic is the atypia seen in the lymphocytic infiltrate in the interstitium (H&E, ×400).

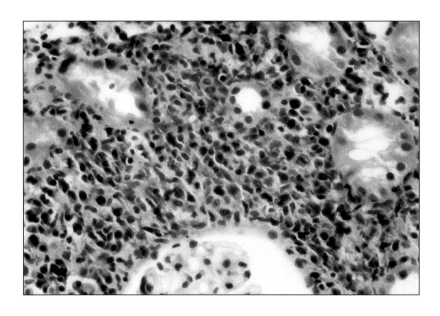

Fig. 4.24 Acute pyelonephritis. Infection of the allograft can mimic acute rejection by the presence of a diffuse interstitial infiltrate with tubulitis (H&E, ×100).

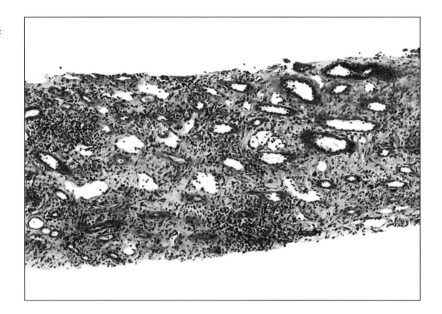

associated with a lymphocytic infiltrate and significant tubulitis may be present. Furthermore, the cytologic features of regeneration can mimic those of viral infection. The presence of plasma cells also poses a diagnostic dilemma as they can be a prominent component of the interstitial infiltrate in patients who have been non-compliant with their therapy.

Fig. 4.25 Acute pyelonephritis. The major distinguishing feature is the presence of polymorph nuclear leukocytes in both the tubular lumina and in the interstitium (H&E, ×200).

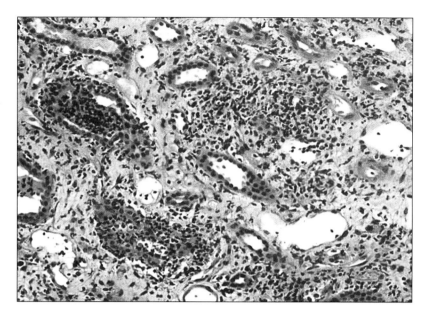

Fig. 4.26 Viral infection. Graft failure may be the result of viral infection by viruses associated with immunosuppression. They can be identified by the presence of nuclear inclusions. Epithelial necrosis and tubulitis may mimic acute rejection (H&E/silver, ×400).

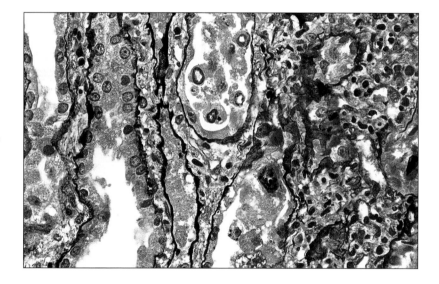

The principal finding associated with polyoma virus infection among renal transplant patients is a viral interstitial nephritis. Intranuclear basophilic viral inclusions without a surrounding halo are present. CMV has cytoplasmic inclusions, as noted above and has both intranuclear and cytoplasmic inclusions. With electron microscopy, intranuclear viral inclusions (with a particle diameter

Fig. 4.27 CMV. Cytomegalovirus infection is characterized by the presence of large cytomegalic cells and a homogeneous ground glass nucleus (H&E, ×600).

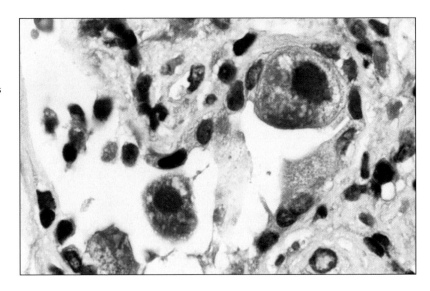

Fig. 4.28 CMV. The presence of cytomegalovirus infection can be confirmed by histochemical staining specific for the viral antigen (Anti-CMV, ×200).

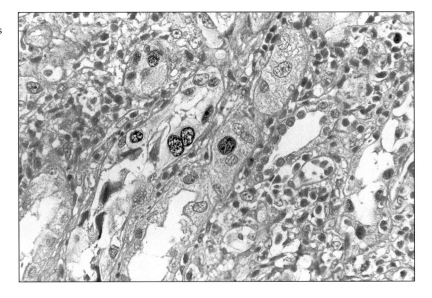

size of 30–50 nm) and tubular damage characterized by tubular cell necrosis, prominent lysosomal inclusions, and luminal cellular casts can be seen.

While these standard histologic markers are satisfactory for current evaluation, it is anticipated that newer molecular biological

Fig. 4.29 CMV. Electron microscopy may also be helpful demonstrating viral particles in the nucleus (TEM, ×16,000).

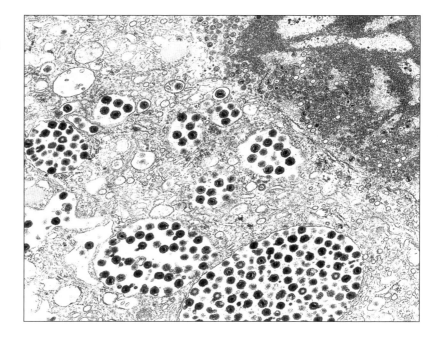

Fig. 4.30 Viral infection. Polyoma virus infection characterized by stratification of irregular epithelium associated with pleomorphic nuclei with amphophilic inclusions (H&E, ×400).

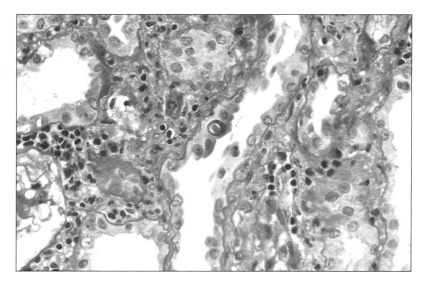

techniques and more specific characterization of the lymphocytic infiltrate will aid the diagnosis and evaluation of renal allograft biopsies in the future.

Fig. 4.31 Polyoma virus. This is best confirmed by histochemical staining for the large T antigen of SV40 seen here in glomerular cells (anti-SV40 immuno-staining, ×200).

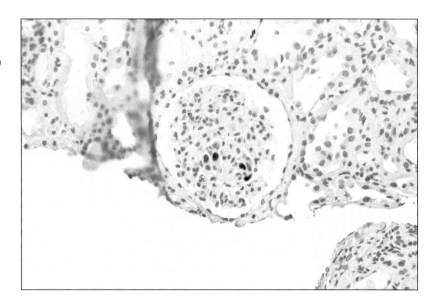

Fig. 4.32 Polyoma virus. Electron microscopy is also helpful by the demonstration of intranuclear viral particles (TEM, ×16,000).

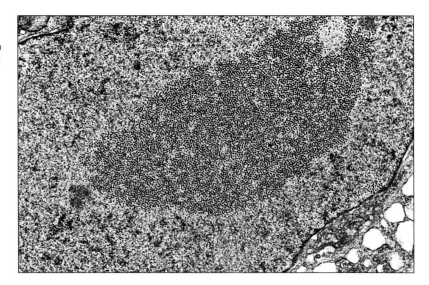

Selected reading

Racusen L C et al 1999 The Banff 97 Working Classification of Renal Allograft Pathology. Kidney International 55:713–723.

Colvin R B et al 1997 Evaluation of the pathologic criteria for acute renal allograft rejection: Reproducibility, sensitivity and clinical correlation. Journal of the American Society of Nephrology 8:1930–1941.

Cystic Diseases of the Kidney

References to **Brenner & Rector's** *The Kidney* **7th edition** are given in parentheses below.

Introduction

While single simple cysts of the kidney are relatively common and have little clinical implication, there are a group of hereditary cystic diseases which are of importance because of their contribution to the development of end stage renal disease. Each of the diseases has its own genetic abnormality and each of the diseases has their own characteristic clinical presentation. The exact mechanisms by which the genetic abnormalities result in the physiologic and pathologic abnormalities are still incompletely identified. Cystic diseases are classified according to the genetic presentation and according to the regions of the kidney which are involved. This is summarized in Table 5.1.

Autosomal dominant polycystic kidney disease

Autosomal dominant polycystic kidney disease affects between 1 in 500 to 1 in 1000 individuals. It is found in all racial and ethnic groups and is seen throughout the world. It is the most common of

TABLE 5.1   Classifications of cystic diseases

1. Autosomal dominant polycystic kidney disease (adult)
2. Autosomal recessive polycystic kidney disease (infantile)
3. Medullary cystic disease
4. Medullary sponge kidney
5. Cystic renal dysplasia
6. Acquired polycystic disease

genetic polycystic kidney disorders. As its name implies, autosomal dominant polycystic kidney disease is inherited in autosomal dominant pattern with complete penetrance. Thus, a child of an affected parent has a 50% chance of inheriting the abnormal gene. About half the patients affected are unable to give a family history consistent with autosomal dominant polycystic kidney disease. Autosomal dominant polycystic kidney disease was previously termed adult form of polycystic kidney disease because it may not become clinically apparent until the third or fourth decade of life. While 100% of gene carriers will show evidence of the disease only about 50% progress on to renal failure.

Pathology

Autosomal dominant polycystic kidney disease (ADPKD) results in kidneys which are enlarged and diffusely cystic (Figs 5.1–5.4). It is important to note that whereas the cysts appear to involve the entire kidney, only a portion of the total number of nephrons in the kidney are cystic (Figs 5.5–5.8). The cysts range in size from barely visible to several centimeters in diameter. Microdissection studies have demonstrated the cyst to be spherical dilatations or outpouchings from existing renal tubules (Fig. 5.9). As the cysts enlarge, they appear to become detached from their tubule of origin. In the early stages of the disease, the non-cystic parenchymal elements remain normal but as cysts increase in number and grow in size, the residual normal tissue becomes atrophic and non functional and results in the development of end stage renal disease. The disease is a systemic one and can produce cysts in other organs including liver, pancreas and lung,

Fig. 5.1 Autosomal dominant polycystic kidney disease (ADPKD). The kidneys are markedly enlarged and consist of numerous cystic structures bulging throughout the surface. Many of the cysts contain dark material.

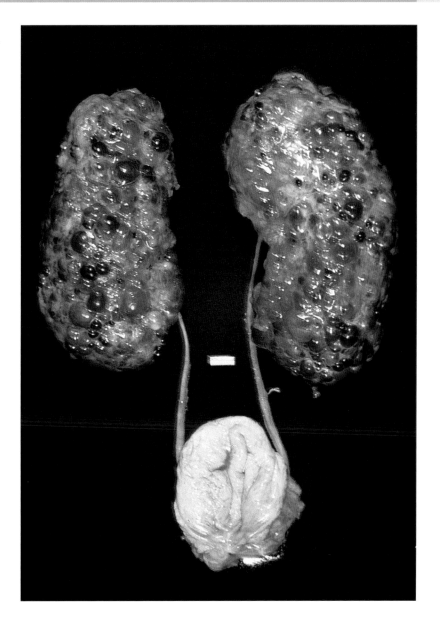

Fig. 5.2   ADPKD.

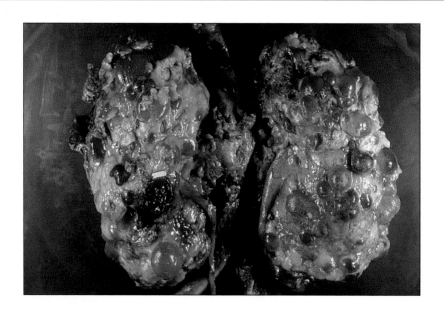

Fig. 5.3   ADPKD.

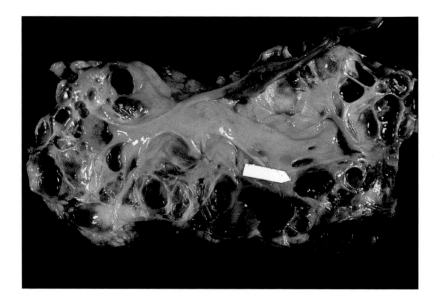

Fig. 5.4 ADPKD. Cut surface shows that the cysts are interspersed by fibrous tissue.

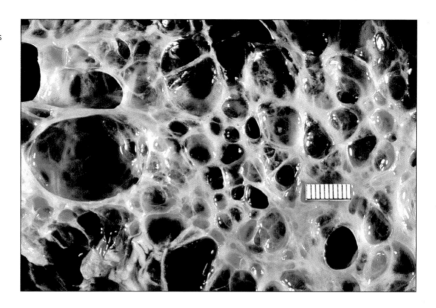

Fig. 5.5 ADPKD. Microscopic examination reveals the cysts to be lined by flattened epithelium and the interstitial tissue to consist predominately of fibrous tissue with small capillaries and atrophic tubules (H&E, ×400).

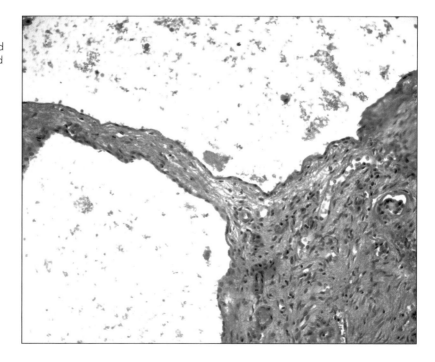

Fig. 5.6   ADPKD. In some areas, the cysts can be seen to displace normal tubular structures (H&E, ×200).

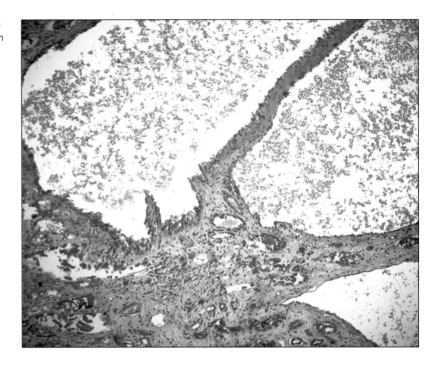

Fig. 5.7   ADPKD. Only a minority of the nephrons are involved by cystic formation. Normal tubular structures are scattered throughout the interstitial fibrous tissue (H&E, ×200).

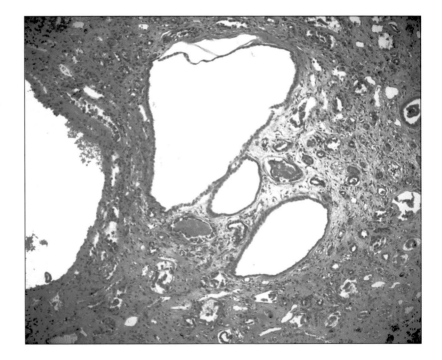

Fig. 5.8 ADPKD. Cysts involve both cortex and medulla and are seen extending into the inner medullary region (H&E, ×200).

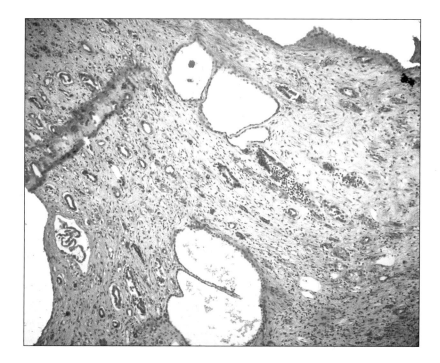

Fig. 5.9 ADPKD. The cysts initially begin as saccular aneurysmal dilatations of the tubule which then separate from the tubule itself as is seen here in a microdissected specimen.

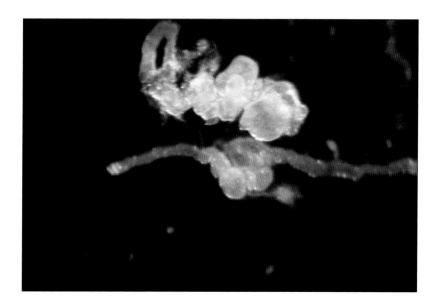

Autosomal recessive polycystic kidney disease

Autosomal recessive polycystic kidney disease is a rare disorder that occurs in 1 in 6000 to 55 000 live births. It was previously termed infantile polycystic disease in that it manifests itself at birth and results in significant perinatal mortality. In approximately three quarters of the cases, autosomal recessive polycystic disease results

Fig. 5.10 Autosomal Recessive Polycystic Kidney Disease (ARPKD). The kidneys are shown *in situ* occupying almost the complete abdominal cavity of a new born infant.

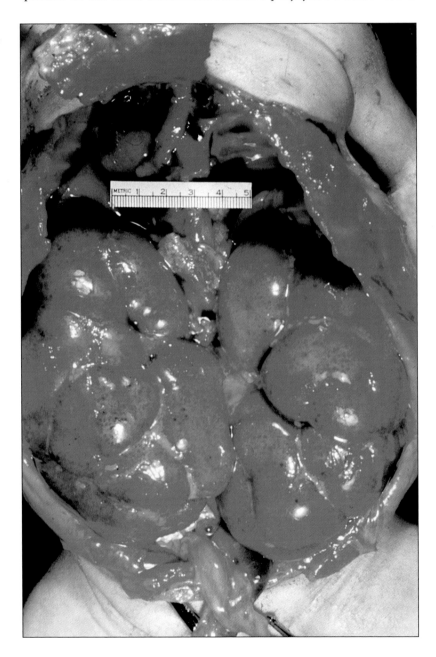

in death within a few days of birth. Occasional patients have survived through adolescence.

Pathology

Autosomal recessive polycystic kidney disease (ARPKD) affects both the kidneys and liver in approximately equal proportions. The kidneys are grossly enlarged and may fill the entire abdomen at the time of birth (Figs 5.10, 5.11). They are markedly enlarged and demonstrate numerous elongated fusiform cylindrical cysts that

Fig. 5.11 ARPKD. Cut surface of the kidney demonstrates that both the cortex and medulla are completely replaced by a sponge like appearance.

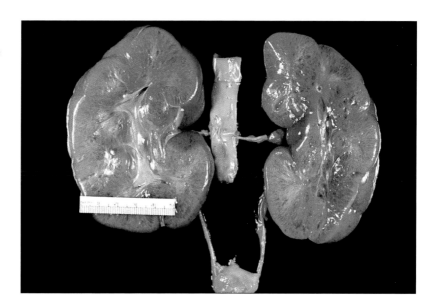

occupy the entire kidney. The cysts are lined by a flattened cuboidal epithelium and histochemical and specific binding studies have demonstrated that they appear to be dilated terminal branches of the collecting ducts.

The kidneys in these disorders have a similar morphological pattern (Fig. 5.12, 5.13).

Fig. 5.12 ARPKD. Microscopic examination shows the cysts to be elongated tubular structures, which reach from the cortical surface and extend into the medulla (H&E, ×200).

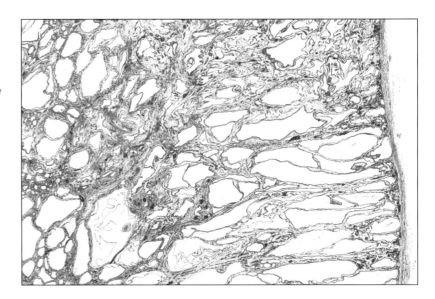

Fig. 5.13 ARPKD. The dilated tubular structures are separated by loose connective tissue with glomerular structures interspersed.

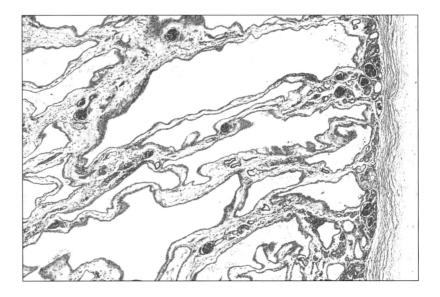

Medullary cystic disease

Medullary cystic disease has been described under two names: juvenile nephronophthisis and uremic medullary cystic disease. Juvenile nephronophthisis is an autosomal recessive disorder that usually presents in childhood. Uremic medullary cystic disease on the other hand is an autosomal dominant disorder, which usually presents in adults. Aside from the hereditary features and ages of presentation, the two conditions appear essentially similar morphologically.

Pathology

In longitudinal sections of the kidney, the cysts are present at the cortical medullary junction (Fig. 5.14–5.16). The cysts can vary in size from microscopic to 1–2 cm in diameter. The cortex is spared

Fig. 5.14 Medullary cystic disease (MCD). The cortex is preserved and the medulla appears somewhat blunted. Cysts are present at the junction of the cortex and medulla and in this example measure up to 4 cm in diameter (×5).

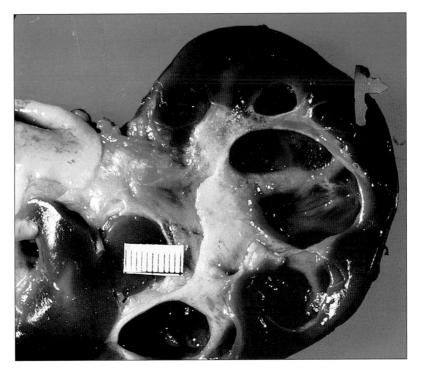

Fig. 5.15 Medullary cystic disease (MCD). Another example demonstrates the presence of cysts at the cortical medullary junction. In this example, cysts vary in size from less than 1 mm to over 1 cm in diameter.

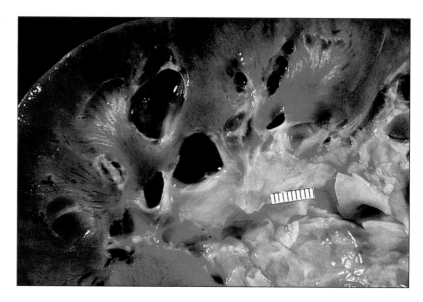

Fig. 5.16 Medullary cystic disease (MCD). The cysts are confined to the cortical medullary junction and the cortex appears atrophic (H&E, ×1).

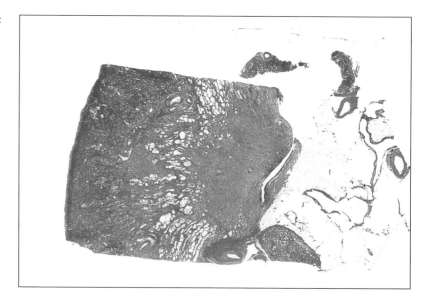

Fig. 5.17 Medullary cystic disease (MCD). The cyst is lined by flattened epithelium and surrounded by some relatively normal appearing tubular structures (H&E, ×200).

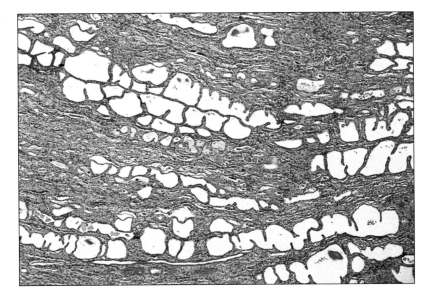

Fig. 5.18 Medullary cystic disease (MCD). The adjacent tubules show evidence of atrophy and there is the presence of interstitial fibrosis. There is no significant interstitial infiltrate (H&E, ×100).

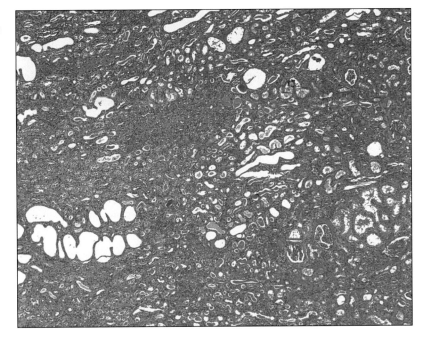

from cyst formation but non-specific glomerular hyalinosis and interstitial fibrosis with tubular atrophy is present (Figs 5.17–5.19). The microdissection studies have shown that the nephrons are altered by numerous small diverticula, highly variable in size involving the late distal tubule and collecting duct.

Fig. 5.19 Medullary cystic disease (MCD). End stage disease. The cortex proximal to the cysts shows marked atrophy with interstitial scarring and glomerulo-sclerosis. There is also marked hyalin and arteriolosclerosis (H&E, ×200).

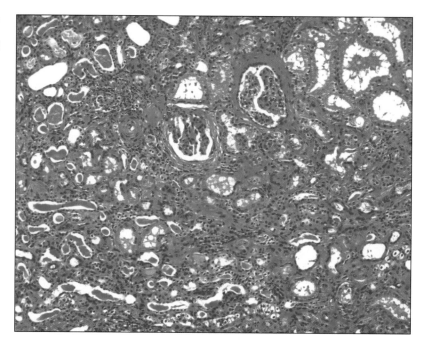

Fig. 5.20 End stage of medullary sponge kidney. The cortex is grossly atrophic and the prominent finding is the presence of shortened papillae with foci of calcification.

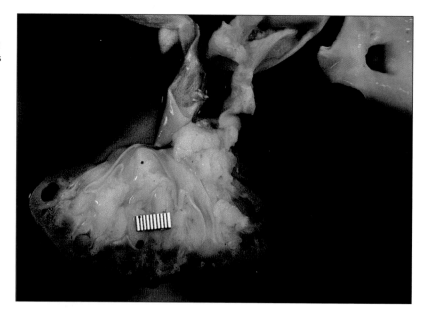

Medullary sponge kidney

Medullary sponge kidney is usually not recognized until late in life when secondary calcification of the medulla is associated with recurrent infection. The incidence of this disease is approximately 1 in 5000.

The only visible abnormality in this disease is the presence of irregular enlargement of the medullary and inner papillary portion of the collecting duct. The papillary are often calcified and shed to form renal calcinosis. Obstruction and infection are common secondary changes (Fig. 5.20).

Etiology/pathogenesis

Autosomal dominant polycystic kidney disease (PKD) is caused by genetic mutations in chromosome 16 for PKD1 and chromosome 4 in PKD2. PKD1 and PKD2 encode proteins called polycystins that appear to be members of a group of transmembrane molecules that transmit signals from the extracellular matrix to regulate cellular proliferation, differentiation and transport. Numerous mutations including deletions, substitutions and frame shifts have been identified in the genes encoding the polycystins, all of which however appear to diminish cellular function and alter cellular physiology and cell proliferation/cell/matrix interaction leading to cyst formation. The phenotype produced by these abnormal proteins is essentially identical in morphology and the clinical presentation is similar except that PKD2, the less common genotype, progresses to end stage renal failure at a slower rate. A spectrum of mutations have been identified in autosomal recessive polycystic disease. Juvenile nephronophthisis is linked to at least three different loci, called NPH1-3. Nephrocystin, the gene product of NPHP1, may function in signaling at focal adhesions. Medullary cystic disease is caused by mutation in one of two loci, MCKD1 or 2.

Selected reading

Bennett W B 1976 Kindred coexistence of medullary sponge kidney and medullary cystic disease. Annals of Internal Medicine 85:829.

Bergmann C, Senderek J, Sedlacek B et al 2003 Spectrum of mutations in the gene for autosomal recessive polycystic kidney disease (ARPKD/PKHD1). Journal of the American Society of Nephrology 14:76.

Hildebrandt F, Omram H 2001 New insights: nephronophthisis–Medullary cystic kidney disease. Pediatric Nephrology 16(2):168–176.

Hildebrandt F, Rensing C, Betz R et al 2001 Establishing an algorithm for molecular genetic diagnostics in 127 families with juvenile nephronophthisis. Kidney International 59:434.

Igarashi P, Somlo S 2002 Genetics and pathogenesis of polycystic kidney disease. Journal of the American Society of Nephrology 13:2384.

Qian F, Germino F J, Cai Y et al 1997 PKD1 interacts with PKD2 through a probable coiled-coil domain. Nature Genetics 16:179.

Acquired cystic disease

With the advent of long-term renal maintenance therapy, it has been observed that individuals on relatively long periods of dialysis develop multiple cysts in their remnant kidneys. This phenomenon is known as acquired cystic disease (ACD). An additional feature in acquired cystic disease is the occurrence of renal tumors. Papillary adeno-carcinomas of small size are common and larger tumors have a definite propensity for metastases.

The pathology of the kidneys is variable (Figs 5.21, 5.22). On section, the kidneys demonstrate cysts involving the cortex and medulla of the kidney in an irregular fashion. The cysts vary in size and are sometimes as large as those seen in adult polycystic kidney disease.

Selected reading

Fick G M, Gabow P A 1994 Hereditary and acquired cystic disease of the kidney. Kidney International 46:951.

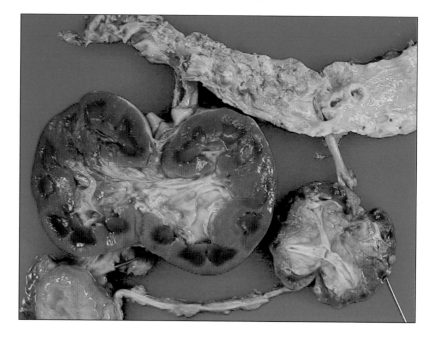

Fig. 5.21   Acquired cystic disease (ACD). This image demonstrates both end stage native kidney and transplanted kidney from a patient with longstanding renal failure. The native kidney is atrophic and demonstrates acquired cystic disease involving the cortex.

Fig. 5.22 Acquired cystic disease (ACD). There are randomly distributed cysts of irregular shaped lined by flattened epithelium (H&E, ×100).

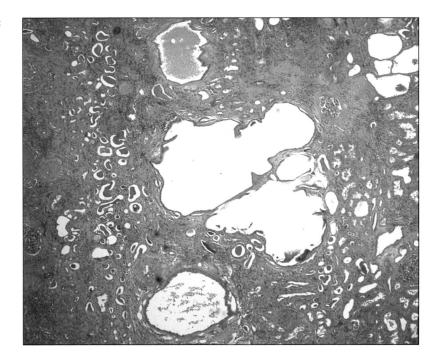

Cystic renal dysplasia

The term cystic renal dysplasia implicates a developmental disorder that occurs during the development of the embryo and its maturation. Renal dysplasia includes a spectrum of renal defects, which are often associated with abnormal collecting systems.

Dysplastic kidneys are grossly deformed in an irregular fashion. Histologically, they have a characteristic of having irregular cysts of varying size surrounded by primitive mesenchyme which in some instances is variably differentiated (Figs 5.23–5.28).

Etiology/pathogenesis

Cystic renal dysplasia may be syndromal or nonsyndromal and has multiple possible etiologies, all due to abnormal development of the kidney and urinary tract during development.

Fig. 5.23 Unilateral renal cystic dysplasia. This image demonstrates cystically altered kidney with multiple cysts proximal to the kidney. There is evidence of obstruction of the ureter. The distal ureter is dilated suggesting ureterovesical obstruction as well.

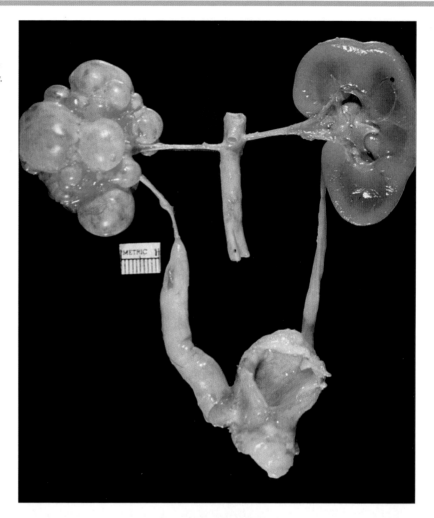

Fig. 5.24 The cysts in multicystic dysplasia are irregular in size and are distributed throughout the parenchyma.

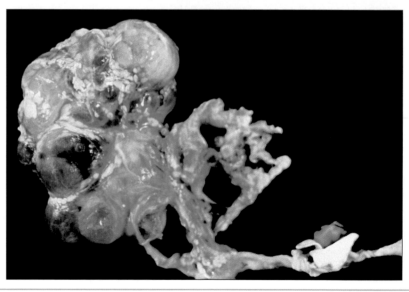

Fig. 5.25 Multicystic dysplasia. Cross section demonstrates obstruction at the ureteral pelvic junction with dilatation of the pelvis and multiple cysts involving the residual cortex.

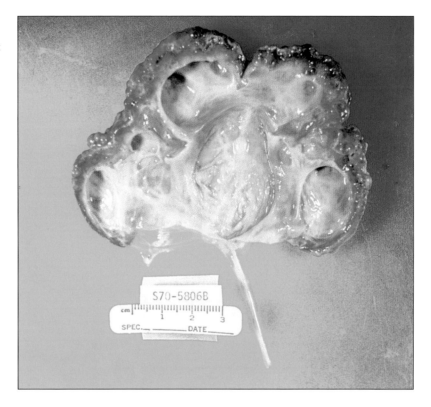

Fig. 5.26 Renal dysplasia. There is immature mesenchyme in the interstitium and cysts of varying sizes are distributed randomly throughout the parenchyma. Glomeruli are seen scattered in the interstitium (H&E, ×200).

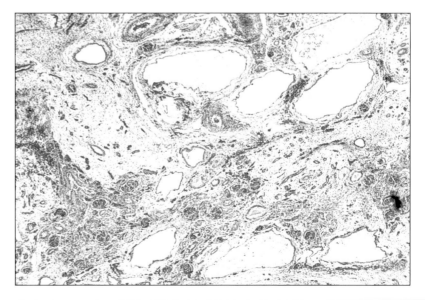

Fig. 5.27   Renal dysplasia. Loose primitive mesenchyme in the interstitium sometimes resembling cartilage is present (H&E, ×200).

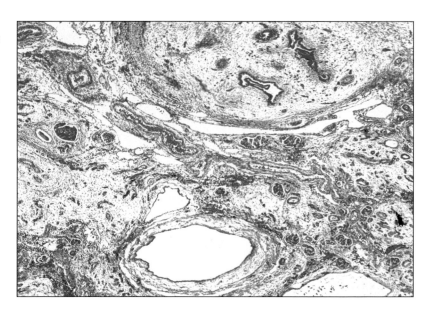

Fig. 5.28   Renal dysplasia. Cysts may also involve the glomeruli and abortive glomerular structures are seen here with cystic dilatation of Bowman's space (H&E, ×400).

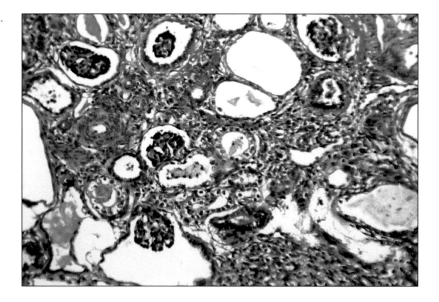

Selected reading

Matsell D G, Bennett T, Armstrong, R A et al 1997 Insulin-like growth factor (IGF) and IGF binding protein gene expression in multicystic renal dysplasia. Journal of the American Society of Nephrology 8:85.

Renal Neoplasia

References to **Brenner & Rector's** *The Kidney* **7th edition** are given in parentheses below.

Introduction

Primary neoplastic lesions of the kidney can be divided into the age group that is affected. Renal tumors in children in general resemble the nephrogenic tissues of embryogenesis and include Wilms' tumor and clear cell sarcoma. Renal cell carcinomas are the major neoplasia of the kidney in adults. They have been classified on the basis of the histologic appearance, but recent studies have determined that they also can be stratified according to cytogenetic characteristics. These are summarized in Table 6.1. In addition to the tumors involving the renal parenchyma, the collecting system is also subject to neoplasia which histologically fit into the same categories as those involving the ureters and bladder and are variants of transitional cell carcinoma.

Renal cell carcinomas

Renal cell carcinomas range widely in size ranging from one to two centimeters to several to massive tumors weighing several times the weight of the normal kidney. They are typically solid, ovulated masses which bulge into the renal parenchyma. While they may appear circumscribed, they frequently have infiltration of the perinephric

TABLE 6.1   Pathologic classification of renal neoplasms

Carcinoma	Growth pattern	Cell of origin	Cytogenetic characteristics		Incidence (%)
			Major	Minor	
Clear-cell	Acinar or sarcomatoid	Proximal tubule	3p –	+5, +7, +12, –6q, –8p, –9, –14q, –Y	75–85
Chromophilic	Papillary or sarcomatoid	Proximal tubule	+7, +17, –Y	+12, +16, +20, –14	12–24
Chromophobic	Solid, tubular, or sarcomatoid	Intercalated cell of cortical collecting duct	Hypodiploidy	–	4–6
Oncocytic	Typified by tumor nests	Intercalated cell of cortical collecting duct	LOH 1p,14q		2–4
Collecting-duct	Papillary or sarcomatoid	Medullary collecting duct	LOH 8p,13q	–	1

tissues and invade the vasculature, predominately the venous structures. The orange-yellow coloration is typical of the clear cell type, which often has foci of necrosis and scattered areas of hemorrhage. Chromophilic tumors may give a more friable, crumbling appearance. Microscopically, renal cell carcinomas have a great diversity of patterns. They may be diffuse, tubular, cystic, papillary or sarcomatoid. As the kidney is derived from mesenchyme, the sarcomatoid tumors have features that resemble leiomyo- or fibro-sarcomas. Ultrastructurally, clear cell renal carcinoma contains abundant lipid and glycogen whereas chromophobe renal cell carcinoma is characterized by the presence of abundant intracytoplasmic vesicles (Figs 6.1–6.16).

Other renal epithelial tumors

A rare form of renal cell carcinoma is that which arises in the collecting ducts and has been termed collecting duct carcinoma. Histologically, this has a pattern of branching tubules surrounded by an abundant stroma. Another important variant of renal cell tumors is

Fig. 6.1 Renal cell carcinoma. There is a lobulated yellow/orange mass with foci of hemorrhage typical of conventional (clear cell) renal cell carcinoma.

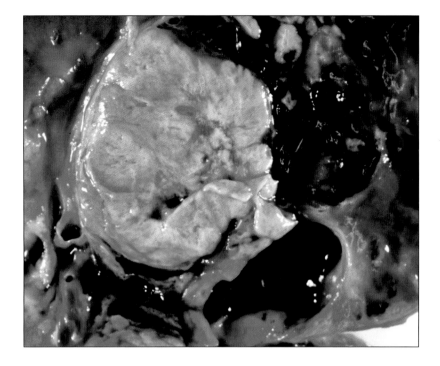

Fig. 6.2 Renal cell carcinoma. There is a prominent delicate vasculature throughout the tumor with strands of fibrosis. The cells are clear with dark central nuclei (H&E, ×100).

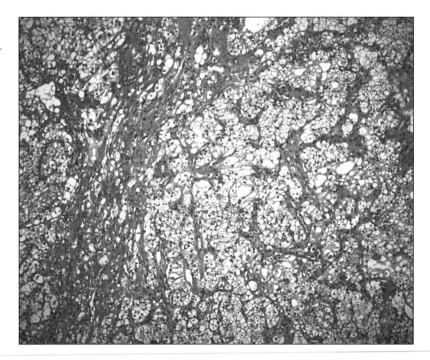

Fig. 6.3 Renal cell carcinoma. Higher power demonstrates the fibrovascular core and the nature of the clear cells (H&E, ×200).

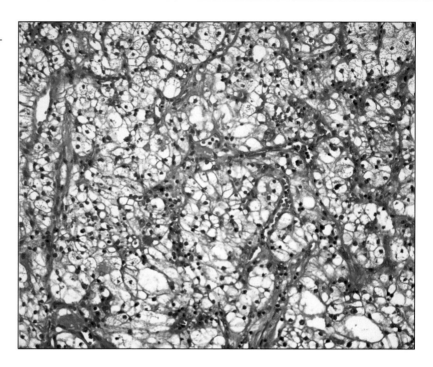

Fig. 6.4 Renal cell carcinoma. Delicate fibrovascular stroma surrounds cells with clear cytoplasm and excentric dark nuclei (H&E, ×400).

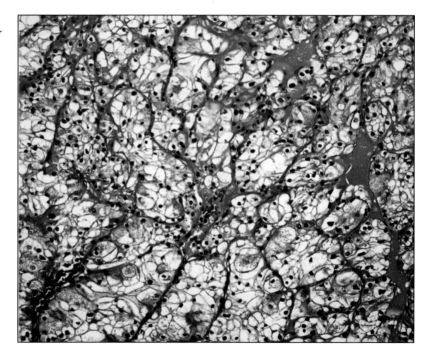

Fig. 6.5 Renal cell carcinoma. Electron microscopy reveals cytoplasm of clear cell tumors containing abundant glycogen (TEM, ×8,000).

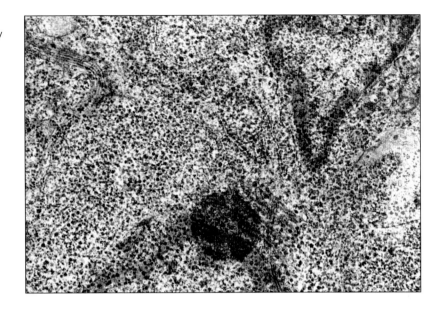

Fig. 6.6 Renal cell carcinoma. Periphery of conventional (clear cell) carcinoma demonstrates invasion of the perinephric adipose tissue (H&E, ×100).

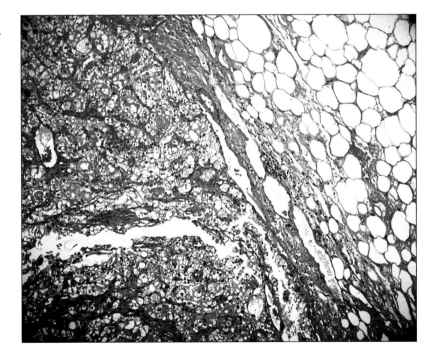

Fig. 6.7 Renal cell carcinoma. Invasion of the capsule is also evident with abundant vascular formation (H&E, ×100).

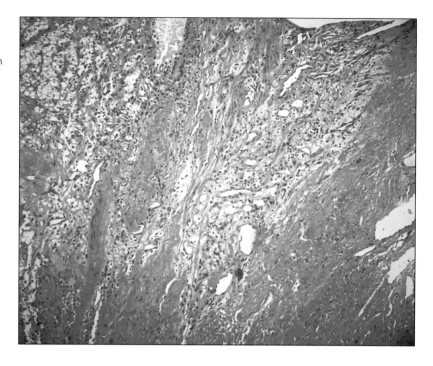

Fig. 6.8 Renal cell carcinoma. The invasive component sometimes has a sarcomatous appearance with elongated fibroblast like tumor cells with irregular hyperchromatic nuclei (H&E, ×200).

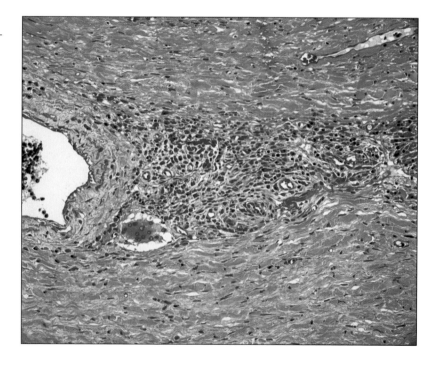

Fig. 6.9 Chromophilic carcinoma of the eosinophilic type. The cells are arranged in a pseudo-papillary pattern in this islet of tumor, which has eosinophilic cytoplasm and central nuclei (H&E, ×100).

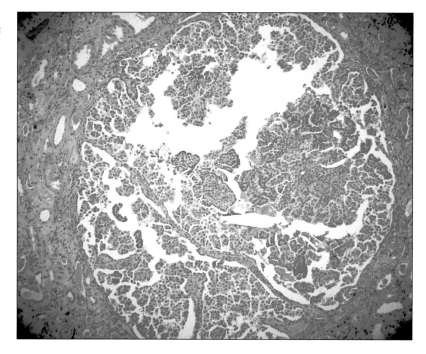

Fig. 6.10 Chromophilic (papillary) renal cell carcinoma. There is an obvious papillary pattern with papillae with a central fibrovascular core and surface lining of tumor cells (H&E, ×200).

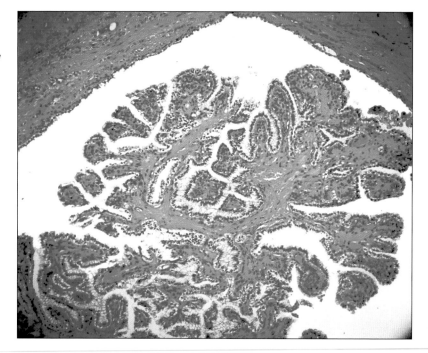

Fig. 6.11 In chromophilic renal cell carcinoma with the papillary pattern, the tumor cells contain basally located nuclei with an eosinophilic cytoplasm (H&E, ×400).

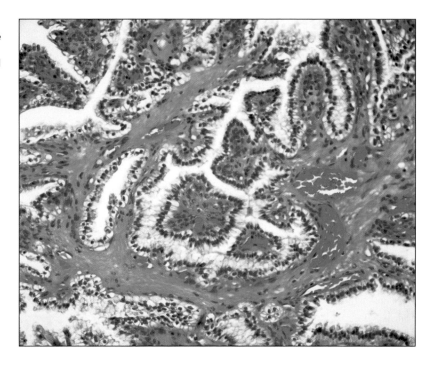

Fig. 6.12 Basophilic renal cell carcinoma can present in a more solid pattern. The cells have a scant cytoplasm and prominent nuclei which appears to give a basophilic appearance (H&E, ×400).

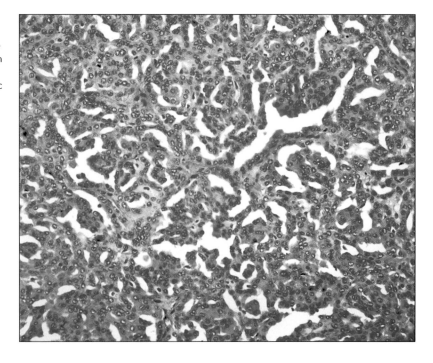

Fig. 6.13 Chromophobe carcinoma. The tumor consists of sheets of cells, with a thin fibrovascular stroma. The cytoplasm is prominent and has a pale staining pattern (H&E, ×100).

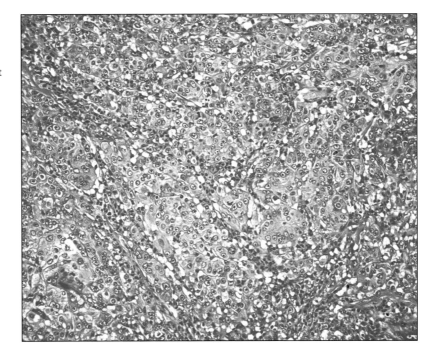

Fig. 6.14 Chromophobe carcinoma. The cytoplasm of the cells contains large numbers of minute intracytoplasmic vesicles which gives a pale reticular or flocculent appearance to the cytoplasm (H&E, ×400).

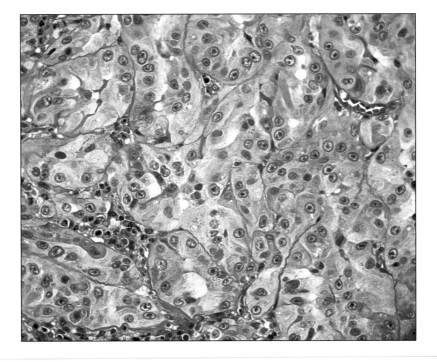

Fig. 6.15 Chromophobe renal carcinoma. Some solid variants of the chromophobe type have a more eosinophilic appearance than typical chromophobe carcinoma cells (H&E, ×100).

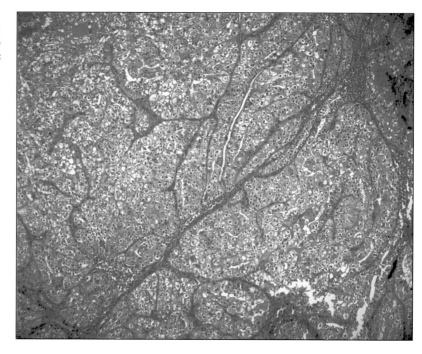

Fig. 6.16 Chromophobe renal carcinoma. The fibro-vascular stroma surrounding islets of tightly packed tumor cells with slightly eosinophilic cytoplasm is shown (H&E, ×100).

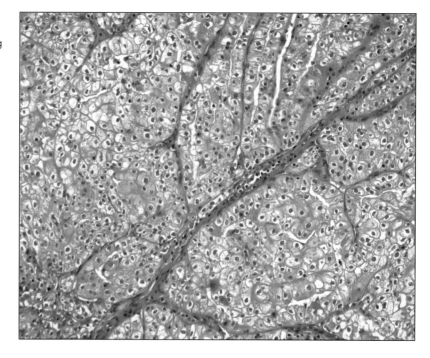

the so-called renal oncocytoma. This is of importance in that the prognosis of oncocytomas is much more favorable than that of renal cell carcinoma. Renal oncocytomas have a homogeneous dark brown appearance and histologically cells have a finely granular eosinophilic cytoplasm. Electron microscopy reveals abundant mitochondria (Figs 6.17–6.20).

Fig. 6.17 Renal oncocytoma. The brown color is typical of the oncocytoma. It also demonstrates a central fibrous core.

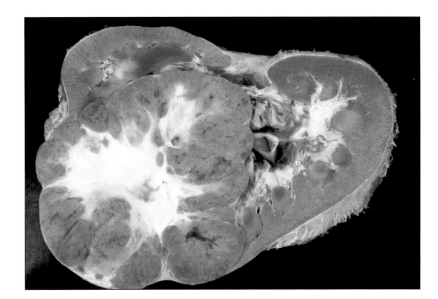

Fig. 6.18 Oncocytoma. The cells of the oncocytoma are arranged in diffuse sheets or islands of tumor cells with a background of edematous connective tissue (H&E, ×100).

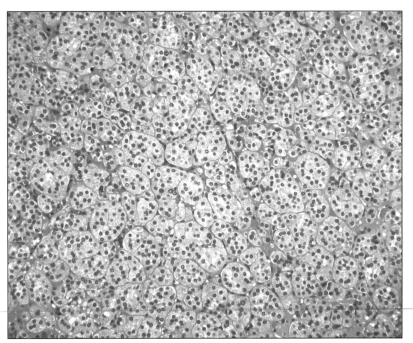

Fig. 6.19 Oncocytoma. There is relatively even pattern of cells with uniform nuclei and granular eosinophilic appearance of the cytoplasm (H&E, ×400).

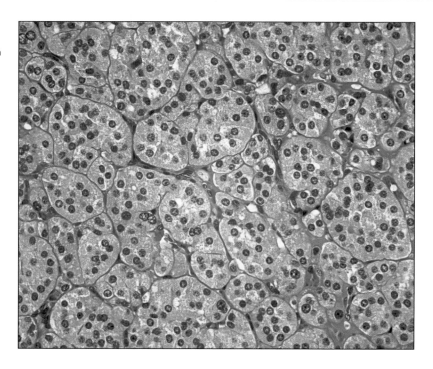

Fig. 6.20 Oncocytoma. There are abundant mito-chondria that give the granular appearance by light microscopy (TEM, ×8,000).

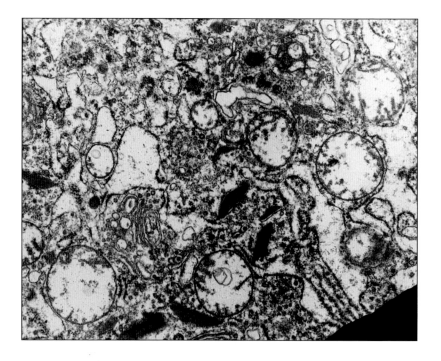

Selected reading

Kennedy S M, Merino M J, Linehan W M et al 1990 Collecting duct carcinoma of the kidney. Human Pathology 21:449–456.

Morra M N, Das S 1993 Renal oncocytoma: A review of histogenesis, histopathology, diagnosis and treatment. Journal of Urology 150:295–302.

Thoenes W, Storkel S, Rumpelt H J 1986 Histopathology and classification of renal cell tumors (adenomas, oncocytomas and carcinomas): The basic cytological and histopathological elements and their use for diagnostics. Pathology, Research and Practice 181:125–143.

Wilms' tumor

Wilms' tumors comprise more than 80% of renal tumors of childhood. They are mostly identified in children 2–4 years of age and are often associated with congenital anomalies, which fall into syndromic patterns. Of these, the so-called Denys–Drash syndrome is of particular interest in that it is associated with the presence of focal and segmental glomerulosclerosis in the non-neoplastic renal tissue. Histologically, Wilms' tumor consists of sheets of small cells with inconspicuous cytoplasmic hyperchromatic nuclei and frequent mitotic figures. The cells may be present in a variety of patterns sometimes showing abortive glomerulogenesis and in other areas, showing tubular structures (Figs 6.21–6.26).

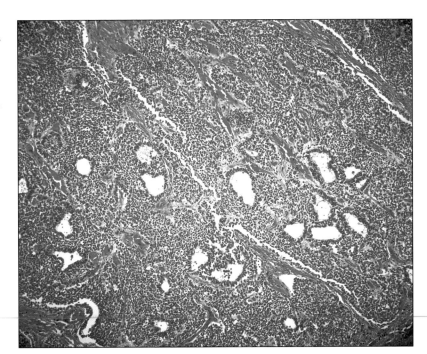

Fig. 6.21 Wilms' tumor. Histologically Wilms' tumors are composed of various mixtures of primitive renal blastema, epithelium and stroma. Blastema here appears as sheets of uniform small blue cells, which surround abortive tubular structures composed of epithelium and supported by a dense fibrovascular stroma (H&E, ×100).

Fig. 6.22 Wilms' tumor. The blastema consists of randomly arranged densely packed small cells with dark blue nuclei with frequent mitotic figures and a relatively inconspicuous cytoplasm (H&E, ×200).

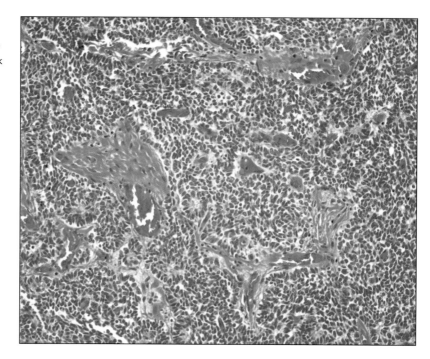

Fig. 6.23 Wilms' tumor. In some areas, the blastema has a serpentine appearance with an elongated spindle cell pattern (H&E, ×200).

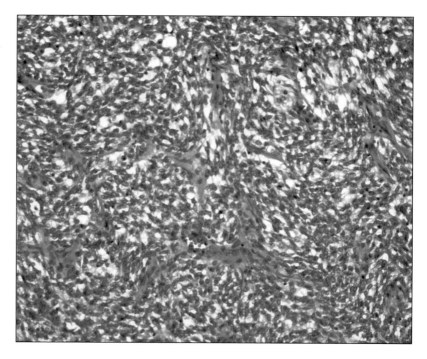

Fig. 6.24 Wilms' tumor. Abortive tubular structures with a differentiated epithelial lining can be found surrounded by more primitive blastema (H&E, ×400).

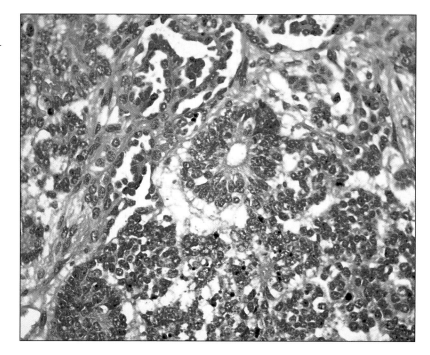

Fig. 6.25 Wilms' tumor. Electron micrograph demonstrates a primitive tubule made up of blastema epithelial cells forming a lumen (TEM, ×2,000).

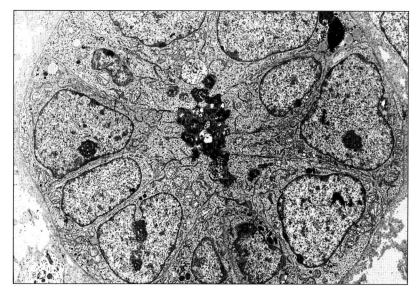

Etiology/pathogenesis

Wilms' tumor is thought to be the result of abnormal proliferation of metanephric blastema, without normal differentiation into tubules and glomeruli. A number of genetic aberrations have been implicated in the pathogenesis of Wilms' tumor. The chromosomal deletion of

Fig. 6.26 Wilms' tumor. Abortive glomerular structures are also identified within the mass of blastema. True capillary lumina are not present (H&E, ×400).

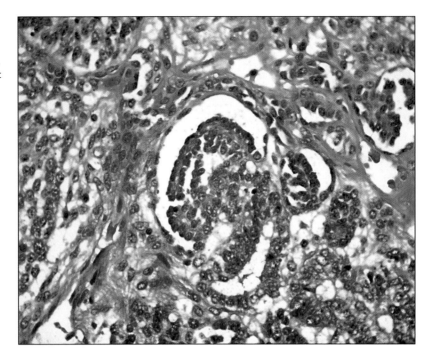

the WT1 gene located within the short arm of chromosome 11p13 often leads to the combination of Wilms' tumor and aniridia, genitourinary malformation, and mental retardation (i.e. WAGR syndrome). Other Wilms' tumor genes include WT2 at 11p15.5 linked to Beckwith–Wiedemann syndrome, deletion of chromosome 16 and duplication of chromosome 12.

Interestingly, in nonsyndromal Wilms' tumor, the WT-1 gene itself is only rarely mutated. Rather, abnormalities of e.g. imprinting affecting WT-1 function are thought to be involved.

Selected reading

Ritchey M L, Azizkhan R G, Beckwith J B et al 1995 Neonatal Wilms' tumor. Journal of Pediatric Surgery 30:856–859.

Transitional cell carcinoma of the renal pelvis

Primary transitional cell carcinoma (TCC) of the renal pelvis or ureter accounts for less than 5% of all renal tumors. Tumors of the upper urinary tract are twice as common in men, and the peak incidence occurs between age 50 and 60 years. Transitional tumors of the renal pelvis and ureter are histologically identical to bladder

Fig. 6.27 Papillary transitional cell carcinoma of the pelvis. The appearance of the tumor is similar to that seen in papillary transitional cell carcinoma of the bladder. There are fibrovascular cores surrounded by a stratified transitional epithelium (H&E, ×100).

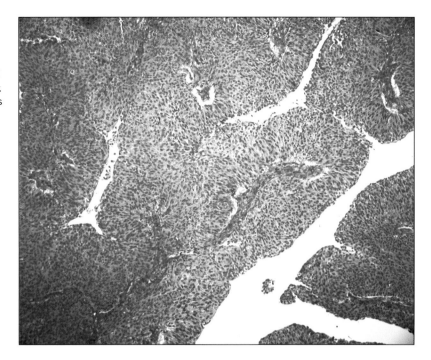

Fig. 6.28 Papillary TCC. The epithelium has pleomorphic nuclei, which vary in size and shape and vary in degree of differentiation (H&E, ×200).

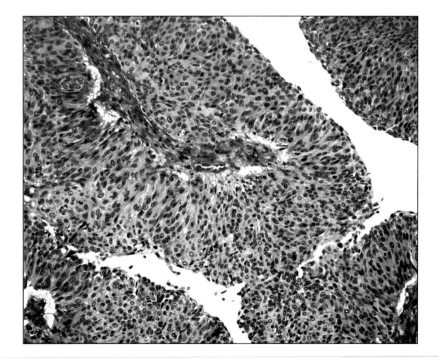

epithelial tumors. Morphologically, these tumors can be papillary or solid in configuration, and they may have associated carcinoma *in situ* (Figs 6.27–6.28).

Etiology/pathogenesis

The surface epithelium (urothelium) that lines the mucosal surfaces of the entire urinary tract is exposed to potential carcinogens that may be excreted in the urine, or activated in the urine by hydrolyzing enzymes. Environmental exposures are thought to account for most cases of urothelial cancer.

Selected reading

Munoz J J, Ellison L M 2000 Upper tract urothelial neoplasms: incidence and survival during the last 2 decades. Journal of Urology 164:1523–1525.

Index

M

X